Praise for **Heal Faster**

'No matter your age, health, mindset or experience, Dr Maizes provides the ideal roadmap to recovery for just about any situation your body might encounter. I know I will turn to it time and again and encourage you to do the same.'   Arianna Huffington, Founder & CEO, Thrive Global

'*Heal Faster* is a must-read for anyone seeking to unlock the body's innate power to repair, restore, and thrive. Dr Maizes brings together the best of conventional science and integrative wisdom to show how healing is not just about treating disease – it's about creating the conditions for health. With compassion, clarity, and deep medical insight, she offers practical, evidence-based strategies to accelerate recovery from illness, surgery, or injury. This book is a roadmap to resilience and vitality that empowers both patients and practitioners alike.'
Dr Mark Hyman, *Sunday Times* bestselling author of *Young Forever* and *The Pegan Diet*, host of The Doctor Hyman Show

'Like having a trusted doctor friend with a vast repertoire of experience in optimizing healing, who you can consult in detail whenever you need to.'
Jon Kabat-Zinn, founder of MBSR (Mindfulness-Based Stress Reduction) and author of *Full Catastrophe Living*

'Whether you have a mild cold or are facing major surgery, *Heal Faster* is an invaluable resource to ensure a smooth, complete recovery. Drawing on her scientific knowledge and decades of experience in treating patients, Victoria Maizes shows us that, with the right approach and support, the body really can heal itself. Read this groundbreaking book to find out how.'
Dr Andrew Weil, #1 *New York Times* bestselling author and founder of the Andrew Weil Center for Integrative Medicine at the University of Arizona

'*Heal Faster* offers profound insight into our natural power to heal ourselves.'
Rachel Naomi Remen, MD, *New York Times* bestselling author of *Kitchen Table Wisdom*

'This reader-friendly volume distils the medical wisdom and experience accumulated over decades by veteran physician and Integrative Medicine pioneer Victoria Maizes. Avoiding jargon or abstruse theory, and covering topics ranging from the common cold and anxiety through cancer and heart disease, *Heal Faster* is a practical manual for prevention and recovery in many crucial aspects of physical and mental health.'

Gabor Maté, *Sunday Times* bestselling author of *The Myth of Normal*

'An essential operating manual for how to get well and stay well. I learned so much from this book.'

James Nestor, *Sunday Times* bestselling author of *Breath*

Heal Faster

Unlock Your Body's Rapid Recovery Reflex

Victoria Maizes, MD

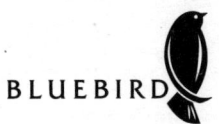
BLUEBIRD

First edition published 2026 by Simon & Schuster

First published in the UK 2026 by Bluebird
an imprint of Pan Macmillan
The Smithson, 6 Briset Street, London EC1M 5NR
EU representative: Macmillan Publishers Ireland Ltd, 1st Floor,
The Liffey Trust Centre, 117–126 Sheriff Street Upper,
Dublin 1 D01 YC43
Associated companies throughout the world

ISBN 978-1-0350-3500-7

Copyright © Victoria Maizes 2026

This publication contains the opinions and ideas of its author. It is intended to provide helpful and informative material on the subjects it addresses and does not constitute medical advice, nor is it a substitute for professional help or therapy. It is sold with the understanding that the author and publisher are not engaged in rendering medical, health, or any other kind of personal professional services in the book. Readers are advised to consult their own licensed medical or healthcare advisors and must obtain specific medical advice before starting, stopping, amending any course of treatment or medication, adopting any of the suggestions in this book or drawing inferences from it. Any reliance on the information contained in this book is strictly at your own risk. The author and publisher specifically disclaim all responsibility for any liability, loss or risk, personal or otherwise, which is incurred as a consequence, directly or indirectly, of the use and application of any of the contents of this book.

The rights of Victoria Maizes to be identified as the author of this work has been asserted in accordance with the Copyright, Designs and Patents Act 1988.

Interior design by Ruth Lee-Mui

All rights reserved. No part of this publication may be reproduced, stored in a retrieval system, or transmitted, in any form, or by any means (including, without limitation, electronic, mechanical, photocopying, recording or otherwise) without the prior written permission of the publisher.

Pan Macmillan does not have any control over, or any responsibility for, any author or third-party websites (including, without limitation, URLs, emails and QR codes) referred to in or on this book.

1 3 5 7 9 8 6 4 2

A CIP catalogue record for this book is available from the British Library.

Printed and bound in the UK using 100% Renewable Electricity by CPI Group (UK) Ltd

This book is sold subject to the condition that it shall not, by way of trade or otherwise, be lent, hired out, or otherwise circulated without the publisher's prior consent in any form of binding or cover other than that in which it is published and without a similar condition including this condition being imposed on the subsequent purchaser. The publisher does not authorize the use or reproduction of any part of this book in any manner for the purpose of training artificial intelligence technologies or systems. The publisher expressly reserves this book from the Text and Data Mining exception in accordance with Article 4(3) of the European Union Digital Single Market Directive 2019/790.

Visit **www.panmacmillan.com/bluebird** to read more about all our books and to buy them.

*To all who have been told, "You have to take these medicines for the rest of your life," but kept on searching.
It takes courage!*

*To anyone approaching surgery or cancer treatment determined to do everything within their power to achieve a better outcome.
Bravo!*

To anyone who believes there is a better way to get healthy than what is commonly offered in conventional medical care.

May you find guidance within these pages on your journey to health.

Contents

Introduction: You Can Recover   1

Part One
Recovery from Short-Lived Conditions

1. Conquering Colds and Vanquishing Viral Infections — 13
2. Soothing the Gut — 27
3. Sleeping Soundly — 41
4. Unwinding Anxiety — 57
5. Mending Musculoskeletal Pain — 77
6. Supporting Healthy Skin and Hair — 96
7. Preventing PMS and Upholding Urogenital Health — 116
8. Mastering Menopause — 133

Part Two
Recovery from Longstanding Conditions

9. Healing Heart Disease — 151
10. Deactivating Pain Signals — 169
11. Reversing Type 2 Diabetes — 199
12. Easing Asthma — 215
13. Building Stronger Bones — 230
14. Defeating Depression — 246
15. Taming Post-Traumatic Stress Disorder — 266
16. Overcoming Long Covid — 286

Part Three
Recovery from Surgery

17	Setting Yourself up for a Successful Surgery	301
18	Your Surgical Prehab	306
19	Your Post-Op Experience	322
20	Recovery from Orthopedic Surgery	337
21	Recovery from Heart Surgery	346
22	Recovery from Breast Cancer and Its Surgery	359
23	Recovery From Minimally Invasive Surgery	375
24	Final Considerations	383
	Your Rapid Recovery Toolkit	387
	How to Choose a Supplement	401
	Acknowledgments	403
	Index	405

Full references for *Heal Faster* are available online at www.DrVictoriaMaizes.com/Resources

Introduction: You Can Recover

Are you happy with your health? I hope that the answer is a resounding *Yes!* But, if you are not, I intend to guide you back to robust health. Maybe you have been recently diagnosed with a medical disorder, or perhaps you experience aches and pains that seem to last just a little longer than they once did. Your sense of your body's "normal" might have shifted over time.

Does your new "normal" include a diagnosis of prediabetes, high blood pressure, or depression? Do you find yourself taking one, two, or even three prescription drugs daily? We're generally led to believe this is just the way of normal aging. We're encouraged to adhere to medications rather than to strive to reverse the conditions that necessitate their use. All told, your new normal may not seem very normal at all, but what can you do other than endure it?

In this book I will show you there is in fact quite a lot you can do. It begins with thinking differently about your health. I want you to challenge the notion that illness is your destiny. Consider that in general we have access to advanced healthcare systems with modern technology. In the United States, doctors can choose from among twenty thousand prescription medications to treat their patients,[1] or one of the tens of millions of surgical procedures conducted each year.[2] Despite all these interventions, and despite spending more than 17 percent of our GDP on healthcare[3]— more than that of any other wealthy country[4]—we are less healthy and live shorter lives than people in other developed countries.

As an example, a 2024 analysis published by the Commonwealth Fund found that among the ten wealthiest countries in the world, the United States has the lowest life expectancy—more than four years less than the ten-country average.[5] The U.S. also ranks last in preventable deaths. Of course, many factors contribute to this poor performance, including inequities, lack of access to care or health insurance, and not enough primary-care doctors. But another reason is complacency; in many countries we have put our trust in medicines and surgeries instead of enlisting our body's remarkable recovery capacity.

Let me tell you about one of my patients, whom I will call John. (All patient names in this book are pseudonyms, and I have altered details to protect their identities.) A few years ago, John's doctor on the East Coast referred him to me. He was not doing well. Three years earlier, John had a bad case of viral gastroenteritis, or stomach flu. Severely dehydrated, John was given IV fluids at the hospital and sent home the next day. He felt better for a few weeks, but then he experienced tingling in his extremities, which snowballed into partial paralysis. After a lumbar puncture, John was diagnosed with Guillain-Barre syndrome, a disorder in which the immune system attacks the body's own nerves.

John's doctors threw the kitchen sink at him. Hoping to "reboot" his immune system, first they tried plasmapheresis, whereby the liquid part of the blood—plasma—is separated from the cells and replaced with saline. John immediately got worse and remained in the hospital for two weeks. Unable to walk, he was sent to a nursing home, where he was administered powerful pain medications to treat his nerve pain and intravenous immunoglobulin to treat the Guillain-Barre. None of it worked. By the time he turned sixty, John was effectively bedridden.

Finally, John's doctor threw up his hands. "I think you should go to Arizona," he said. "The desert air might help."

When John showed up for his appointment with me at the Andrew Weil Center for Integrative Medicine in Tucson, Arizona, he calmly explained that he was considering killing himself. He was weak, overweight, and depressed, and just getting out of his wheelchair required herculean effort. He was sick and tired of taking medications and treatments that seemed to only make him worse. I explained to John that as an integrative-medicine doctor, I would do my best to partner with him in the healing process.

"Something seems to be preventing your body from healing," I said. "Let's work to figure out what it is." I explained we would explore all the factors that could be influencing his health: mind, body, spirit, and even his relationships. We would harness a wide range of approaches, from conventional to alternative medicine, to kick-start his body's innate healing response.

Instead of simply prescribing more medication, I asked John to walk me through his day. What time did he wake in the morning and when did he go to sleep at night? What did he usually eat and at what time? What kind of music did he listen to? Anything from the food we eat to the way we breathe can aid the recovery process—or arrest it. When I heard his story, I made a variety of recommendations. At first, John was resistant, balking at my suggestions of a juice fast or the use of guided imagery. But he did agree to an elimination diet, a mainstay of integrative medicine that identifies food intolerances, sensitivities, and allergies by removing one or more items from your diet.

John rolled out of my office in his wheelchair, and six weeks later he walked back in. His crippling morning pain was gone. His depression had lifted. He could move around comfortably with a cane. He had steadily reduced his battery of medications. After diligently removing foods from his diet, John had discovered three pain triggers: garlic, ginger, and, worst of all, black pepper. Black pepper contains a compound called *piperine*, which in sensitive individuals can cause an inflammatory condition called *leaky gut*, whereby large molecules that would normally be prevented from crossing the intestinal lining enter the body. Once on the verge of suicide, after eliminating these foods, John was hopeful for the first time in three years.

John's experience serves as an example of our magnificent ability to recover. In simple terms, *recovery* means a return to normal after a disturbance, whether it's a viral infection, type 2 diabetes, or heart surgery. The scientific term for this is *homeostasis,* from the Greek words for "similar" (*homoiós*) and "standing still" (*stasis*). Sometimes, like with a simple paper cut, recovery takes place in just a few hours. Healing from surgery generally takes months, and it can take a year for a broken bone to fully mend. In each circumstance, your body has activated an innate ability to restore a normal state. How quickly—and how completely—your recovery activates, what impedes it, and the remarkable degree of control we have over it are the subjects of this book.

The urge to return to homeostasis is the result of an ancient *recovery reflex* inside all of us that can heal everything, from the common cold to type 2 diabetes, to a surgical procedure to psychological trauma. Think of your recovery reflex as your body's built-in reset button—an automatic response system that kicks in to bring you back to homeostasis whenever something throws you off. It's your body's internal first responder, always on call to restore equilibrium in real time.

Sometimes this process is obvious, such as when your recovery reflex urges your heart to beat faster and pump more blood as you race up the stairs. Other times it's invisible, like when your natural killer cells hunt down cancer cells before they multiply. When your blood sugar rises after a meal, your recovery reflex signals the pancreas to secrete insulin to help your cells absorb excess glucose.

Your recovery reflex's healing ability is miraculous. Consider that even if 70 percent of your liver is removed, it can rebuild itself within a few weeks. Your intestines regenerate their entire lining, called the *epithelium*, every five to seven days due to the constant wear and tear of digesting food. Your skin sheds and regrows between thirty and forty thousand cells daily. If you've been a lifelong smoker, your recovery reflex stimulates the lungs to regrow their tiny hair-like cilia after your last cigarette, significantly improving your blood circulation and reversing chronic cough and shortness of breath. The body's resilience even extends to emotional wounds. The mind can heal from profound grief and trauma, often emerging stronger and more compassionate.

As we'll see in this book, your recovery reflex plays a critical role even during surgery. Your body heals a large incision by constricting blood vessels to reduce blood loss, moving platelets into the incision site to form a temporary "plug," and knitting a mesh that serves as a scaffold for cell migration and tissue repair. Then, your recovery reflex launches an inflammatory response to clear any debris and prevent infection.

Most often, your recovery reflex activates on its own and your body heals completely and uneventfully. Being healthy dramatically enhances your reflex, and lifestyle choices improve—or inhibit—its potency. For instance, a study of ninety-four moderately heavy drinkers reveals that those who abstained from alcohol for a month showed improvements in insulin resistance, blood pressure, and weight compared to a control group that did not give up drinking.[6] They also experienced improved sleep and mood, less depression and anxiety, and healthier skin and microbiome. Countless other factors influence your recovery reflex, including genetics, age, how well nourished or hydrated you are, physical activity levels, how many environmental toxins you are exposed to, sleep habits, how much stress are you under, your outlook on life, and even the altitude you live at. We do not have control over all these variables, but you may be surprised to learn in every chapter of this book how many can indeed be altered.

I am frequently struck by how often people are able to activate their recovery reflex and "snap back" from debilitating illnesses. For instance, later in this book you will meet another one of my patients, Vivian, who resolved her debilitating menopausal hot flushes, heavy menstrual bleeding, and painful leg nodules by throwing away her coffee pot, which we discovered was leaching plastic chemicals. Other patients of mine have activated their recovery reflex by using a light box, instituting a fourteen-hour overnight fast, taking a supplement, or practicing guided imagery.

My goal is for you to discover novel approaches to awaken your recovery reflex and restore your health. Consider that nearly 20 percent of Americans suffer from chronic pain that interferes with their daily activities.[7] Many people consider this their new normal—but it does not have to be. You have a tremendous untapped ability to control the strength and speed of your recovery, and this book will cover the latest science and medical insights to help you recover from nearly anything that life throws at you. Along the way, we will see that rapid—and just as important, *complete*—recovery is possible not just from a bout of the flu but also from longstanding illness, surgery, and poor mental health.

An Integrative Approach to Health

This probably sounds familiar: You go to your doctor complaining of a problem, and you are referred to a specialist. Sometimes it can feel like your body is not a unified whole, but rather a collection of isolated parts, each requiring separate attention. Cardiologists focus on the heart, neurologists on the brain, gastroenterologists handle the digestive system, dermatologists specialize in the skin, and so on. While this depth of expertise can be invaluable, too often we fail to see, and therefore fail to treat, the whole person—mind, body, and spirit. Think of Humpty Dumpty: Without taking a step back and examining how the individual pieces fit together, he can never be made whole again.

Conventional medicine, also commonly called *Western medicine*, is what most people receive when they see their doctor. When you are ill, your body is evaluated from a biophysical perspective, and doctors rely on treatment methods that have been shown to be effective across large populations. Western medicine excels in certain domains, including trauma (such as treatment after a car accident), surgery, infectious diseases, and some cancers. But if you need to recover from, say, a nagging illness, a sports injury, or a longstanding disease like type 2 diabetes, there are better science-backed approaches. The treatment options you will find in this book apply what I see as the very best and most scientifically sound conventional and alternative approaches. This is called *integrative medicine*.

Integrative medicine neither rejects conventional medicine nor accepts alternative therapies uncritically. It takes account of the whole person (body, mind, and spirit), including all aspects of lifestyle, and it prioritizes less invasive, more natural interventions whenever possible. It is a pragmatic, larger paradigm, focused on the philosophy of restoring health with the safest, least toxic methods possible.

I have spent close to thirty years as an integrative-medicine doctor at the University of Arizona's Andrew Weil Center. Every day I see patients return to health who have been struggling with both short- and long-standing conditions. Many of them have been told there's nothing they can do to reverse their heart disease, diabetes, osteoporosis, or arthritis. They accept a long-term condition because "it runs in the family." In fact, even with a genetic disposition, the vast majority of your health is based on your lifestyle choices. Rather than accepting "there is nothing you can do," this book will guide you toward healing by revealing how much you actually *can* do.

Consider the Ornish program,[8] founded by the cardiologist Dean Ornish. He enrolled patients with moderate to severe heart disease and had them eat a less-than-10-percent-fat vegetarian diet and engage in regular exercise, stress-reduction practices, and group support. Within a year, the intervention group saw blockages in their arteries decrease by 37 percent, while the control group (who did not make any lifestyle changes) saw blockages *increase* by over 8 percent. The intervention group also experienced 91 percent less chest pain (angina) after one year, compared to a 186 percent increase for the control group. Integrative nephrologists have even told me about patients with end-stage kidney disease on the verge of dialysis who regained kidney function by adopting plant-forward diets.

Make no mistake: This is not a vegan diet book. While I will often point out the benefits of eating plant-based foods, I will also note when eating more animal protein and fat is the optimal approach. For instance, I observe with awe when a vegetarian diet completely reverses one of my patient's type 2 diabetes, while another's diabetes responds to the opposite approach: a ketogenic diet based on eating meat. This is an example of biochemical individuality, or the concept that each person has unique needs and health considerations based on their genetics, lifestyles, heritages, traditions, and preferences. The integrative-medicine philosophy is that recovery is not one-size-fits-all; rather, it should be tailored to your unique circumstances. Thus, in this book I will help you determine what foods, medicine, and treatments are appropriate to activate *your* recovery reflex.

Integrative medicine also produces what I have termed "side benefits." Watch any TV commercial for the latest medication, and you may hear the narrator breeze through a laundry list of side effects, such as diarrhea, constipation, skin rashes, dizziness, drowsiness, headache, insomnia, and even abnormal heart rhythms. A "cure" for one ailment sometimes causes trouble elsewhere in the body. In contrast, when I prescribe daily walks to treat elevated blood pressure, my patients frequently notice *side benefits* like reduced stress levels, weight loss, and improved joint function. I practice 4-7-8 breathing to reduce my stress—breathing in for four counts, holding for seven counts, exhaling for eight counts—and my side benefits include sleeping better, being less prone to startling, and having warmer hands and feet.

As I will make clear in this book, integrative medicine sometimes leads with medication and surgery, such as with a cancer diagnosis or a broken hip. In these scenarios, integrative therapies can enhance Western medicine. At other times, an integrative approach will eliminate the need for a surgery or medication by introducing other therapeutic approaches. These can include dietary changes, addressing stress, restoring restful sleep, using appropriate supplements, or acupuncture and body work. The synergism of these gentle treatment approaches can make a profound difference for your health. If you are having uncomfortable side effects from medications, integrative medicine may help you get off those medications. An integrative plan will prioritize options that fit with your preferred treatment course with a goal to activate your recovery reflex and restore your health. I will show how I recommend treatments to my patients, although make sure to talk to your own doctor before beginning a new practice or stopping an existing one.

What to Expect in this Book

I will draw from forty years of medical experience as a practicing doctor, a medical school professor, and the founding executive director of the Andrew Weil Center for Integrative Medicine, where I train doctors to practice medicine in new ways by emphasizing the body's vast healing systems. I will encourage you to use these same strategies to recover faster and more completely.

But, first, as I do with my patients, I want you to reflect for a moment on everything you are already doing right. Perhaps it is the way you nourish your relationships, your commitment to eating a healthy diet, the way you attend to your stress, how you prioritize sleep, or your regular exercise routine. Keep up these healthy practices and celebrate all you are doing well!

Now, consider a recent study that analyzed data from two long-term population studies that found participants who followed five specific lifestyle habits[9]—eating lots of fruits and vegetables and avoiding processed foods; not smoking; getting at least three and a half hours of exercise per week; drinking in moderation; and maintaining a healthy body weight—had much lower incidences of heart disease and cancer. The researchers found that following all five habits from age fifty onward extended life span by more than a decade, compared to following none of those habits.

These are just five lifestyle choices you can make to improve health and enhance your recovery reflex. We are going to explore many more of them in this book. For instance, the latest circadian-medicine research—an emerging field that focuses on how biological rhythms, driven by the body's internal clock, influence health and disease—reveals the value of *when* we eat or sleep, not just how much we get of either. I've seen patients who follow a time-restricted eating pattern reverse their diabetes, lose weight, and dramatically improve their immune response. We'll also see how the mind–body connection can be harnessed to heal, including, for example, how hypnosis can treat irritable bowel syndrome or how guided imagery hastens recovery from surgery.

Heal Faster is divided into three parts. Part One addresses rapid recovery from short-lived conditions—everything from the common cold, to urinary tract infections, anxiety, and trouble sleeping. Part Two addresses recovery from stubborn health problems, those longstanding diseases that doctors often tell us are irreversible. We'll see how rapid recovery methods can arrest or reverse conditions including heart disease, diabetes, and low bone density as well as mental health challenges such as depression and PTSD. Part Three focuses on recovery from surgery. If you are scheduled for surgery, you'll see how rapid recovery practices can maximize the speed of recovery and help get you feeling your best self. Of course, you likely do not require recovery from many of the ailments in this book, but you may have friends and loved ones who do and will benefit from your knowledge.

Sickness or injury can occur unexpectedly. The secret to a rapid recovery is immediately responding to whatever ails you. This means keeping your house well stocked with what I call "Your Rapid Recovery Toolkit," which is appendix 1. This includes items that range from the well known—think heating pads and elastic bandages for musculoskeletal injuries—to the less widely known, such as raw garlic and zinc for colds. I also include items that may not "physically fit" into your toolkit, but that are equally essential tools for any recovery, such as information on the Mediterranean diet and on deep-breathing exercises. Lastly, I provide direction on how to choose dietary supplements.

• • •

In this book, I want to challenge any negativity you may experience when you see your doctor. Sometimes it seems that doctors are so fixated on not creating false hopes that they may actually create false despair. Their busyness and burnout reduce their curiosity about promising new treatments. So many of my patients who have had success with integrative medicine report that their doctor never asked for detailed information so that other patients could benefit. Take the neuroscientist Jill Bolte Taylor, PhD, for instance, who made a full recovery from a devastating stroke using mindfulness techniques and later wrote a bestselling book, *My Stroke of Insight,* detailing her experiences. "In twenty-two years, not one doctor has asked how I had a full recovery from my stroke," she said.[10]

In *Heal Faster,* I encourage you to be curious about your body's incredible ability to heal. I want you to aim high, ask questions, get to the root of what ails you, and ultimately discover therapeutic treatments to restore your health. I firmly believe in the healing potential of the human body. I want you to, as well. You have access to an amazing rapid recovery reflex; now is the time to unlock it and unleash it.

Part One

Recovery from Short-Lived Conditions

1

Conquering Colds and Vanquishing Viral Infections

Everyone is familiar with the common cold: runny or stuffy nose, sore throat, coughing, sneezing, perhaps a low-grade fever, and generally feeling *bleh*. These symptoms result from a viral infection of the upper respiratory tract. Of all the places you can witness the human body's incredible recovery mechanisms, this may be the most discernible. Your body knows exactly how to vanquish a virus, and integrative medicine can speed up the process.

Colds can be caused by more than two hundred different types of viruses,[1] with rhinovirus the most common. As any parent or teacher will know, colds are highly contagious, spreading easily through infected droplets in the air when someone coughs or sneezes, or through contact with contaminated surfaces or an infected person's hands. The average adult comes down with two to three colds each year.[2] While they are less severe than many other conditions in this book—most colds usually resolve within a week—they are unpleasant and disruptive, leading to seventy million missed work days annually and costing the U.S. economy some $40 billion.[3] Western medicine does not offer any medications that speed a cold along, but there are many integrative strategies at your disposal that can. They work by supporting your rapid recovery reflex, both preventing colds and accelerating your return to feeling well again.

For example, my thirty-five-year-old patient Lydia is a kindergarten teacher who complained of constantly catching whatever cold was circulating around her classroom; she effectively had one long cold from November through April. "What can I do to give my immune system a boost?" she asked me. I recommended that she chop a clove of fresh garlic every morning and spread it on her toast. (Garlic has potent antiviral and antibacterial qualities, but only when cut or pressed.) I also recommended a mixed-mushroom supplement and a daily effervescent vitamin C supplement in conjunction with frequent handwashing. Lydia was delighted to report in a follow-up visit three months later that she had not had a cold since instituting her antiviral regimen.

The flu, which I will discuss in this chapter, is a much more severe illness caused by the influenza virus that infects up to forty-one million Americans each year.[4] It comes on suddenly and can present with fever, body aches, cough, a sore throat, fatigue, and headaches.[5] While fever and body aches are uncomfortable, they signal that the body is amping up its recovery systems to fight the infection. Having a fever means your white blood cells are activating to kill harmful bacteria; the fever also activates other cellular defense mechanisms, including macrophages, natural killer cells, and dendritic cells.[6] Indeed, fever is a key component of your recovery reflex, so it is worth skipping the paracetamol (acetaminophen) if you can! Western medicine includes vaccines to prevent the flu and medications to treat symptoms and shorten its duration; integrative medicine delivers further armaments with herbs and supplements that shorten the flu's duration.

With a few simple strategies, you may ensure your recovery reflex functions optimally, thwarting viral symptoms and speeding your recovery from the cold, flu, and herpes. (In the chapter "Overcoming Long Covid," I will cover the viral illness that has captured so much of our attention in recent years: Covid-19.)

Cold and Flu

For as long as humans have existed, we have sought remedies for the common cold. In medieval Europe, it was believed that stuffing onions in sleeping socks could ward off illness.[7] (The strong smell likely only succeeded in warding off other people!) From the "Gogol Mogul" (a Russian beverage combining egg yolk with sugar, milk, and butter) to traditional Chinese lizard soup, every culture has a cold remedy.[8]

The flu is a more serious illness. Consider the 1918 Spanish Flu, which infected a staggering one-third of the world's population and claimed twice the number of lives as World War I.[9] A robust integrative approach can help reduce the severity and duration of both cold and flu symptoms. Here is what I recommend.

Nutrition

A balanced diet can help strengthen your immune system, reduce the severity and duration of symptoms, and support overall health. Here is what to put on your plate.

> **Vegetables and Fruit:** Women who consume more vegetables and fruits reduce the risk of respiratory infections, as demonstrated in one study of more than one thousand pregnant North American women.[10] But even without a specific supportive study, I recommend everyone eat them! Vegetables and fruits are our major source of antioxidants, including vitamin C, which can help boost the immune system, shorten the duration of cold symptoms, and support the production of infection-fighting white blood cells.
>
> **Garlic:** When my children were sick, one of my favorite remedies was to press a clove of garlic and mix it into a bit of cream cheese, then spread it on a bagel. To this day, my kids swear by raw garlic! When garlic is chopped, crushed, or pressed, it produces allicin, a sulfur-containing compound.[11] Allicin is known for its antibacterial, antiviral, and antifungal properties, which help the immune system combat infections. While it may be yummy roasted or cooked, only raw garlic is an effective antimicrobial. Garlic has been shown to help prevent colds from reoccurring. In one double-blind study,[12] 146 people were randomized to receive either a garlic supplement or a placebo. After twelve weeks, sixty-five members of the placebo group had colds, compared with just twenty-four in the garlic group. You can easily add garlic to your morning toast, stir

it into your salad dressing, or throw it in a stir-fry right before serving; I recommend consuming fresh, pressed garlic over taking supplements.

Honey: Honey has a thick, viscous consistency that coats the throat, providing a soothing effect while reducing irritation and discomfort. It was found by Oxford University researchers to be superior to usual care (such as cough syrup and paracetamol/acetaminophen) for improving symptoms of upper respiratory tract infections.[13] Honey is also a yummy and effective cough suppressant.[14] Add it to your tea or simply lick it off the spoon before you go to bed. (Just be sure to brush your teeth afterward!)

Chicken Soup: No, your *grandmother* was not the first person to realize chicken soup is an excellent cold remedy. During the Middle Ages, the Jewish physician and philosopher-scientist Maimonides prescribed chicken soup as a cure for everything from colds to asthma, to weight gain and leprosy.[15] While chicken soup may not be quite the panacea Maimonides claimed, its benefits for colds are substantial. The broth keeps you hydrated, helping to thin mucus and keep your throat moist, while adding spices like garlic and pepper can open nasal passages.[16] If you are a vegetarian, a hot vegetable soup can provide immune-enhancing vitamins and minerals. While it has not been formally studied, the broth likely helps thin mucus as well. I recommend adding chopped astragalus root to either chicken or vegetable soup early in the onset of the viral infection for an immune boost.[17]

Medicinal Mushrooms: Mushrooms have been recognized for their medicinal properties for centuries. Many contain polysaccharides, particularly beta-glucans, which enhance the function of the immune system. Reishi, shiitake, maitake (hen of the woods), turkey tail, and cordyceps mushrooms are all associated with immune-boosting benefits.[18] You can add them to soups, stews, and stir-fries, or brew them into teas. Another easy way to take mushrooms is as an extract or capsule.

Herbal Medicines

An internet search will reveal a plethora of herbal remedies for cold and flu symptoms. Here I will focus on those with the strongest scientific evidence.

Echinacea: A flowering plant in the daisy family, echinacea is also commonly known as coneflower. It has been used as a cold remedy for centuries, particularly by Native Americans.[19] Echinacea is believed to inhibit the replication of viruses while stimulating the activity of immune cells, including macrophages, natural killer cells, and T-cells; as a side benefit, it even reduces anxiety. While it is still unclear whether echinacea reduces the overall severity of cold symptoms, one review of fourteen clinical trials found that echinacea reduced the chance of developing a cold by 58 percent and lessened the cold duration by as many as four days.[20] There are many ways to consume echinacea, and the dose depends on the particular plant variety. This can be confusing. To keep things clear, when you are at the store, I recommend you purchase one of the following:

- A 1:5 tincture (> 60 percent alcohol) of *E. angustifolia* root. Take 9 to 15 ml per day.
- *E. angustifolia* dried root. Take 1 to 3 gm daily.
- *E. angustifolia* root powder. Take 900 mg daily.
- *E. angustifolia* root extract. Take 290 mg (or 6 tablets) daily.

The herbalists I work with recommend the following mixture: Infuse an echinacea tea bag for 10 minutes along with a bag of black tea. Add lemon juice (to help with swelling in your throat), 1 pressed garlic clove, honey, and a pinch of cayenne pepper. While this may sound like an intense beverage to drink, it will soothe your sore throat. Note that echinacea is generally considered safe. However, it may inhibit an enzyme called CYP1A2. Speak to your doctor if you are taking medications that are metabolized by this enzyme, including paracetamol (acetaminophen), amitriptyline, diazepam, estrogen-based medicines, propranolol, and warfarin.

Elderberry: With only three days left before a big international trip, my patient Michael was desperate for fast relief from the flu, which had hit him hard several days earlier. It was too late for an antiviral medication, so I suggested he take elderberry syrup. Michael did, and by the time he arrived at the gate, his symptoms had dramatically improved. Elderberry has been used since ancient Egyptian times to treat fever and rheumatism.[21] The berries contain compounds called *anthocyanins*, which have been shown to inhibit the replication of the cold and influenza viruses. One 2021 study showed that elderberries can reduce the duration of cold symptoms by an impressive two days. In another study,[22] sixty adults with influenza were given either three teaspoons of elderberry syrup or a placebo four times daily for five days; those who took the elderberries recovered more quickly—by an average of four days. Finally, elderberries are also excellent for cold prevention, according to one study of 312 people flying overseas from Australia, who were given either elderberry supplements or placebo ten days before the onset of their travel.[23] Among those who got sick, the elderberry users experienced a two-day shorter duration of the cold and noticeably milder symptoms. Elderberries are delicious, especially in syrup form. I recommend 3 teaspoons four times daily for cold and flu relief.

Andrographis: Andrographis (*Andrographis paniculata*) is an herb traditionally used in Ayurvedic and Chinese medicine to treat respiratory infections, along with constipation, digestion, and snake bites. It has been shown in studies to stimulate the immune system by increasing the production and activity of white blood cells.[24] One meta-analysis found that compared to typical care, andrographis shortened the duration of cough and sore throat symptoms while reducing the number of sick days taken.[25] I recommend taking 3 to 6 grams daily of the powdered herbal extract (containing up to 500 mg of andrographolide constituents) for up to ten days.

Astragalus: Astragalus is a traditional herbal medicine widely used in Chinese medicine. The root of the *Astragalus membranaceus* plant contains carbohydrates called *polysaccharides*, which stimulate the immune system by increasing the production of white blood cells.[26] Astragalus is an adaptogen, meaning it helps protect the body against physical and emotional stress. It is commonly taken by cancer patients to help strengthen their immune system after chemotherapy, and I recommend it to many of my patients to prevent recurrences of upper respiratory infections. Talk to your healthcare team before taking astragalus. The typical dose is a 500 to 1,000 mg capsule twice daily; alternatively, you can chop astragalus root and add it to winter soups.

Supplements

A number of supplements have been shown to reduce the severity and duration of cold and flu symptoms. Here is what I recommend.

Vitamin C: If you walk into your local drug store, you may see an entire shelf devoted to vitamin C supplements. But do they actually work? The evidence suggests a modest benefit. One study found that adults who take 1 to 2 grams of vitamin C per day have an 8 percent faster recovery from colds.[27] While this degree of improvement is not dramatic, vitamin C supplements are inexpensive and rarely cause side effects. I recommend effervescent vitamin C tablets, which are added to water and have a pleasant fizzy taste; or liquid sachets of vitamin C; or supplements by trusted sources that use high-quality ingredients.

Probiotics: Probiotics are live microorganisms found in foods such as yogurt, kimchi, sauerkraut, kefir, and kombucha. They support your recovery reflex and alleviate cold symptoms by stimulating the production of antibodies and boosting the activity of immune cells. One randomized trial found that compared to a placebo, people taking probiotics had 30 percent fewer cold recurrences after an infection.[28] And a meta-analysis of twenty randomized controlled trials found that probiotics reduce the duration of illness among children and adults.[29] Current evidence suggests that probiotic formulations containing *Lactobacillus rhamnosus* and *Lactobacillus casei rhamnosus* may be the most effective organisms, depending on the condition being treated and individual patient factors.[30] You can find the most up-to-date U.K. recommendations at https://probioticguide.uk.

Zinc: Zinc is an essential mineral that supports the immune system and is thought to interfere with the cold virus's ability to reproduce and spread. One meta-analysis reported that patients who took zinc got over their colds about a day faster compared to those on a placebo.[31] Note that the studies generally show zinc is most effective when started soon after the onset of symptoms. I recommend my patients begin sucking on low-dose 5 to 7 mg zinc lozenges at the very first hint of a cold, as often as every 2 to 3 hours while awake, until symptoms subside. Don't exceed more than 50 mg per day. You can find zinc lozenges in pharmacies and online.

Nasal Decongestion

When a cold or flu virus infects the nasal passages, the body's rapid recovery system responds by releasing inflammatory compounds, including histamines, cytokines, and leukotrienes, which help fight the infection. Blood flow increases in the nasal passages, delivering more immune cells to the infection site, but also causing swelling of the nasal tissues—in other words, a stuffy nose. I recommend rinsing your nasal passages with saline using either a neti pot or another form of sinus rinse or nasal irrigation.[32] These nasal-irrigation systems will shrink the swollen nasal passages, dramatically clearing out mucus and making it easier to breath.

You can purchase pre-mixed salt packets buffered with bicarbonate of soda, or do it yourself by adding 1/4 teaspoon of table salt and a pinch of bicarbonate of soda to a glass of room-temperature distilled water. (You can make your own distilled water by boiling tap water for up to 5 minutes and letting sit until lukewarm.) Follow the irrigation instructions on the label. After each use, wash the neti pot with soap and water and allow to air-dry. Periodically disinfect the neti pot with a solution of 1 percent sodium hypochlorite (bleach) or by microwaving it. While many of my patients are initially reluctant, they quickly become believers! In one trial involving 143 people with an acute upper-respiratory infection,[33] symptoms like nasal congestion and runny nose were significantly reduced among those using a nasal saline spray when compared to usual supportive care.

There are a few common over-the-counter nasal decongestants available. However, I typically do not recommend using over-the-counter nasal decongestants as they can cause a fierce rebound congestion if used for more than one to two days.

Saunas for Cold Prevention

There is some evidence that regular use of a sauna can halve the incidence of colds.[34] In one study of fifty participants, one group used a sauna once or twice a week for six months while a second group avoided all hyperthermic treatments. The sauna users first took a warm shower, then sat or lay down for up to twelve minutes in the 80–90°C (175–200°F) sauna room; this was followed by fifteen minutes cooling off with cold water and twenty minutes of rest. This cycle was repeated two or three times, followed by a final rest period. Three months into the experiment, the frequency of colds among the sauna users dropped significantly; they had just nine colds compared to twenty-three colds among the abstainers.

Antiviral medication

After a long flight, my patient Sandy came down with flu symptoms: fever, runny nose, congestion, and body aches. "I feel like I've been hit by a truck," she told me. Because it had been just sixteen hours since the onset of her symptoms, I prescribed oseltamivir, a neuraminidase inhibitor. Neuraminidase is an enzyme on the surface of the influenza virus that allows the virus to be released from infected cells and spread to new cells. By inhibiting this enzyme, oseltamivir prevents the virus from spreading within the body. Within twenty-four hours, Sandy was feeling significantly better.

When taken within the first forty-eight hours of the onset of symptoms, oseltamivir is one of the antiviral medicines that can reduce the duration of the flu by one to two days while lessening the fever, chills, muscle aches, sore throat, and fatigue. If you come down with a bad case of the flu, I highly recommend taking an antiviral medication.[35] Side effects, which may include nausea, vomiting, and headache, are generally mild and are mitigated by taking the medication with food.

Boosting the Potency of the Flu Vaccine

Did you know you can increase the potency of your annual flu vaccine by getting it in the morning, after a good night's rest and after pumping some iron beforehand?

Indeed, the flu vaccine leads to a significantly higher antibody production when injected in the morning compared to later in the day,[36] reflecting the importance of circadian rhythms on immune function. Your immune response will also be stronger after a good night's sleep and if you exercise your biceps and deltoid muscles in the hours prior to injection.[37] Lastly, taking probiotics has been shown to improve the uptake of the flu vaccine and may be especially beneficial in anyone who is immunocompromised or elderly.[38]

Herpes

Perhaps it will seem odd to combine herpes in the same chapter as the common cold, but there is significant overlap when it comes to activating your recovery system. And herpes is very common, affecting some four billion people worldwide.[39] There are multiple different herpes viruses, but I will focus on the most common: herpes simplex virus type 1 (HSV-1), which leads to cold sores or fever blisters around the mouth and face, and herpes simplex virus type 2 (HSV-2), which typically causes sores and blisters in the genital area. As we'll see, dealing with both is straightforward, and I hope to help you let go of any feelings of shame or stigma.

My thirty-year-old patient Roberta reported monthly bouts of soreness around her vulva and pain urinating after contracting genital herpes from her husband. She was also extremely embarrassed. I acknowledged her feelings, but emphasized she had nothing to be ashamed of. What she was experiencing was common, and I reassured her there was a great deal we could do to reduce the frequency and intensity of her outbreaks.

I suggested she increase her intake of lysine, an amino acid that inhibits replication of the herpes virus, by adding a supplement. We discussed the importance of managing stress, which is another common trigger. I prescribed acyclovir (an antiviral medication) to be taken as a preventive medication. Finally, I advised her to begin using propolis, a resin-like material made by bees, to help the sores heal more quickly. With time,

Roberta's outbreaks became rare, and she was able to discontinue daily use of acyclovir, instead taking it only to treat the occasional outbreak.

Herpes is spread primarily through direct contact with an infected person. There are two types: HSV-1, which is spread through saliva (by kissing or even sharing a utensil or glass), and HSV-2, which is contagious through sexual contact. After the initial infection, the virus can remain dormant in the body and reactivate at a later point. These reactivations are often, but not always, triggered by factors within your control. Both types are also much more common than you think: As many as 80 percent of American adults have been infected with HSV-1,[40] and about one in six has HSV-2.[41] People with HSV-1 generally have less than one outbreak per year, while HSV-2 can cause four or five outbreaks a year.

High stress levels are strongly associated with herpes outbreaks. If you or a loved one carries the virus, I encourage you to read the chapter "Unwinding Anxiety," where we explore potential strategies to manage anxiety.

Nutrition and the Herpes Virus

Essential amino acids play a significant role in protein synthesis, tissue repair, and nutrient absorption. There are nine "essential" amino acids, meaning your body cannot synthesize them on its own; they must be consumed in your diet. Two are linked to HSV-1 and HSV-2 outbreaks: lysine and arginine. High-lysine foods include cheese, fish (especially cod and sardines), eggs, soybeans, pulses (legumes), beef, pork, and poultry. Arginine-rich foods include white rice and white flour, deep-fried foods, processed meats, chocolate, corn, and peanuts. Be aware that many protein powders are rich in arginine as well.

Lysine and arginine compete with each other for absorption and utilization in the body. When lysine levels are high, that inhibits the uptake of arginine, and vice versa. This matters because arginine provides the raw materials the herpes virus needs to reproduce, leading to an increased risk of outbreaks. Effectively, you can reduce the odds of an outbreak by eating foods rich in lysine and low in arginine.

Aciclovir

Aciclovir (sometimes acyclovir) is an antiviral medication used to treat oral and genital herpes by inhibiting the replication of the virus. Studies show that it can significantly shorten healing time, reduce pain, and limit the spread of the virus.[42] The standard seven- to ten-day regimen is prescribed either as a five-times-daily dose of 200 mg or a three-times-daily dose of 400 mg; begin within seventy-two hours of the onset of symptoms, for best results. Aciclovir is also prescribed to prevent outbreaks.[43] Two similar antiviral prescription medications are famciclovir and valaciclovir.

Vitamins, Minerals, Supplements, and Herbal Medicines

In addition to the supplements like vitamin C and zinc described earlier in this chapter, several supplements have been proven to shorten the duration and frequency of herpes outbreaks. Here is what I recommend.

> **Lysine:** As noted earlier, eating lysine-rich foods can reduce herpes outbreaks, though a lysine supplement may be the easier route for most people. In one randomized controlled trial,[44] participants who took a little over 1,200 mg of lysine daily had significantly fewer herpes outbreaks over twenty-four weeks, compared to those who took half that dose or were on a placebo. Other studies have shown that taking a lysine supplement also reduces the severity and healing time of outbreaks when they do occur.[45] I recommend taking 1 gram orally three times daily. (Higher doses may cause stomach discomfort.[46])
>
> **Lemon Balm:** Known for its antiviral properties, lemon balm has long been used to help manage herpes symptoms. It contains the compounds rosmarinic acid, caffeic acid, and eugenol, which inhibit the replication of the herpes simplex virus. In a study of sixty-six patients with recurrent oral herpes, using lemon balm within two days of an outbreak significantly reduced the severity and duration of blisters.[47] Another study showed that applying lemon balm two to four times daily for ten days provided the fastest healing. I recommend looking

for a lemon balm product available as a cream, salve, or essential oil for treating cold sores.

Propolis: As we saw earlier with Roberta, propolis has antiviral properties that can help heal herpes lesions. Propolis contains bioactive compounds like flavonoids, phenolic acids, and esters, which have been shown to inhibit the replication of herpes simplex virus.[48] Propolis can be applied directly to herpes sores in the form of an ointment, cream, or lip balm. Apply it to the affected area three to four times a day. In one study of 189 people, propolis ointment was found to be more effective than acyclovir ointment in healing cold sores.[49]

Self-Hypnosis for Herpes Outbreaks

The mind–body connection can be harnessed to reduce herpes recurrences. In one study,[50] people with genital herpes who practiced six weeks of self-hypnosis using an audiotape saw a 40 percent reduction in further herpes outbreaks. I recommend downloading an audio track from Hypnotic World (www.hypnoticworld.com).

Your Rapid Recovery Prescription for Conquering Colds and Vanquishing Viral Infections

Your rapid recovery reflex helps you bounce back from colds and viral infections, and there are things you can do to boost it. Following are ways to help speed up your recovery from a cold, the flu, and herpes viruses. People respond differently to treatments, so please experiment to find one that works best for you.

For Cold and Flu

1. Amp up your consumption of vegetables and fruits, medicinal mushrooms, raw garlic, and honey.

2. Experiment with herbal medicines, and determine whether echinacea or andrographis is most effective for you. If you get the flu, elderberry can help shorten its duration. I also recommend astragalus.
3. Take vitamin C, probiotics, and zinc lozenges at the very first hint of a cold or the flu—all of which can reduce the severity and duration of cold symptoms.
4. For nasal decongestion or post-nasal drainage, rinse your nasal passages with saline using a neti pot, sinus rinse, or other nasal irrigation system.
5. If you have the flu, take elderberry and talk to your doctor about whether to get a prescription for an antiviral medication. Take both within the first forty-eight hours of the onset of symptoms.

For Oral and Genital Herpes
1. Consider whether stress is a trigger for you. If it is, amp up your centering practices (see the "Unwinding Anxiety" chapter).
2. Reduce the odds of an outbreak by eating foods rich in lysine and low in arginine, or by adding a lysine supplement.
3. Experiment with supplements that shorten the duration and frequency of herpes outbreaks, including vitamin C, zinc, lemon balm, and propolis.
4. Take acyclovir if needed to treat genital herpes. Begin taking the medication within seventy-two hours of the onset of symptoms. If you have frequent outbreaks, consider a smaller preventative dose. In conjunction with the strategies listed here, you can greatly reduce the frequency of outbreaks.

2

Soothing the Gut

One day, a twenty-nine-year-old man named Mike came to see me complaining of severe acid reflux, also known as heartburn or *gastro-oesophageal reflux disease* (GORD, or sometimes GERD), a condition in which stomach acid flows back up into the esophagus, causing a burning sensation. The pain was so bad that he was downing dozens of antacids every day. He knew that there were more powerful medicines available, but he had a strong preference to go "natural."

As I took Mike's history, I realized he had an erratic eating history, with frequent late-night snacking. "Let's experiment with keeping your meals in a ten-hour window." I said, explaining that time-restricted eating can decrease heartburn and regurgitation symptoms. I also asked him to stop eating at least three hours before bedtime, as food consumption in this window increases the risk of GORD sevenfold.[1] After following this structured eating plan for two months, Mike's symptoms vanished entirely. As a side benefit, he lost 3 kilograms (7 lb)—mostly the stubborn belly fat from around his waist he'd been struggling to get rid of for years. He told me at our follow-up visit that he felt "terrific."

More than two thousand years ago, the Greek physician and philosopher Hippocrates famously declared that "all disease begins in the gut."[2] Somehow this wisdom got lost, and the link between gut health and overall well-being is only gradually being re-acknowledged today. The gut, which comprises the mouth, esophagus, stomach, small intestine, colon, rectum, and anus, is an incredibly complex "tube" responsible for countless functions, including the digestion and absorption of nutrients; elimination of waste and toxins from the body; and provision of a physical barrier to prevent harmful substances and pathogens from entering the bloodstream. The gut is also host to the trillions of beneficial bacteria, fungi, and viruses that make up our microbiome and keep us healthy.

There are also some six hundred million neurons embedded in the walls of your GI tract,[3] which are collectively known as the *enteric nervous system* (ENS). In fact, there are more neurotransmitters in your ENS than in your brain, including 95 percent of the "feel good" neurotransmitter serotonin.[4] The ENS communicates bidirectionally with your brain—and is therefore often called the *gut–brain axis*—via the vagus nerve, which runs from the brainstem to your abdomen, touching nearly every major organ along the way. Given how critical the gut is to your brain function, it's no wonder we talk about having a "gut feeling" about something!

In this chapter, we are going to examine two common forms of stubborn tummy trouble: GORD, a digestive disorder in which stomach acid flows back up into the esophagus; and IBS, or irritable bowel syndrome, an uncomfortable condition that causes recurring abdominal symptoms like constipation, diarrhea, wind or gas, and bloating. I will begin by covering an extremely powerful integrative tool—the elimination diet—which can identify and eliminate food triggers that cause symptoms of both conditions. Next, we'll see how other integrative-medicine strategies, from Egyptian licorice tea to hypnotherapy, can activate your recovery reflex to help relieve GORD or IBS symptoms while preventing flare-ups.

General Upset Stomach

Lots of folks have the occasional upset stomach. If your stomach is feeling off, I recommend a tea blend with cardamom, fennel and ginger or Egyptian licorice tea. For bloating immediately after meals, I recommend a teaspoon of Angostura bitters with soda water (club soda) or juice before or after meals to stimulate your digestive enzymes. For a mild case of heartburn due to a rare dietary indiscretion, you can chew deglycyrrhizinated licorice (DGL) tablets. (More about DGL later.)

If you travel and note a bit of diarrhea, a probiotic with lactobacillus can help restore homeostasis. For occasional constipation, you can eat prunes or kiwifruit,[5] increase your hydration, and eat more fiber. If, on the other hand, you find tummy trouble frequently plagues you, read on for ways to remove triggers and activate your recovery reflex.

The Elimination Diet

One of the most valuable tools to activate your recovery reflex is an elimination diet. This structured trial helps identify food sensitivities, intolerances, or allergies that may be impeding your recovery reflex from supporting a healthy equilibrium. Elimination diets work by removing potential offenders from your diet and then gradually reintroducing them one at a time, while monitoring symptoms. A well-designed elimination diet is the gold standard for discovering what foods may be impacting your gut health. It is amazing to me how longstanding discomforts can resolve completely when an offending food is removed and equilibrium is restored. Signs that you may want to start an elimination diet are not limited to GI complaints like constipation, diarrhea, bloating, and cramping; they may show up as headache, irritability, fatigue, mood swings, anxiety, joint pain, eczema, inflammation, and more.[6]

Patients often ask me for a blood test to see what they may be sensitive or allergic to, but with the exception of celiac disease (a true autoimmune disease caused by exposure to gluten), blood tests are not reliable. The most effective method is to eliminate the potential food trigger, watching for a response—Is your skin, mood, or GI tract feeling better?—and then reintroduce the food to see if anything changes. I ask my patients to keep a symptom record so they can tell, for example, whether their migraine headaches have decreased in frequency. (See sample following.) I also ask that they be strict during the initial four-week elimination trial.

Sample Symptom Record

Date	Time	Location	What I was Doing	What Happened After	Severity (1-5)	What I said to Myself During	Other

The most common food sensitivity is lactose, the sugar found in milk products. This intolerance is found in 65 percent of the world population, including the vast majority of people of East Asian descent.[7] With the exception of northern Europeans, only 5 percent of whom are intolerant, in adulthood most people lose the ability to digest cow's milk. This intolerance is often obvious, evidenced by abdominal pain, bloating, flatulence, nausea, and diarrhea between thirty minutes and two hours after eating dairy. For instance, my patient Tanisha followed my recommendation to do a trial of eliminating dairy. Three weeks later she had lost 5 kilograms (11 lb) and her longstanding bloating and constipation resolved entirely—a perfect example of how homeostasis can rapidly return after removing an offending trigger!

Other common food intolerances are to wheat, soy, corn, citrus, and eggs. Less common but not rare are tree nuts, peanuts, shellfish, yeast, and alcohol. My twenty-year-old patient Helen reached out to me after returning from a college semester in Italy, where she had gained significant weight. She also felt sluggish, constipated, and irritable. Curiously, she had also developed a bumpy red rash on her upper outer arms, called *keratosis pilaris*.

"I just feel *miserable*," Helen said, explaining that her symptoms, which had been mild in the past, had become progressively worse during her time overseas.

"I have a suggestion," I said, "It's called an elimination diet. And the first thing I want you to stop eating is wheat." When Helen removed wheat from her diet, her rash vanished. Her mood improved markedly, and over the next two years she lost nearly 16 kilograms (2.5 stone/35 lb). The culprit was gluten, a protein found in wheat that was causing an inflammatory response in her gut.

It's critical to strictly adhere to the elimination trial during the initial four-to-six-week period. This requires discipline and pragmatism. Choose a convenient time when you have no exciting social engagements or holidays that might tempt you to "cheat." For detailed instructions on getting started with an elimination diet, see "Your Rapid Recovery Toolkit" (appendix 1).

Gastro-oesophageal Reflux Disease

Commonly known as GORD (or GERD), gastro-oesophageal reflux disease is a digestive disorder in which stomach acid flows back, or *refluxes*, into the esophagus through a ring of muscles called the *lower oesophageal sphincter* (LOS, or sometimes LES), which normally functions as a one-way valve. This backwash of acid irritates the lining of the esophagus and can cause a burning sensation in the chest known as heartburn; it can also cause acid regurgitation into the mouth, difficulty swallowing, chronic cough, often at night, and wheezing.[8]

GORD is common, with as many as 30 percent of Americans experiencing symptoms each year.[9] Anyone can get it, but certain factors,[10] including pregnancy or excess weight (which puts pressure on the abdomen and causes the LOS to relax inappropriately) can raise your risk of its symptoms. Eating large meals, smoking, and drinking alcohol can also relax the LOS. The good news is that in most cases you can activate your recovery reflex and reverse GORD entirely. As we'll see, dietary supplements and stress management can help, as well as paying attention to *what*, *how much*, and *when* you eat.

Treating Minor GORD Symptoms

If you're experiencing GORD symptoms, I highly recommend you begin with an elimination diet, as discussed in the previous section. Fried and fatty foods and alcohol are common triggers, but so are dairy products, spicy seasonings and sauces, tomatoes and tomato-based products, vinegar-based foods, chocolate, caffeinated beverages, and carbonated beverages. I recommend a trial period in which you avoid acidic foods and beverages such as regular or diet soda. One study used a strict acid-free diet in twenty people who had not responded to high doses of medications for laryngopharyngeal reflux, which causes symptoms similar to those caused by GORD.[11] The study found that nineteen out of the twenty participants who avoided acidic foods (specifically those with a pH lower than 5) reduced their symptoms by 95 percent.

When you have the occasional GORD symptoms or general tummy ache, the following can help you recover quickly:

Deglycyrrhizinated Licorice (DGL): DGL is a form of licorice root that has had the glycyrrhizin component removed. (Glycyrrhizin is the compound in licorice that increases blood pressure and causes water retention.[12]) DGL increases the production of mucus in the stomach and esophagus, which acts as a protective barrier that shields the lining of the stomach and esophagus from the damaging effects of stomach acid. A common dosage is one or two 380 mg chewable tablets taken before meals, as needed.[13]

Egyptian Licorice Tea: A cup of Egyptian licorice tea can also soothe GORD symptoms. I recommend infusing the tea bag in hot water with a lid over the cup for 5 to 10 minutes before drinking.

Eat Smaller, Earlier Meals: Eating a large meal stretches the stomach, exerting pressure on the LOS.[14] Eating smaller meals can help lower the risk of GORD symptoms. Note also that midnight snacking increases your risk of GORD fivefold, eating quickly increases the risk fourfold, and eating beyond fullness increases the risk almost threefold.[15]

Adjust Sleep Habits: Wait at least two hours after eating to lie down, allowing ample time for your stomach to empty. If needed, raise the head of your bed by 15–20 centimetres (6–8 in) or get a wedge-shaped pillow, which can help prevent stomach acid from flowing back into the esophagus while you're lying flat.[16]

Use Antacids as Necessary: Over-the-counter antacids can neutralize stomach acid and provide quick relief for heartburn and indigestion. Bismuth subsalicylate, a mild antacid with antimicrobial effects that is used to treat diarrhea, can also be used, especially if you also have diarrheal symptoms. Pay attention to any dietary choices that make you need an antacid. (For me, it's gazpacho!)

Tapering off PPIs

Many people take proton pump inhibitors (PPIs) to manage their GORD. PPIs are among the most commonly prescribed medications in the U.S., with some fifteen million adults taking them.[17] (They are also available over the counter.) A recent large-scale study showed that a majority of American people on PPIs use them daily, and nearly three-fourths have been using them for more than two years.[18]

PPIs work by decreasing the production of acid in the stomach. Stomach acid is an important part of your body's recovery defense mechanism. It initiates the breakdown of food and the release of vitamins from proteins, and it is also a key barrier against harmful microorganisms that may be ingested with food. The most common PPIs are esomeprazole, lansoprazole, and omeprazole). While they are effective at reducing GORD symptoms, PPIs have potential long-term side effects, including an increased risk of liver disease, chronic kidney disease, and bone fracture, particularly of the hip, wrist, and spine. Long-term use of PPIs can also affect the absorption of nutrients,[19] including magnesium, calcium, and vitamin B12. Reduced stomach acid can also increase the risk of GI infections, most notably *Clostridium difficile* (*C. diff*).

While PPIs reduce stomach acid and help heal ulcers or GORD, it can be extremely difficult to stop using them,[20] as people often experience a huge rebound of acid production and GORD symptoms. My patient Santosh took PPIs for fifteen years because of severe heartburn. Every time he tried to wean himself off, his reflux returned with a vengeance. Fortunately, a regimen I commonly use with three supplements—D-limonene, deglycyrrhizinated licorice, and Iberogast—made it possible for him to discontinue his PPI. (More on these supplements soon.) He also discovered and eliminated his dietary triggers: tomato soup and spicy food.

PPIs are usually meant to be taken only for two to eight weeks,[21] with the exception of a few rare conditions such as Barrett's esophagus, where acid reflux has damaged the esophagus lining, increasing the risk for cancer.[22] If you experience rebound acid production whenever you attempt to go off a PPI, consider this protocol to help you taper:

1. **Start Taking a D-limonene supplement.** D-limonene is derived from the peels of citrus fruits, including oranges, lemons, and grapefruits, coupled with dill and bergamot. It has anti-inflammatory and antioxidant effects and may also help reduce stress.[23] I recommend beginning D-limonene supplements before tapering off the PPI. The recommended dose is 1,000 mg every other day.[24]
2. **Add Melatonin:** Melatonin, a hormone primarily known for regulating sleep–wake cycles, has also been shown to protect the mucosal lining of the stomach, help heal ulcers, and increase the tightness of the LOS.[25] One study found it was effective in relieving heartburn.[26] However, it is only available on prescription in the U.K. and your doctor can only prescribe it for sleep problems.
3. **Add Iberogast:** Iberogast is an herbal supplement that contains extracts from nine different medicinal plants. It is useful in treating many gastrointestinal disorders, including GORD.[27] Several of the herbs in Iberogast, such as chamomile and licorice root, have anti-inflammatory properties that can help soothe the lining of the esophagus and stomach by reducing irritation and inflammation caused by acid reflux.[28]
4. **Slowly Reduce PPI Dose:** Instead of stopping PPIs abruptly, gradually reduce the dosage over several weeks. For example, if you are taking 40 mg daily, reduce the dose to 20 mg and then to 10 mg. Alternatively, take 20 mg every other day. You can taper into even smaller doses with a pill splitter.
5. **Use an H2 Blocker for Lingering Symptoms:** H2 receptor antagonists, also known as H2 blockers, are a class of medications that reduce stomach acid production by blocking histamine receptors on the cells in the stomach lining. They are less potent—and much safer—than PPIs. These medications can be helpful to combat the rebound effect common with reducing PPI usage. I recommend 300 mg of cimetidine every 6 hours as needed. Alternatively, take famotidine or nizatidine.
6. **Take Slippery Elm:** Sometimes, when someone is still struggling to taper off a PPI, I recommend slippery elm, which is a powder derived from the inner bark of the slippery elm tree; it contains mucilage, a gel-like substance that becomes slick when mixed with water and can protect the stomach lining.[29] A typical dosage is 1 tablespoon of slippery elm

powder mixed with cold water, taken up to three times a day. You can also use sucralfate, a medication that works similarly by coating the lining of the GI tract,[30] though it will require a prescription.

7. **Gradually Taper off Supplements:** While your immediate goal is to eliminate PPIs, once you have fully resolved your GERD symptoms and stopped eating the foods that trigger symptoms, the next step is to gradually taper off the supplements. Occasional use of DGL is fine, as is melatonin, if you have been prescribed it as a sleep aid.

Irritable Bowel Syndrome

Irritable bowel syndrome (IBS) is a common gastrointestinal disorder, affecting as many as 15 percent of American adults.[31] IBS is characterized by symptoms including abdominal pain, bloating, diarrhea, constipation, and wind or gas that vary in severity and duration. Generally speaking, people with IBS have one of three variations: IBS with constipation (IBS-C); IBS with diarrhea (IBS-D); and IBS with mixed bowel habits (IBS-M), which can present as either constipation or diarrhea.

There is no specific test for IBS, so many healthcare providers use the "Rome IV Criteria" for diagnosis,[32] which includes having belly discomfort averaging at least once per week in the last three months, associated with at least two of the following: defecation, a change in frequency of stool, or a change in appearance of the stool.[33] The cause of IBS is not fully understood and may include gut–brain axis communication issues; abnormal sensitivity to the muscle contractions that move food through the digestive tract; or an imbalance in your microbiome. IBS can make activities like road trips or long hikes stressful because you may not be able plan toilet access. Integrative medicine, in many cases, can restore normal bowel function, provide symptom relief, and improve quality of life.

If you suspect a food is triggering your IBS symptoms, I again recommend you carry out an elimination diet. Maya, the wife of one of my fellows, had terrible IBS for most of her adult life, including six episodes of diarrhea every day for thirty years. When she removed eggs from her diet, her symptoms cleared up entirely. As delighted as I was that she found an answer to her chronic symptoms, I felt sad that she had suffered for decades when the fix was so straightforward.

A More Extensive Elimination: Low-FODMAP Diet

A major advance in the treatment of IBS is the identification of FODMAP foods as a trigger in many people. Fermentable oligosaccharides, disaccharides, monosaccharides, and polyols (FODMAPs) are carbohydrates that are not easily digested and produce excess fluid and wind or gas. As a result, the small intestine draws in extra water to help move FODMAPs into the large intestine, where the fermentation process creates wind and fatty acids, particularly in people with IBS.[34]

Avoiding FODMAP foods reduces the amount of fermentable carbohydrates in the gut, easing symptoms such as bloating, wind, abdominal pain, and diarrhea. The low-FODMAP diet was developed by a research team at Monash University in Melbourne, Australia. Today, a low-FODMAP diet is recommended for those with IBS by other healthcare providers around the world, with studies showing it can significantly reduce IBS symptoms in as many as 75 percent of patients.[35]

I recommend visiting Monash University's website at www.monashfodmap.com for a comprehensive list of high- and low-FODMAP foods, but in the meantime, here's a primer:

	High-FODMAP Foods	Low-FODMAP Alternatives
Vegetables	Artichokes, asparagus, cauliflower, garlic, green peas, mushrooms, onions, sugar snap peas	Aubergine (eggplant), green beans, pak choi (bok choy), green peppers (capsicums), carrots, cucumbers, lettuce, potatoes
Fruits	Apples, apple juice, cherries, dried fruits, mangoes, nectarines, peaches, pears, plums, watermelons	Cantaloupe melons, kiwifruits, mandarin oranges, oranges, pineapples, blueberries
Dairy and Alternatives	Cow's milk, custard, evaporated milk, ice cream, soy milk (made from whole soybeans), sweetened condensed milk, yogurt	Almond milk, brie/camembert cheese, feta cheese, hard cheeses, lactose-free milk, soy milk

Protein	Most pulses (legumes), some marinated meats/poultry/seafood, some processed meats	Eggs, firm tofu, plain cooked meats/poultry/seafood, tempeh
Breads and Cereals	Wheat/rye/barley-based breads, breakfast cereals, biscuits and snack products	Oats, quinoa flakes, quinoa/rice/corn pasta, rice cakes (plain), sourdough spelt bread, wheat/rye/barley-free breads
Sweeteners	Fructose-glucose syrup (high fructose corn syrup, honey), sugar-free confectionery	Dark chocolate, maple syrup, rice malt syrup, table sugar
Nuts and Seeds	Cashews, pistachios	Macadamias, peanuts, pumpkin seeds/pepitas, walnuts

Implementing a low-FODMAP diet is a form of elimination diet. The process begins by identifying high-FODMAP foods in your diet and swapping them out for low-FODMAP alternatives—for instance, eating coarse oats instead of wheat-based breakfast cereal. Continue eating the low-FODMAP diet for four to six weeks. If your IBS symptoms improve, begin reintroducing high-FODMAP foods from one category at a time, which will help you identify specific triggers. Pay close attention to how your body reacts as you reintroduce each food; I recommend keeping a symptom record. Be sure to closely inspect food labels, as processed foods often contain hidden FODMAPs.

After a few months, you will have gained a good understanding of which foods trigger IBS and which you can safely eat.

Hypnosis

In one study, thirty people with IBS were randomly selected to either receive seven sessions of hypnotherapy or seven sessions of psychotherapy plus placebo pills. The hypnotherapy participants were led to envision a normally functioning, healthy digestive system with no cramps, frequency, diarrhea, or constipation. At the end of the study, the psychotherapy group saw a small improvement in symptoms, while the hypnotherapy group saw a dramatic improvement, including zero relapses for three months following the study. This is a beautiful example of a mind–body activation of your innate recovery system.

So how do you get started? Gut directed hypnosis is a structured approach in which a trained hypnotherapist meets with you weekly for up to three months. During these sessions you are guided into a state of deep relaxation by focusing on your breathing and visualizing calming images. Once induced into this deeply relaxed state, the hypnotherapist provides positive suggestions and visualizations aimed at reducing IBS symptoms. If there are no trained hypnotherapists in your area, or if the cost is prohibitive, you can use audio recordings or an app.

Treating IBS Symptoms

Should you have a flare-up, in addition to noting what may have triggered it (and avoiding those foods or better managing the stressor), there are several additional integrative therapies I recommend for relief.

> **Probiotics:** As discussed earlier, people with IBS often have an imbalance of healthy bacteria in their gut. In particular, studies suggest that people with IBS have fewer butyrate-producing bacteria.[36] Butyrate produced by bacterial fermentation of dietary fibers has several important functions, including reducing inflammation and reducing gut permeability. While a normal gut allows only water and nutrients to enter the bloodstream, people with IBS may have a "leaky gut" that allows larger molecules to pass through the intestinal lining. Probiotic supplements contain live bacteria and yeasts that support butyrate-producing bacteria, which are key to gut homeostasis because they help restore the normal gut barrier.[37] I recommend taking *B. Longum* and *L. plantarum* for four to eight weeks; these have been shown to enhance gut barrier function, inhibit pathogen inflammatory responses, restore the microbiome, and decrease the inflammatory response in the gut.[38]
>
> **Peppermint (for IBS-D):** Peppermint oil capsules, a widely used remedy for IBS-D, contain menthol, which has antispasmodic properties.[39] By calming the overactive muscles in the GI tract, peppermint oil can help regulate bowel movements and reduce the urgency and frequency of diarrhea. The typical dosage is one to two capsules taken two to three times daily before meals. Note that you should not take peppermint oil if you have GORD, as its muscle-relaxing effects can cause the lower esophageal

sphincter to relax and worsen heartburn. Choose peppermint capsules that have an enteric coating, meaning they are designed to pass through the stomach intact and dissolve in the intestines. Note that the peppermint may also reach the anus, causing a (completely safe but unusual) burning sensation.

Carminatives (for IBS-C): Carminatives are botanicals that help prevent wind or gas formation in the gut. They also contain compounds that relax the muscles of the gastrointestinal tract, mitigating the spasms and cramps common with IBS-C.[40] Carminatives can be found in nearly all spices and culinary herbs. In particular, I recommend ginger (fresh ginger, ginger tea, or ginger supplements); fennel (you can drink fennel tea or chew fennel seeds after meals); caraway (you can add seeds to foods or drink caraway tea); and cumin (add ground seeds to dishes while cooking). Most of the herbs in the mint and carrot families are also carminatives, including anise, basil, cinnamon, garlic, lemon, and nutmeg.

Chamomile: Chamomile is a flowering plant from the Asteraceae family and is commonly used to treat IBS symptoms, thanks to its antispasmodic properties. I recommend drinking chamomile tea throughout the day.[41]

Acupuncture: A meta-analysis of six randomized, placebo-controlled trials found that acupuncture improved control of IBS symptoms.[42] It works by modulating the autonomic nervous system, which controls the function of the GI tract, improving gut motility (the movement of digested food through the GI tract) and reducing symptoms including diarrhea and constipation.

Your Rapid Recovery Prescription for Soothing the Gut

Not only does "all disease begins in the gut," as Hippocrates declared, but rapid recovery begins there, too. You can tap into the brain–gut connection to soothe even the most stubborn forms of tummy trouble.

The first step for any lingering GI discomfort is an elimination diet, which identifies food sensitivities, intolerances, or allergies.

For GERD
1. Eliminate food triggers and explore the role of stress.
2. Eat smaller, earlier meals, and stop eating at least 3 hours prior to going to bed.
3. Treat occasional GORD symptoms with DGL, Egyptian licorice tea, and antacids as necessary.
4. While PPIs are effective, they can have serious long-term side effects. Taper off them with D-limonene, melatonin (if you have a prescription), Iberogast, H2 blockers, and slippery elm.

For IBS
1. A low-FODMAP diet can dramatically reduce IBS flare-ups.
2. Consulting a hypnotherapist can reduce IBS symptoms.
3. When needed, treat IBS symptoms with probiotics, acupuncture, and chamomile. Use carminatives for IBS-C and enteric-coated peppermint oil for IBS-D.

3

Sleeping Soundly

A few years ago, a thirty-six-year-old woman named Jennifer came to see me. She had just started a new high-pressure job and she was not sleeping well. After taking what felt like forever to fall asleep, she'd wake up at 2 a.m. with racing, anxious thoughts. She'd finally doze off at 5:30 a.m., only to be jolted awake an hour later by her alarm clock.

"My bed feels like a battleground," she told me. Once a place for peace and rest, just thinking about the bedroom now gave Jennifer knots of anxiety. What if she couldn't fall asleep? What if she couldn't stay asleep? *What if . . . what if . . .* Jennifer had begun going to bed at 8 p.m. to make up for her lack of rest.

After hearing her story, I asked Jennifer to wait until 10 p.m. to go to bed so she'd be truly sleepy. I also asked her to go outside first thing in the morning and expose herself to bright light. Lastly, I asked her to limit her time in bed to sleep and lovemaking. If she did not fall asleep (or fall back to sleep, if she awoke in the night) within fifteen minutes, she was to get up, go into another room, and do something else until she felt tired again. Additionally, I recommended avoiding bright lights before bedtime and experimenting with a number of free apps that contain guided imagery, binaural sounds, and boring bedtime stories to help her drift off to sleep. Jennifer also took nightly warm baths with Epsom salts and a few drops of lavender essential oil. Collectively, these steps transformed her battleground into an oasis. Within six weeks, she was effortlessly falling—and staying—asleep.

When you think about it, sleep is a peculiar habit. After all, life is short—why spend one-third of it doing seemingly nothing? In fact, while we sleep, our rapid recovery reflex is hard at work. It's a bit like what happens at a resort during the off-season: The guests are gone, but the rooms are being deep-cleaned and all necessary maintenance work is completed. Your body takes care of a lot of business while you sleep: Your brain clears out waste products, such as beta-amyloid, which is linked to Alzheimer's disease,[1] and it processes and consolidates information from the day, helping to form long-term memories. Your immune system reboots, increasing the production of cytokines,[2] which help fight infections and reduces inflammation. Finally, your metabolism resets, helping you maintain a healthy weight and promoting your overall health and well-being. All told, most adults need seven to nine hours each night and teenagers need eight to ten.

Everyone tosses and turns now and then, but sometimes one sleepless night turns into two sleepless nights and then three. As many as 30 percent of the general population have symptoms of insomnia,[3] a sleep disorder characterized by difficulty falling asleep or staying asleep. When you have sleepless nights, you generate "sleep debt," which is the difference between the amount of sleep you need and the amount of sleep you actually get. The larger your sleep debt, the higher your risk of developing poor health effects.

Data from more than sixty thousand people in the U.K.'s Biobank found that compared to those with poor sleep habits, people who regularly sleep well can have as much as a 48 percent reduced risk of all-cause mortality,[4] including up to 57 percent lower risk of death due to cardiometabolic issues and diabetes, and up to a 39 percent reduced risk of cancer mortality. A study that restricted participants' sleep to four or six hours (compared to the usual seven) for just two weeks found that shorter sleepers had lower scores on all tested metrics, including attention, cognitive thought, working memory, mood, and reaction times.[5] Even the switchover from standard time to daylight saving's time, when we "lose" an hour on the weekend, has an impact on our health. A study that analyzed a broad patient population across most hospitals in Michigan in the U.S. over three years found a 24 percent *increase* in heart attacks on the Monday after the switch, compared with a 21 percent *decrease* in heart attacks after the switch back to standard time.[6]

Through healthy sleep practices, like the kind we'll see in this chapter, your recovery reflex can help pay down this debt. As we'll see, from the surprising benefits of a "power nap" to sleep apps and supplements, you have many tools at your disposal to support your recovery reflex and become a master sleeper.

What is Sleep, Exactly?

Sleep is a highly active and complex process divided into two phases: non-rapid eye movement (NREM) sleep and rapid eye movement (REM) sleep.[7] These two phases cycle through the night multiple times in a predictable pattern, lasting from 70 to 120 minutes.

1. **NREM Sleep:** This stage is critical for physical recovery and memory consolidation. We spend roughly 75 to 80 percent of our total sleep time in NREM sleep, which itself contains three stages progressing from light to deep sleep.[8]
    - **Stage 1 (N1):** N1 sleep, which lasts for one to seven minutes, is the transition between wakefulness and sleep. During this stage your body begins to relax and your eye movements slow.
    - **Stage 2 (N2):** This is light sleep, when your heart rate slows and your body temperature drops. Sleep spindles (sudden bursts of brain activity) and K-complexes (large brain waves) occur, which assist in memory consolidation. N2 lasts between ten and twenty-five minutes during the first cycle and lengthens with each successive cycle.
    - **Stage 3 (N3):** This is deep sleep, most of which occurs in the first part of the night. N3 lasts twenty to forty minutes, during which you are difficult to rouse. N3 sleep is the most important stage for physical restoration and growth, immune function, energy conservation, and clearing out waste products.
2. **REM Sleep:** After around ninety minutes of NREM sleep, your body

enters REM sleep, which in its initial cycle may only last one to five minutes; as the night continues, your REM phases lengthen and may last as long as an hour.[9] REM is when most dreaming occurs. (People typically have multiple dreams each night,[10] though you may rarely remember them.) During REM sleep, your brain activity picks up dramatically as your body experiences atonia, which is the temporary paralysis of your muscles except for those controlling breathing and your eyes, which move back and forth rapidly, as the name suggests. This sleep is essential for cognitive functions, including memory consolidation, learning, and creativity. (One potential impact of a short night's sleep is that your REM sleep may be shortchanged.)

Sleep is largely regulated by the hormone melatonin, which is produced by the pineal gland in the brain and signals to the body it is time to prepare for sleep. Typically, light exposure suppresses melatonin production and darkness triggers it. Among people with conventional sleep patterns, melatonin levels begin to rise two to three hours before bedtime, promoting sleepiness. In the morning, melatonin levels begin decreasing, helping to wake you up.

You can probably see now why sleep *quality* is just as important as sleep duration. Consider that "eight hours" in bed may include thirty minutes to doze off, waking up two to three times during the night, and lying awake due to intrusive thoughts, leaving fewer than seven hours of genuine sleep. In one study, researchers selectively deprived healthy young adults of deep sleep in a lab setting using subtle sounds that interrupted deep sleep.[11] Despite getting eight hours of "sleep," after only three nights, the participants' ability to regulate their glucose levels were significantly impaired.

Developing healthy sleep hygiene begins with understanding your unique circadian rhythm—that is, your personal biological clock. You've heard the old adage about early birds and night owls, and most people identify as one or the other. The most recent science suggests there could be between five and seven different preferences for sleeping and waking times, known as chronotypes. There are early birds and night owls, yes, and there are also late-morning bears, late-evening wolves,[12] and some who don't fall neatly into any one category.

To determine your chronotype, I recommend taking a Morningness-Eveningness Questionnaire (MEQ), which is available for free at https://qxmd.com. The quiz includes questions like, "What time would you get up if you were entirely free to plan your day?" and "How alert do you feel during the first half-hour after you wake up in the morning?" I always thought of myself as a morning lark, but I'm in fact closer to a moderate morning person. Knowing your chronotype helps you identify (or confirm) when you are naturally most alert and productive, and when your body would prefer to begin shutting down for the day. The Composite Scale of Morningness (CSM)[13] and the Morningness-Eveningness Stability Scale improved (MESSi)[14] tools are also effective at determining your chronotype.

It can also help you time your medications more effectively. A large trial revealed that night owls who took their blood-pressure medication at night had a 34 percent lower risk of heart attack, while taking the same dose of medication in the morning increased the risk of heart attack by 62 percent.[15] Chronotherapy is a relatively new area of study that explores how *when* a drug is taken impacts its effectiveness and side effects.[16] Such timing is increasingly studied for cancer medications[17] and some anti-inflammatory medicines.[18] In some cases, it may be better for women to take a drug at a different time than men,[19] so ask your doctor or pharmacist about the ideal schedule for taking your medication.

While knowing your specific chronotype will help you refine the ideal timing to go to bed, strategies for how to fall asleep—and how to stay asleep—are also relevant. This begins with understanding the fundamentals of a good night's sleep.

Setting Yourself up for Successful Sleep

Dr. Matthew Walker is a professor of neuroscience and psychology at the University of California, Berkeley, and the director of its sleep and neuroimaging lab. After studying the mechanics of sleep extensively for his book *Why We Sleep: Unlocking the Power of Sleep and Dreams*,[20] Dr. Walker developed what he considered the essential components of healthy sleep:

Keep a Consistent Sleep Schedule: Go to bed and wake up at more or less the same time every day, even on the weekends. A consistent sleep schedule helps regulate your circadian rhythms while promoting regular secretion of hormones, including melatonin and cortisol (which promotes wakefulness). Studies routinely show that a large sleep variability—that is, frequently changing bedtime and wake-up times—is associated with poorer health outcomes.[21]

Maintain a Cool, Dark, and Quiet Sleep Environment: To fall asleep and stay asleep, your core body temperature needs to drop. Keeping your bedroom at 18–20°C (65–68°F) will help (more on this later).[22] Research shows that exposure to artificial light, especially blue light from screens, inhibits melatonin production in the hours leading up to bedtime. Consider using a sleep mask or blackout curtains if you live in a place that does not get dark until very late in the evening. You can minimize noise by using earplugs or white-noise machines.

Get Daytime Light Exposure: Expose yourself to sunlight first thing in the morning as you are waking up and throughout the day. Daytime light exposure helps synchronize your internal clock, ensuring your sleep–wake cycle is aligned with the day–night cycle. Morning light exposure also helps suppress melatonin, promoting wakefulness.

Use the Bed for Sleep and Intimacy Only: Avoid using your bed for activities like watching TV, working, or eating. This helps strengthen the mental association between bed and sleep. I admit that I enjoy reading and the occasional cup of coffee in bed; small rituals like these are fine if you do not have insomnia, but if you do struggle to fall or stay asleep, strive to reserve your bed for sleep and lovemaking.

Avoid Coffee and Alcohol Before Bedtime

We all have that friend: After a long, delicious dinner out, just as you're about to call for the check, they ask the waiter: "Can I have a coffee, please?" When the server inquires, "Decaf?" your friend replies, "No, regular." Even though it's 9:30 p.m.! "Caffeine doesn't affect me," they insist. It is true that there are people with a fast-metabolizing gene,[23] and it's possible that caffeine impacts your friend significantly less than it does you. Still, that late-night dose of caffeine is likely to impair your friend's sleep.

Caffeine, a stimulant found in everything from coffee and tea to chocolate, energy drinks, and some medications, works by inhibiting adenosine, a chemical that induces drowsiness and prepares the body for sleep. That's not necessarily a bad thing in the morning, when you're trying to kick-start your day. But consuming caffeine, especially close to bedtime, can shorten total sleep duration. In particular, caffeine is thought to reduce precious deep sleep while causing more frequent awakenings during the night.

The half-life of caffeine (the time it takes for the body to eliminate half the caffeine consumed) ranges from about three to seven hours,[24] but it can be longer depending on individual differences and factors like age, genetics, liver function, and pregnancy. Owing to its long half-life, caffeine consumed hours before bedtime can be present in your system at levels sufficient to disrupt sleep when you're ready to call it a night. For this reason, I recommend you don't drink (or eat) caffeine within ten hours of going to bed.

What about another nightcap favorite, alcohol? On one hand, alcohol, which is a sedative, can make you feel sleepy. However, research generally shows that having alcohol in your system disrupts normal sleep architecture by inhibiting REM and deep sleep.[25] This can lead to frequent waking and fragmented sleep overall. Alcohol can also relax the throat muscles, aggravating sleep apnea (more on this condition later), and relax the esophageal sphincter, worsening acid-reflux symptoms.

Sleep Trackers

In today's age of wearable technology, you no longer have to guess how efficiently you are sleeping. A wearable sleep tracker can monitor your sleep patterns, including sleep latency (how long it takes you to fall asleep), awakenings, heart rate, breathing patterns, core temperature, heart-rate variability, and sleep efficiency, which is the percentage of time you spend in bed truly sleeping. There are even apps that can detect if you snore!

By analyzing your sleep data, you can make informed changes to your habits and track your progress. For instance, while I always considered myself a good sleeper, my sleep tracker revealed the impact of alcohol and food on my sleep patterns and heart-rate variability. This knowledge has helped me make better decisions. For example, when I do drink alcohol, I opt for a cocktail at 5 p.m., rather than a nightcap at 8 p.m.

There are many sleep trackers on the market, but the most popular are smartwatches, fitness bands, and sleep rings. The data suggest that the Oura Ring, which you wear on your finger, and the Whoop, which uses a wrist band, may be the most accurate.[26] Both are combined with a smartphone app. Other good options include Fitbit and Apple Watch.[27]

Finish Dinner Early

When do you have your last meal of the day? Whether it's a late dinner or that midnight bowl of ice cream, you may still be digesting food when you go to bed. Dr. Satchin Panda, a researcher at the Salk Institute and the author of *The Circadian Code*, explains that we have internal clocks that govern different biological functions. For instance, when we eat, the body initiates a series of cellular processes to put us into "digest mode," during which we metabolize nutrients. But at night, we are supposed to enter "repair mode," to reboot and rejuvenate our organ systems.[28] To optimally support our recovery reflex, it is important to avoid eating for two to three hours before bedtime.[29] Eating late can also lead to indigestion and heartburn, making it harder to fall and stay asleep.

Understanding the Role of Body Temperature

Research has long shown that the ideal bedroom temperature is at 18–20°C (65–68°F).[30]

Typically, your body temperature follows a daily pattern, rising during the day to around 36.8°C (98.2°F) and falling at night to about 36.2°C (97.2°F). Just as you turn down the thermostat in your house at night, so does your brain. A drop in body temperature signals it is time to prepare for sleep, helping to initiate drowsiness and promote deeper sleep stages.

There are several strategies you can deploy to cool down your core body temperature. While it might seem counterintuitive, I recommend taking a hot bath or shower before bedtime. The hot water stimulates your body's recovery reflex, activating thermoregulatory mechanisms that circulate the blood away from your core to your hands and feet, thereby dropping your core temperature.[31]

To reduce your core temperature while in bed, I recommend wearing what I like to call "sleeping socks," which are loose fitting and made of natural fibers, like wool or cotton, that allow your feet to breathe. They also have little to no elastic, which can constrict circulation. Warming your feet with socks causes the blood vessels to dilate, improving blood flow to your extremities. Other pleasurable options include placing a heating pad or a hot water bottle near your feet.

Finally, as the melatonin leaves your body in the morning and the cortisol rises, your body will begin to warm up. There are steps you can take to support your innate physiological mechanisms to facilitate this process and wake up faster. Your morning coffee is one good way, as caffeine helps raise your core temperature.[32] Drinking a cup of hot tea or hot water will warm your core, as well. Washing your face with cold water has the opposite effect of a hot bath: it constricts your blood vessels, reduces peripheral circulation, and raises core body temperature.

Cognitive Behavioral Therapy for Insomnia

Needless to say, anxiety and sleep issues frequently go hand in hand, and they can be difficult to separate. A bad night's sleep can exacerbate anxiety, and vice versa. I discuss anxiety in depth in the "Unwinding Anxiety" chapter, and one valuable strategy described there—cognitive behavior therapy (CBT)—has also been well researched for the treatment of insomnia.

Cognitive behavioral therapy for insomnia (CBT-I) is a structured, evidence-based program designed to help people who struggle with insomnia by changing thoughts and behaviors that negatively impact sleep. CBT-I creates a customized plan for you based on your sleep patterns and challenges.

Ideally you would see a therapist for six to eight sessions to learn CBT-I.[33] If you do not have access to a specialist in your area (there are a limited number of trained CBT-I therapists), a number of apps can help you get started, including ShutEye and Sleepio. Another excellent—and free—choice is Insomnia Coach, which was developed by the U.S. Department of Veterans Affairs.[34] (It is helpful for anyone with sleep trouble, not just veterans.) CBT-I helps you replace anxious, negative thoughts about sleep with more positive and realistic ones. Many people with insomnia dread being in the bedroom, as they associate it with difficulty falling or staying asleep; CBT-I can help you reassociate calm, upbeat feelings with the bedroom and reclaim it as a place for peaceful sleep.

Your CBT-I program will give you feedback unique to your sleep circumstances. One surprising technique involves creating "sleep hunger" and building up the urgency to sleep. For instance, you may be instructed not to go to bed until 11 p.m., even if you feel tired at 8 p.m. This builds up the need to sleep and reduces sleep-onset insomnia. Practicing healthy sleep hygiene, as discussed earlier in this chapter, is also an element of CBT-I. Another important CBT-I tool is reframing—gradually helping you reassociate the bed with tranquility instead of tossing and turning.

Julie Morgenstern, a productivity consultant and author of *Time Management from the Inside Out,* points out that we are more likely to push sleep off in favor of other activities—watching a TV series, reading a book, and so on—because we view sleep as the last thing we do at night. Instead, she suggests, use bedtime to get a head start on the upcoming day. In other words, reframe sleep as a new beginning, not an end.[35]

Sleep Apps

Using your phone to fall asleep might seem counterintuitive; after all, I previously suggested you avoid blue light before bedtime. However, apps for sleep do not require gazing at a screen and can be highly effective in helping you fall and stay asleep. Your healthcare provider may recommend a specific sleep app. Here are my favorites.

Insight Timer: Insight Timer is my all-time favorite app because it has a library of over two hundred thousand free tracks from psychologists, mindfulness teachers, and spiritual leaders. Once you download the app, you will discover an entire section with sleep meditations, bedtime tales, nature soundscapes, and sleep music. I recommend experimenting with several different tracks; once you find one that resonates with you, use it consistently. Over time, your neuroplastic brain will learn to associate that sound with falling asleep.

Calm: Calm has a wide range of stories, meditations, and soundscapes that are available for free for the first week and then for a monthly charge. It has a section called "Sleep Stories" that features actors such as Matthew McConaughey reading bedtime tales to help you fall asleep.

Reveri: Reveri is a self-hypnosis app with a robust sleep section developed by Stanford University psychiatrist Dr. David Spiegel. The app works by first playing you a series of instructions to get you into a focused state of attention. Afterward, you're given hypnotic suggestions to reduce stress and help you drift off to sleep. You can try it out for free before you commit to a subscription.

National Institutes of Health: The National Institutes of Health offers a free guided meditation for sleep at https://clinicalcenter.nih.gov.

Spiritual Practices

Many people take the time to pray or meditate before going to bed, and most religious traditions have prayers meant to be said before sleep. For example, a Jesuit prayer begins:

Dear God, as I lay me down to sleep, relax the tension of my body; calm the restlessness of my mind; still the thoughts which worry and perplex me. Help me to rest myself and all my problems in your strong and loving arms.[36]

And a Jewish prayer offers this comforting message:

May it be Your will, Lord my God and God of my ancestors, that I lie down in peace and that I arise in peace . . . May I have a night of tranquil slumber. May I awaken to the light of a new day, that my eyes may behold the splendor of Your light. . . .[37]

Yoga Nidra, meanwhile, is an ancient practice that combines guided imagery with the savasana (or corpse) pose from yoga. Most of the apps listed earlier offer this practice.

Another spiritual practice that may settle your consciousness in a joyful way is that of gratitude. One study involving eighty-eight people found that participants who kept a gratitude journal slept thirty minutes longer per night and woke up feeling more refreshed, compared to those who didn't practice gratitude.[38] Another idea is to list three things each evening you feel grateful for. (The challenge is to come up with three new things every time!) These things do not need to be big. For example, a recent list of mine included seeing a prickly pear cactus in full bloom, witnessing a beautiful sunset, and having a wonderful call with an old friend. If you share a bed with someone, consider sharing this practice before going to sleep.

Recovery Napping

You've almost certainly experienced this phenomenon: After a big lunch, you get back home or to the office and . . . you want to curl up and go to sleep. Big meal or not, feeling tired between the hours of 1 and 4 p.m., often referred to as the "afternoon slump," is a common experience for many people.

If you typically resist the urge to take a nap, you may want to reconsider.

In 1995, the National Aeronautics and Space Administration (NASA) found that drowsiness was increasingly a problem for its pilots. Instead of devising ways to keep their pilots awake, NASA gave them an opportunity to take a nap during flight while the co-pilot had the controls. The results of an extensive survey found that pilots who napped for twenty-six minutes showed alertness improvements of up to 54 percent and job-performance improvements of up to 34 percent, compared to pilots who did not nap.[39] Thus, the "NASA nap"—or "power nap"—was born. Given its tremendous physical and psychological benefits, I like calling it a "recovery nap."

Recent studies confirm the benefits of a short, mid-afternoon recovery nap. A 2023 study involving thirty-two young adults found that naps ranging from ten to sixty minutes improved mood and memory encoding, and alleviated self-reported sleepiness for up to four hours.[40] As for the ideal length of a nap, the results confirm what NASA found: about thirty minutes. Beyond that, you may experience some "sleep inertia" by entering N3 deep sleep, which makes waking up more challenging.

Some important caveats: First, if you have insomnia, I do not recommend a recovery nap, as it can interfere with the build-up of sleep hunger at bedtime. Second, if you feel the urge to nap every day because of excessive daytime sleepiness, you might have obstructive sleep apnea (OSA), which occurs in the U.S. in approximately 30 percent of men and 11 percent of women between the ages of thirty and seventy.[41] In OSA, the upper airway collapses during sleep, leading to intermittent oxygen deprivation and awakenings from sleep.[42] If you have a bed partner, they may witness snoring, gasping, or pauses in your breath. Sleep apnea is diagnosed with a sleep study, nowadays frequently carried out with portable equipment at home. Remarkably, as many as 90 percent of people who have sleep apnea don't know it![43] So, if you suspect you might have sleep apnea, bring it up with your doctor.

Sleep Meds and Supplements

Many of my patients ask me about taking medication for their sleep trouble. However, these medications alter normal sleep patterns and architecture, sometimes leading to incomplete arousal from deep sleep, potentially resulting in sleepwalking and other complex sleep behaviors.[44]

A friend who is a criminal-defense lawyer told me an unsettling story about a client who was pulled over in the middle of the night for speeding. When the police officer looked inside the car, he found the man naked and completely bewildered. He could not remember getting in the car; the last thing he remembered was taking his sleep medications and going to bed. Even though the medications were prescribed by his doctor, the man was charged with a DWI. Most of the approximately 18 percent of U.S. adults who use some type of sleep medication will not get in their car in the middle of the night,[45] but sleep eating, sleep cooking, and other behaviors are known to occur.[46]

What about over-the-counter sleep aids? These medications usually contain antihistamines. While many people use them, they are minimally effective in inducing sleep, can reduce sleep quality, and may cause residual drowsiness. Worse still, your body quickly develops a tolerance to their sedative effects,[47] necessitating larger doses over time. Other side effects include dry mouth, constipation, and urinary retention. Some studies have also shown a link between long-term use of sleep aids and an increased risk of dementia.[48]

The good news is there are several supplements that are safe to take. Here is what I recommend:

> **Valerian:** The scientific name *Valeriana officinalis* is derived from the Latin *valere*, meaning "nice and healthy." This is apt, given that the root of valerian—a genus of tall, flowering grass—has been used since the times of ancient Greece and Rome to reduce anxiety and insomnia.[49] I recommend a dosage of 300 to 600 mg of valerian root extract taken 30 minutes to 2 hours before bedtime. Be sure to buy the capsule rather than the liquid to avoid its pungent smell!
>
> **Melatonin:** This supplement increases melatonin levels in the blood, similar to the rise in melatonin that occurs naturally in response to darkness. Melatonin supplements are believed to be non–habit forming and have a half-life of just thirty minutes, so you won't feel a hangover effect the next day. If you frequently wake up in the middle of the night (a phenomenon called *sleep-maintenance insomnia*), you can take a dose of

melatonin to help you fall back asleep. The American Academy of Family Physicians recognizes melatonin as a first-line therapy for insomnia.[50] Ask your doctor to prescribe melatonin, preferably as a sublingual tablet as this is more rapidly absorbed than the oral form.

Magnesium: In one study of older adults with insomnia, magnesium supplements were found to reduce the time it takes to fall asleep by seventeen minutes.[51] I recommend a dosage of 400 mg taken one or two hours before bedtime. Alternatively, experiment with adding a cup of Epsom salts to your nightly bath.

To Reset Your Circadian Rhythm, Go Camping

I sometimes see patients who stay up extremely late and are desperate for a way to "reboot" their sleep schedule to more reasonable hours. Here's a novel solution to help your rapid recovery reflex reset your circadian rhythm: go camping.

Kenneth Wright, an integrative physiology professor at the University of Colorado at Boulder, had a simple question: Can someone "reset" their circadian rhythm to align closer with sunrise and sunset? After taking volunteers on a one-week summer camping trip in the Rocky Mountains, Dr. Wright showed that by the end of the trip, the campers' bodies began releasing melatonin around sunset. By sunrise, their bodies had stopped releasing it and they were much less groggy.[52]

Of course, not everyone can—or let's be honest, *wants*—to go for a weeklong camping trip in the wilderness. (I know, I know, I'm an outlier.) But a shorter window may work as well. In a follow-up study, Dr. Wright brought fourteen campers into the wilderness for just two days. Sure enough, the campers' melatonin levels began to rise more than an hour earlier than before they left.[53]

The take-home point is that you can indeed reset your inner clock, and being away from all artificial lighting is one way to do so!

Your Rapid Recovery Prescription for Sleeping Soundly

You do not have to view your bedroom as a battlefield. With time, you can reassociate it with peace, tranquillity, and a good night's sleep. Here is how to get started:

1. Use the MEQ, CSM, or MESSi questionnaires to determine your chronotype. This will help you learn your ideal timing to go to bed.
2. Set yourself up for successful sleep by maintaining a consistent sleep schedule; creating a cool, dark, and quiet sleep environment; ensuring daytime light exposure; and using the bed for sleep and lovemaking only.
3. Finish dinner two to three hours before bedtime and avoid late-night coffee and alcohol.
4. Use a sleep tracker to monitor your sleeping patterns.
5. Cool down your body temperature before bedtime by warming your feet (such as with sleeping socks) or by taking a hot shower or bath.
6. Use CBT-I to better understand your sleep patterns and change negative thoughts and behaviors that affect your sleep.
7. Experiment with an app that offers sleep meditations, soundscapes, or stories to help you fall asleep.
8. Before bedtime, consider adding a spiritual or religious practice, or the ritual of noting three things you are grateful for.
9. If you do not have insomnia, a thirty-minute midday nap can improve mood and alertness and help you avoid the "afternoon slump."
10. Avoid sedative-hypnotic and over-the-counter sleep medications. Instead, if you wish to use a sleep aid, prioritize valerian or magnesium.

4

Unwinding Anxiety

My patient Louise struggled with anxiety. She was constantly berating herself for being overreactive, which only fed a downward spiral: *Why do I get anxious so easily? Why am I so sensitive to everything?* It didn't help that she taught yoga, which is supposed to make you feel calm and at peace. Was she not breathing properly? Was she not practicing the poses correctly? Louise felt like an imposter in her classes as she attempted to be the model of the serene instructor who had it all together, when in fact she was a bundle of nerves.

As I took her history, I learned that Louise was also a harpist in the local symphony. Her fingers and brain were wired to detect the slightest differences in vibration and tone, which meant her nervous system was highly attuned. As Louise spoke, she suddenly had an "Aha!" moment and exclaimed: "The sensitivity that makes me anxious is also what makes me a talented harpist! It is a fundamental part of me!" This positive reframe—that her exquisite sensitivity made her a gifted musician—did not eliminate all her anxiety, but it meant she could more easily quiet the critical voice in her head.

Anxiety is part of the human experience, and it originates from the most ancient parts of our brains: the amygdala and the limbic system.[1] These areas process emotions and are fundamental to our stress response, which is the evolutionary mechanism that helps humans respond to danger. For millions of years, our ancestors evolved to notice threats, like a predator hiding in the brush or a treacherous cliff overlooking certain death. Our recovery reflex revs up our nervous system to respond to high-risk situations. Unfortunately, the brain is not good at distinguishing genuine mortal threats from modern agita like taxes, college admissions, and annoying bosses, so our nervous system can overreact and cause chronic states of anxiety.

It is common for people to feel anxious because of a challenging situation at work, school, or when public speaking. In contrast, generalized anxiety disorder (GAD) is more pervasive and lasts for at least six months. It manifests as excess worry that is disproportionate to the situations that trigger it, and it is often accompanied by physical symptoms like muscle tension, fatigue, irritability, feeling on edge, and difficulty concentrating or sleeping. Other, more severe forms of anxiety include panic disorder and phobias (including agoraphobia and social phobia). These more extreme manifestations will also be helped by the strategies in this chapter, along with psychotherapy or, in severe cases, medication.

Our nervous system has two major automatic reaction strategies: the sympathetic (SNS) and the parasympathetic (PNS); together they are called the *autonomic nervous system*. The SNS reaction, often referred to as "fight or flight," prepares your body to address stressful or emergency situations by increasing alertness and physical performance. Specifically, it increases heart rate, raises blood pressure, dilates muscles in the lungs to allow in more air, secretes adrenaline and norepinephrine, inhibits digestion to direct blood flow to the heart and muscles, and dilates your pupils to allow in more light and improve vision. As its name suggests, the SNS response prepares you to fight back against a threat or run away. Once a stressful situation passes, the PNS counteracts the SNS's effects, restoring equilibrium. Cortisol levels drop, and the body shifts to a "rest and digest" state.

Stress can be positive, tolerable, or negative. Positive stress refers to short-lived and rapidly deactivated stress—such as butterflies in your stomach before you play in a sporting event or speak in front of many people—that focuses your attention and improves performance. Tolerable stress is potentially damaging, but it can also build protection against future stressors. For example, you may experience this kind of difficult, but manageable stress when preparing for a big job interview. You really want the job, the stakes feel high, but you are not overwhelmed and your stress hormones enhance your performance. Moreover, overcoming such a challenge helps build resilience, and your next high-stakes interview may be less stressful. Toxic stress, however, conveys a damaging stress response as a result of adversity or trauma, combined with a lack of coping resources.[2]

Sometimes the SNS stays in the "on" position and continually releases stress hormones, even long after the threat has passed. Such is the case for the millions of people who struggle with chronic anxiety.[3] Anxiety is the great equalizer: It transcends age, gender, socioeconomic status, cultural backgrounds, and even celebrity. In 1967, while performing a concert in New York's Central Park, Barbra Streisand bungled the lyrics to several of her songs. "I forgot the words in front of 125,000 people, and I wasn't cute about it or anything," she reflected. Her anxiety was so great—what if she forgot the lyrics again?—that she didn't perform in front of an audience for another twenty-seven years![4]

Life gets messy, despite our best efforts. Worries cling to our brains even as we try to push them aside. So the strategies we discuss here are about diffusing anxiety when it does occur. The good news is that the same brain that creates anxious thoughts can also subdue them. As Dr. Victor Frankl, the famed psychiatrist and Holocaust survivor, reportedly said, "Between stimulus and response there is a space. In that space is our power to choose our response. In our response lies our growth and our freedom."[5]

The Importance of Community

Can a study about the stress response in women give us clues about how best to cope with anxiety?

Dr. Shelley Taylor, a researcher at the University of California, Los Angeles, challenged the notion that women respond to stress solely with fight or flight.[6] In her research, she found human female responses to stress are frequently characterized by a pattern she named "tend and befriend." Because females traditionally have played a greater role in caring for young children, responses to threats that protected offspring as well as the self would be more successfully passed on. In fact, "tending," which involved quieting and caring for offspring and blending into the environment, may have been more effective for addressing threats than fight-or-flight responses, which would have been challenging with young children. In addition, affiliating with a social group, or "befriending," means creating relationships that provide resources and protection for the female and her offspring.

This theory introduces the first important strategy for managing anxiety and activating your recovery reflex in the twenty-first century: nurturing a community of friends who comfort and support you during difficult times. This is true for both women and men. Before you read through this chapter, consider where you get your strength during times of challenge. Perhaps you turn to the love of family or friends, your faith community, a spiritual practice, or time in nature. Maybe it's something entirely different. Putting into action the things that you know soothe your spirit and restore your equilibrium is step one for unwinding anxiety.

Turn Knots in Your Stomach into Bows

Harvard Business School researcher Dr. Alison Wood Brooks tested a novel hypothesis: Can you transform anxiety into a positive feeling? Sometimes when we get anxious, people in our lives may unhelpfully tell us to "calm down" or "relax!" Most people find this quite challenging to do. Dr. Brooks took a different tack. Rather than asking participants to move from their high negative-energy state (anxious) to a low positive-energy state (relaxed), she experimented with having them move instead to a high positive-energy state: excitement. Simply, Dr. Brooks asked her subjects to use the following three words: *I am excited.*

In one experiment, Dr. Brooks subjected participants to a series of stressful tasks, including singing karaoke, speaking in public, and taking a complex math test under time pressure.[7] She instructed them to say out loud either "I am anxious," "I am excited," or nothing at all. It turns out the "excited" participants performed better every time, no matter the task: They sang better based on a measurement of their volume and pitch, they were more persuasive speakers, and they even answered more problems correctly on the math test. As Dr. Brooks found, just by saying "I am excited," you can transform your anxiety into enthusiasm.

Eight years ago, when my daughter was preparing for her destination wedding, I felt quite anxious. I am an introvert, and the mere thought of all the large gatherings felt overwhelming. Never mind having to make a toast! Recalling Dr. Brooks's study, I made a conscious effort to reframe my anxiety into something positive. *My daughter is getting married! I love my future son-in-law! And I am so happy for them!* This simple shift made a big difference, and I began anticipating the big event with joy. See if you can apply the same strategy the next time you have an event coming up. Or, as Dr. Brooks put it, "Turn the knots in your stomach into bows."[8]

Of course, we cannot always transform anxious feelings into something positive. Dealing with a serious medical problem, for instance, is never going to be something to get excited about. So, let's look at some strategies that can help in more challenging situations.

Use Cognitive Behavioral Therapy to Reframe Your Stress

My friend Suzie is deathly afraid of snakes. For this reason, she is apprehensive when visiting me in Tucson, which has a robust rattlesnake population. For us locals, rattlesnakes are commonplace and rarely a cause for concern, but visitors are frequently unnerved when they come across one. I knew I was unlikely to convert Suzie's anxiety into excitement, so I used another strategy to help her reframe her fears.

I described a "stress equation" in which the numerator (top of the fraction) is "overestimation of danger" and the denominator (bottom of the fraction) is "underestimation of coping strategies." I explained to Suzie that she was overestimating the limited danger of the snakes and underestimating her ability to avoid a snake bite.[9] For example, she could avoid walking at dusk when the light is dim and the snakes are active, or she could carry a torch. Rattlesnakes don't want to attack humans, I explained; they just want us to leave them alone. In fact, it is at least six times more likely that someone will die from a lightning strike than a snake bite.[10]

"I get it, she agreed. "They just want me to stay away from them."

As for me, for close to forty years I have had a recurrent anxious thought when rapidly descending the steps in hospitals I work at: *What if I trip and fall and knock out my front teeth?* Like Suzie, I sometimes catch myself inflating the numerator of my stress equation and shrinking the denominator. When this happens, I tell myself what I tell my patients: I can reduce my anxiety by considering both the true danger and my coping strategies. *I've walked down thousands of steps in my life*, I remind myself, *and I've never once fallen, so I am clearly overestimating the danger*. Or, I can slow down, hold on to the banister, and engage my coping skills. This form of reframing is a staple of cognitive behavior therapy (CBT), which teaches people to change their negative thought patterns to more effectively manage their emotional responses. Here is how to get started:

1. **Identify Anxiety-Provoking Thoughts:** Identify the automatic thoughts that occur when you face a stressful situation. Sometimes we run away from these anxious feelings; identifying them can make them more manageable.
2. **Challenge These Thoughts:** Once you've identified these thoughts, the next step is to challenge their validity. Ask yourself questions like:
   - Is this anxious thought based on facts or assumptions?
   - Are there other ways to look at this situation?
   - What would I tell a friend who had this thought?
   - Is this thought helpful?
3. **Develop More Positive Thoughts:** Replace the original anxiety-provoking thoughts with more balanced thoughts. For example, instead of thinking, *This project is going to be a disaster*, you might reframe it to, *There certainly are challenges, and I am going to plan carefully and ask for support*.
4. **Practice Mindfulness:** Anxiety is almost always focused on an uncertain future. Mindfulness, which, according to Jon Kabat-Zinn, PhD, founder of the Stress Reduction Clinic at the University of Massachusetts, means paying attention on purpose, in the present moment, and

nonjudgmentally.[11] For instance, set an intention, such as for more happiness or peacefulness. Notice what is happening right now. Don't criticize yourself if your mind wanders. Instead, gently bring it back to the present. One study found that mindfulness and the antidepressant escitalopram were equally effective in reducing anxiety.[12] Participants in the study practiced seeing thoughts and sensations as transient and not necessarily a reflection of reality. Asking yourself, *What am I feeling right now?* or *How am I doing right now?* can bring you back to your present experience, which often does not provoke anxious feelings.

Potential Anxiety Triggers

Anxiety can be triggered by an incredibly wide range of factors that vary from person to person based on past experiences, the current situation, and specific personal sensitivities. Life presents us with countless stressors, from moving to a new home to changing jobs, dealing with a medical problem, or interacting with difficult coworkers. Some of us seem wired to worry, and it can feel impossible to stop.

While some worrying is inevitable, many triggers are avoidable. Indeed, some may be sneakily turning your limbic system up to 11 as you go about your day, making you wonder, *Why am I SO stressed out right now?* Here are some possibilities you may not have considered.

Caffeine: Caffeine is a stimulant that works by blocking the action of adenosine, a chemical that builds up over the course of the day and gradually increases our drive to sleep. Caffeine increases arousal, alertness, and focus. This is probably why 67 percent of Americans drink coffee every day.[13] Still, many of us have experienced the uncomfortably wired feeling associated with having too much caffeine, which mimics the physiological symptoms of anxiety: increased heart rate, elevated blood pressure, and heightened alertness or nervousness.[14] Caffeine can also stimulate the adrenal glands to release stress hormones.[15]

Aspartame: Aspartame is a common artificial sweetener found in diet sodas, sugar-free products, and many processed foods. The body metabolizes aspartame into several chemical components, including phenylalanine, aspartic acid, and methanol. Studies suggest that consuming these substances can disrupt the balance of neurotransmitters in the brain, leading to mood changes and anxiety.[16]

Attention-Deficit/Hyperactivity Disorder (ADHD) Medications: ADHD medications are stimulants that increase the activity of the central nervous system by boosting the levels of neurotransmitters or their receptors. Side effects of ADHD medicines can include anxiety and disrupted sleep.[17]

Asthma Medications: Short-acting beta agonists like albuterol, which is used for quick relief of asthma symptoms in "rescue" inhalers, are stimulants that can cause side effects that mimic anxiety, such as an elevated heart rate.[18] Systemic corticosteroids, used to control severe asthma, can also have side effects including mood swings and increased anxiety.

Poor Sleep: Insufficient sleep can affect the brain's ability to regulate emotions and lead to increased irritability. Worse, you may have more trouble sleeping when you're anxious, creating a vicious cycle that worsens your sleep debt over time. (See the "Sleeping Soundly" chapter for ways to develop better sleep habits.)

Breath Work

How we breathe has a profound effect on our physiology. Our brain associates different emotions with different breathing patterns. Research shows that when we are happy, we take regular and steady breaths, and when we're anxious or fearful, our breathing becomes erratic, shallow, and fast.[19] By changing our breathing patterns—specifically slowing it down and extending the exhale phase—we can reassure our nervous system that danger has passed.

For instance, many years ago I was scheduled to give a lecture in Phoenix, Arizona, which is about a two-hour drive from my home in Tucson. As I often did when working on a weekend, I brought my two daughters along with me, promising them a shopping trip in the bigger city. An hour and a half into the drive, we were diverted off the highway because of construction. I quickly got lost in the sprawling Phoenix suburbs, and—this being in the days before GPS and satnavs—called a friend for directions. We arrived at the conference with less than ten minutes to spare and sprinted to the auditorium. My heart was racing and I was a bundle of nerves. Realizing I was about to take the stage anything but centered, my daughters stopped me and said, displaying a calming presence beyond their years, "Mom, *breathe!*" I took several deep diaphragmatic breaths and felt my heart settle. I got on stage, gave my talk, and we had a lovely time shopping afterwards.

Many of the most effective breathing techniques are based on Pranayama, a yogic breathing practice that originated thousands of years ago in India. Quieting breaths all emphasize breathing more slowly, regularly, and deeply. Instructions for three of my favorites—Box Breathing, 4-7-8 Breathing, and Five-Finger (Starfish) Breathing—are in Appendix 1.

Every now and then, a patient tells me that attempting to take a deep breath when they feel anxious actually makes them feel worse. Instead, I ask them to hum, chant, or sing. These actions similarly activate the vagus nerve—the long, cranial nerve that extends from your brainstem all the way to your pelvis and plays a crucial role in stimulating the parasympathetic nervous system.

Spiritual Practices

A spiritual practice I often recommend to my patients for anxiety is the "loving kindness meditation," also known as the Metta meditation. Begin with directing loving kindness as a blessing for yourself. Slowly and silently repeat these phrases:

May I be safe.
May I be peaceful.
May I be healthy.
May I take care of myself easily.

Next, bring to mind someone you love and direct loving kindness toward them:

May you be safe.
May you be peaceful.
May you be healthy.
May you take care of yourself easily.

Finally, generalize your attention to a larger group and bring to mind your family, your community, or even all beings on the planet, and repeat the following:

May we be safe.
May we be peaceful.
May we be healthy.
May we take care of ourselves easily.

During a particularly stressful period of my life, I used this loving kindness meditation throughout the day. Even though I sometimes never got past the first sentence—"May I be safe"—it still helped. I have heard similar feedback from my patients. You can find a soothing fifteen-minute version of this guided meditation from internationally renowned Buddhist teacher Sharon Salzberg on the app Insight Timer.

Countless patients have told me they turn to prayer, meditation, or attending services as a way to unwind anxiety. They find the antidote to their anxiety in their faith in God. Some say, "God wouldn't give me more than I can handle" or "This is my cross to bear." And at their best, religious services also provide the support of a caring community.

Exercise

When my kids were little, they always seemed to know when I was feeling stressed. They would ask me, "Mom, is it time for your thirty-minute walk?" They are not the only ones who have noticed how a little bit of exercise can do wonders for our mental health. Later, in the "Defeating Depression" chapter we will see how regular exercise is one of the best ways to recover from depression; there is also good evidence that it settles anxiety.

Exercise decreases muscle tension, which has a side benefit of reducing psychological tension. It also activates the frontal regions of the brain,[20] which helps you reason with anxious thoughts and put them in a larger context, while tamping down the SNS. Even minimal activity is helpful. The Irish Longitudinal Study on Ageing tracked more than 7,600 participants, finding that people who walked briskly for ten minutes five days a week had significantly lower odds of anxiety than those who were sedentary.[21]

I also highly recommend yoga, which combines the benefits of physical activity with breath work. I have practiced yoga since medical school, and I find it a wonderful centering practice; while I may show up with a busy mind, by the end of the class I feel calm and centered. Studies have found that hatha yoga in particular is beneficial for reducing anxiety and stress.[22] A meta-analysis revealed that yoga is most helpful for the folks with elevated levels of anxiety who practiced frequently.[23] Another moving meditative practice that has also been shown to be beneficial for reducing anxiety is tai chi,[24] which incorporates a series of slow, dance-like movements that flow into one another. A side benefit is improved balance and reduced falls.[25]

Supplements

Like so many people in the early days of the Covid-19 pandemic, my twenty-seven-year-old patient Roxanne struggled mightily with anxiety. First, she lost her job; then she lost her apartment and had to move in with her parents. She came to see me with a rapid heart rate (tachycardia), an inability to sleep or eat, and nonstop shaking. Roxanne had wrestled with some anxiety in the past, but now she felt it 24/7. Daily walks helped center her to an extent, but they weren't sufficient, and she was opposed to taking any kind of prescription medication. Fortunately, there were many supplements at her disposal that she could use in addition to her therapy sessions, 4-7-8 breathing, and daily walks.

I recommended she take L-theanine capsules, a compound found in green tea, on an as-needed basis, and inositol to help her sleep at night. I also asked her to take 2 grams of omega-3 fatty acids and a B50 vitamin complex daily. Gradually, she noted positive changes. The constant shaking of her hands got better. The tachycardia became less frequent. She began sleeping through the night. She was able to eat more regularly. Eventually, Roxanne found that the anxiety that had torn her life apart had melted away. After getting vaccinated, she found a new job and a new apartment.

As Roxanne discovered, there are multiple supplements that can be used to help manage anxiety. Some are intended to be taken regularly (such as B vitamins and omega-3) while others can be used on an as-needed basis (L-theanine). Here are some of the most effective.

B Vitamins: B vitamins are vital for the production and regulation of neurotransmitters, including serotonin, dopamine, and GABA (gamma-aminobutyric acid), all of which play significant roles in mood regulation. One study found that people who took a high dose (100 mg) of vitamin B6 every day for a month reported feeling less anxious and depressed.[26] I prefer that people take the full complement of B vitamins in a B50 dose. There is also evidence that B vitamins can help prevent PTSD (see "Taming Post-Traumatic Stress Disorder" chapter).

Omega-3 Fatty Acids: These essential fatty acids support brain health and reduce anxiety. Taking enough is necessary, as people often do not take a sufficient dose to improve mood. One meta-analysis of nineteen trials totaling 2,240 participants from eleven countries found that those taking at least 2,000 mg of EPA and DHA daily saw reduced overall anxiety levels.[27] A dose below 2,000 mg did not achieve this effect. Choose an omega-3 supplement with EPA and DHA in about a 1:1 ratio. (See "Your Rapid Recovery Toolkit," appendix 1, for more information about omega-3s.)

Kava Kava: Kava has been used for centuries as a ceremonial drink to promote a state of relaxation. The active ingredients in kava are called *kavalactones*, which have calming effects that can help relieve anxiety,[28] protect neurons from damage, and improve sleep. You may encounter kava when travelling to other countries, but the sale and supply of kava has been banned in the U.K. and some other countries due to health concerns. If you decided to drink kava tea when traveling, do so only in moderation. If you stay on it for weeks at a time, please have tests done to check your liver function. Unlike prescribed benzodiazepines, kava is not addictive, nor is it associated with withdrawal symptoms.[29] Kava kava can have rare but serious side effects, including nausea and headache, so talk to your doctor to see if it's right for you.

L-Theanine: Found primarily in green tea, L-theanine is an amino acid that can help promote relaxation without drowsiness. This is a terrific quick fix when you feel especially anxious. It can also be used longer term. L-theanine is thought to work by increasing levels of the neurotransmitters GABA, serotonin, and dopamine.[30] The dose is 200 to 400 mg daily.[31]

Lavender: Lavender is well known for its soothing properties as an essential oil and is widely used in aromatherapy. Diffusing lavender oil or inhaling it directly can have immediate calming effects on the central nervous system. While most essential oils are not meant to be taken orally, an exception is lavender—in a particular formulation called Silexan which is sold under different brand names, for example, Kalms Lavender One-A-Day and Nature's Way CalmAid. It has been found in hundreds of studies to reduce anxiety levels comparable to the effect of benzodiazepines.[32]

Inositol: Often referred to as vitamin B8, inositol influences hormones associated with mood and cognition.[33] It is naturally found in small amounts in fruits, beans, grains, and nuts, and it can be taken as a dietary supplement to treat anxiety and panic attacks. When my patient Amanda reported frequent bouts of anxiety interfering with her sleep, I recommended she take powdered inositol at bedtime, in addition to her regular walks and yoga practice. I started her on a dose of 4 grams per day and gradually increased it to 18 grams over a four-week period. Amanda's overall anxiety improved markedly. I recommend buying a bottle of powdered inositol rather than the 500 mg capsules, which will be used up very quickly. Stir the powder into water or juice; it is slightly sweet and pleasant tasting.

Magnesium: About 50 percent of Americans do not consume the recommended amounts of magnesium in their diet, which, as I will discuss in later chapters, is linked to high blood pressure, diabetes, and heart disease. It can also be an underlying cause of anxiety.[34] Oral magnesium supplements have been found to be effective in reducing anxiety; I recommend CALM by Natural Vitality. Take 400 mg daily of magnesium citrate or glycinate. I also recommend adding 1 cup of Epsom salts, which is magnesium sulfate, to a hot bath. Taking a bath before bedtime is relaxing in and of itself, and the magnesium from the Epsom salts is absorbed through your skin. You can also add a few drops of lavender essential oil for further relaxation.

Adaptogens: Adaptogens are a unique class of herbal medicines that help the body adapt to stressful situations. They have been used in traditional medicine systems throughout the world and are thought to help balance the body's stress-response system. Here are two adaptogens that I frequently recommend to my patients who are going through stressful moments in their lives:

- Ashwagandha (*Withania somnifera*): Known for its restorative properties, ashwagandha helps reduce anxiety, lowers cortisol levels, and can improve sleep. One randomized trial of sixty-four participants with a history of chronic stress found a "significant reduction" in stress scores and reduced cortisol levels.[35] The dose is 300 mg twice daily of Ashwagandha extract.[36] Unlike other adaptogens, which tend to be energizing, ashwagandha is unique in that it helps people who are "wired, yet tired" get to sleep.
- Holy Basil (*Ocimum tenuiflorum*): Holy basil, also known as tulsi, is a revered herb in Ayurveda, the traditional medical system of India. It is also considered sacred in Hindu culture, where it is associated with the goddess Lakshmi and regarded as an "elixir of life" believed to promote longevity.[37] It is known for its therapeutic properties, including reducing anxiety and emotional stress. It is thought to reduce anxiety by normalizing levels of stress hormones like cortisol—and, indeed, randomized trials have confirmed its effectiveness.[38]

Other Common (and Uncommon) Remedies for Stress Relief

Apps: I recommend mind–body apps to virtually every patient I see. The number of resources at our literal fingertips is remarkable! As discussed earlier in this book, my favorite app is Insight Timer. Additionally, I recommend Unwinding Anxiety, which was developed by psychiatrist and mindfulness researcher Jud Brewer, MD, PhD, to help users identify and unlearn the habit loops that lead to anxiety. In one study, participants who used the app over a two-month period saw a 67 percent reduction in anxiety compared with 14 percent in the control group.[39] The NNT (number needed to treat) was 1.6, meaning that 62 percent of people who use the app will have success.

Weighted Blankets: These typically weigh between 2.25–13.5 kilograms (5–30 lb). A meta-analysis found that 63 percent of people using them reported a reduction in anxiety symptoms.[40] The right weight for you is a matter of individual preference; per the studies, it can be up to 10 percent of your body weight.

Vagus Nerve Stimulating (VNS) Devices: Sensate is a palm-sized device you position over your sternum. The device's vibrations resonate throughout your chest and sync with a companion app that plays a soundscape of your choosing. Sensate works by toning the vagus nerve, and I have found it highly effective for my patients who complain of anxiety.[41] Another VNS device that has been FDA-cleared for use in anxiety is Alpha-Stim, which clips onto the earlobe. It is available in the U.K. online (The Veterans Administration medical director in the U.S.A. told me it has been given out to eighty-five thousand veterans.) GammaCore is a third vagus nerve stimulator that delivers mild electric signals to the neck. It is available on the NHS for cluster headaches and it received European Union authorization for the treatment of anxiety. Before using any of these devices, do talk to your doctor or cardiologist if you have a pacemaker or another implanted device.

Cannabis

The use of cannabis as a medicine dates back to ancient Chinese, Tibetan, and Indian cultures. Today, cannabis is increasingly being used to manage symptoms of anxiety.[42] The plant's two primary active compounds, THC (Delta-9-Tetrahydrocannabinol) and CBD (cannabidiol), have different effects.

One important thing to note about cannabis is that it is highly idiosyncratic; while some people find it dramatically improves anxiety, others report it exacerbates anxious feelings.[43] A large-scale Canadian study surveyed more than two thousand medicinal cannabis users and found that 44 percent reported using it to treat anxiety.[44] Of that cohort, about half were able to replace either an antidepressant or a benzodiazepine, and 61 percent were able to completely eliminate a prescribed drug. An important caveat: In this large study, the cannabis products that relieved anxiety contained THC; CBD alone was not found to be effective at reducing anxiety. However other research suggests that CBD alone is effective for anxiety at a dose of 300 mg daily.[45]

At the time of this writing, cannabis is legal in twenty-four U.S. states and the District of Columbia for recreational and medical purposes, and in an additional fourteen states for medical use alone.[46] In the U.K., recreational use of cannabis is illegal and it is only available on prescription for medical use for a limited number of conditions.

What About Prescription Medications?

Medication is frequently prescribed for anxiety. Selective serotonin reuptake inhibitors (SSRIs) and serotonin-norepinephrine reuptake inhibitors (SNRIs) are antidepressants also used to treat persistent anxiety. While these antidepressants have been found effective,[47] they take several weeks to work and can have problematic side effects, including transient headaches, nausea, drowsiness, weight gain, and difficulty achieving orgasm. The NNT for SSRIs is 5.15,[48] which means that fewer than one in five people who are prescribed one for generalized anxiety will experience symptom relief. For these reasons, I prefer to reserve them for more severe cases of anxiety, such as generalized anxiety disorder (GAD), panic disorder, and phobic disorder.

Benzodiazepines are the oldest class of medication used to treat anxiety,[49] and are among the most widely prescribed medications worldwide.[50] They include alprazolam (only through private prescription, not the NHS), lorazepam, diazepam, and clonazepam, which provide rapid relief of anxiety symptoms. They are highly effective in acutely stressful situations, such as a surgical or dental procedure, fear of flying, or when you are shaken up after a car accident. However, it is best to confine their use to the short term, owing to risks of dependence, sedation, and tolerance.[51] They can be difficult to wean off of and are associated with falls in older people, as well as cognitive problems. For these reasons they are usually prescribed for only a limited period.[52]

Finally, while beta blockers are primarily used for treating hypertension and other heart conditions, they can relieve some of the physical symptoms of anxiety, including a rapid heart rate. They block the effects of adrenaline, helping to ease nervousness. Beta blockers can be useful in situations in which a racing heart could impact your performance, such as a job interview or delivering a speech in front of a large audience. Early in my career, all of the first-year residents in my class took advantage of our prescribing privileges and used beta blockers to quiet our nervous systems when we were assigned to give talks to the entire department. I've since come a long way in managing my public-speaking anxiety, and I no longer rely on beta blockers for public speaking. Nevertheless, I believe it's fine to request a prescription from your doctor for occasional use of beta blockers, as they safely reduce the physical effects of anxiety, such as tremor, palpitations, and perspiration. Once these symptoms resolve, it is easier to achieve a calmer state. (Note that beta blockers are not effective for GAD or panic disorder.[53])

Rapid Recovery from a Panic Attack

A panic attack is a sudden and intense episode of fear or anxiety that triggers physical reactions so severe that many first-time sufferers fear they are having a heart attack!

The former *Nightline* and *Good Morning America* anchor Dan Harris once had a public panic attack live on *Good Morning America*, which was witnessed by five million viewers. He said "It felt like the world was ending. My heart was thumping. I was gasping for air. I had pretty much lost the ability to speak. And all of it was compounded by the knowledge that my freak-out was being broadcast live on national television."[54] Interestingly, this public meltdown ultimately led him to his larger calling: teaching mindfulness. Dan is now the author of the bestselling mindfulness book *10% Happier*, and he created a popular app with the same name.

Panic attacks, as Dan attested, are extremely distressing; they can occur unexpectedly or be triggered by specific situations. Many of the strategies listed earlier in this chapter can help restore your equilibrium, especially CBT, which is also considered an effective long-term treatment for panic attacks. Here are some of the principles.

> **Recognize and Acknowledge:** The first step in managing a panic attack is to recognize it's happening. This is not as obvious as it may sound. Many people go to the hospital with a panic attack because their symptoms are so extreme they think they are about to die. Once you understand you are having a panic attack, you can acknowledge that what you are experiencing is not life threatening. Remind yourself that the sensations are temporary and will pass.
>
> **Find a Safe Place:** If possible, find a safe and comfortable place where you can sit down and focus on regaining control of your breathing and thoughts.
>
> **Focus on Your Breathing:** Use your favorite breathing technique from the list given earlier. Concentrate on consciously shifting your breath so it is slower, deeper, and more regular. During moments of extreme anxiety, we sometimes lose our sense of control. Deliberate breathing helps you regain that sense of control over your body. If it feels impossible to take a deep breath—which happens—see if you can hum or sing.
>
> **Ground Yourself:** While breathing, engage in a physical grounding exercise to bring your focus to the present moment. You can roll your foot gradually

up and down from heel to toe, alternating back and forth between your feet. Another common method is the 5-4-3-2-1 technique, as follows:

- Identify five things you can see around you.
- Identify four things you can touch.
- Identify three things you can hear.
- Identify two things you can smell.
- Identify one thing you can taste.

If you are prone to panic attacks, I recommend that you practice these techniques daily while you are feeling calm. This way, if you do have an attack, you can more readily access them.

Finally, one supplement that has specifically been studied in people with panic disorder is inositol. A regimen of 12 grams per day for four weeks was shown to reduce episodes of panic from an average of 10 per week to 3.5.[55] In a second study, inositol was compared to an SSRI and found to have a greater reduction in panic attacks per week (four fewer compared to 2.4 for the SSRI) and fewer overall side effects.[56]

Your Rapid Recovery Prescription for Unwinding Anxiety

Anxiety is a common human experience. It is likely you have already learned some healthy strategies to center yourself and soothe your spirit. In addition to these practices, the following integrative strategies can help diffuse anxiety, should it occur. Using more than one can often have a synergistic effect.

1. Avoid isolation and reach out to your community of loved ones for support.
2. Turn the knots in your stomach into bows in situations when you can reframe your stress into excitement.
3. Use mindfulness or CBT to alter negative thought patterns and manage your emotional response more effectively.

4. Reduce anxiety triggers, including caffeine, aspartame, and poor sleep. Discuss potential alternate medications for ADHD and asthma with your doctor.
5. Learn to use your breath. By focusing on and controlling your breathing patterns, you can shift your physiology into a relaxed state. I recommend starting a daily practice of 4-7-8 breathing, box breathing, or five-finger breathing techniques.
6. Regular exercise of any kind, including walking, running, yoga, or Tai Chi, can reduce anxiety.
7. When the going gets rough, there are supplements that can help. B vitamins, omega-3 fatty acids, magnesium, and adaptogens are meant to be used regularly for a period of time. L-theanine, lavender, and inositol can be used regularly or on an as-needed basis.
8. I prefer to reserve SSRIs for more severe forms of anxiety and to limit benzodiazepines to short-term treatment, owing to their potential side effects.

5

Mending Musculoskeletal Pain

The U.S. men's water polo team for the upcoming 2024 Paris Olympics had a problem: One of their star players, Hannes Daube, was refusing to do squats in the weight room. Leg strength is everything in water polo, allowing players to tread water and execute powerful movements. If the team had any hope of winning an Olympic medal, the players had to be in peak physical form.

When Dr. Naresh Rao, a sports medicine specialist and team doctor to the U.S. water polo Olympic team, asked Daube what was wrong, the twenty-three-year-old explained that his knee hurt whenever he descended below 45 degrees. He had seen every specialist in the Los Angeles area and undergone every scan imaginable, but no one had an answer for him. After examining Daube and watching him squat, Dr. Rao saw the problem: a condition called *patella alta*. The patella (kneecap) normally sits in a groove at the front of the femur, but in Daube's case, the patella sat above the groove, creating pain when he descended below 45 degrees. Over the course of a few days, Dr. Rao worked on Daube's hip alignment with osteopathic manipulation. This allowed the femur to be positioned more optimally and the patella to track more smoothly. He then assigned Daube a set of preventive "prehab" exercises, including clamshells and glut bridges, which he performed religiously. Fast-forward a few months, and Dr. Rao received a text from Daube: "Doc, I am the squatting master!" His pain was gone, he was training fully, and the U.S. men's water polo team won the bronze medal at the 2024 Paris games.

The moral of this story is this: Alignment matters! As Daube discovered, proper musculoskeletal alignment can reduce excessive stress on joints, reducing pain and granting them smooth and free motion. By distributing forces evenly, alignment helps prevent excessive wear and tear on the joints and prevents acute injuries and longer-term arthritis. In this chapter, we're going to see how alignment, flexibility, and strength tune the equilibrium of your musculoskeletal system to keep it in the best possible shape. I will examine some of the most common musculoskeletal injuries, including ligament and fascial damage, muscle and tendon strains, and fractures. I will explain why traditional advice like icing and bedrest may actually be slowing your recovery, and when newer treatments like platelet-rich plasma injections can expedite it. Finally, we'll see how weekend warriors can reduce the risk of injury with some simple precautions.

Ligament Injuries

Every year, three million people show up in U.S. emergency rooms with an ankle sprain,[1] which is among the most common musculoskeletal injuries. They happen to everyone, from Olympic athletes to pick-up-basketball players and pickleball enthusiasts. Approximately thirty thousand Americans sprain their ankle every single day.

A sprain is an injury that occurs when ligaments—the fibrous tissue connecting bones and joints to each other—are stretched or torn. While I will focus on ankle sprains in this chapter, as they are most common, sprains can affect just about any joint in the body. The information here is relevant for any ligament injury.

Ankle sprains are classified into three grades based on the severity of ligament damage.[2] Grade I (mild) sprains are due to stretching or slight tearing of ligament fibers. Mild sprains may cause minor pain or tenderness, some swelling or bruising, and sometimes difficulty walking or bearing weight. Your recovery reflex will activate and resolve these symptoms within a few days. Grade II (moderate) sprains typically involve partial tearing of the ligament, and you will likely have moderate pain and tenderness, noticeable swelling or bruising, and possibly some instability in the joint. (It may feel like your ankle is about to give way when you put weight on it.) Finally, grade III (severe) sprains involve a complete tear or rupture of an ankle ligament. Significant pain and swelling are common, along with instability in the ankle. Recovery takes considerably longer, and you may need surgery.

The majority of ankle sprains heal without surgical attention, but as many as 40 percent of people have symptoms that persist for a year or longer, including pain, swelling, instability, and sprain recurrences.[3] This is unfortunate, as there are integrative strategies that can help improve the speed and success of recovery.

Use the PEACE and LOVE Method

For many years, the prevailing advice for ankle sprains was RICE: rest, ice, compression, and elevation. However, recent research and clinical practice have raised questions about the accuracy of this age-old advice. Your recovery reflex depends on fresh blood bringing oxygen and nutrients to the damaged ligament. Dr. Rao notes that excess icing delays the healing process by reducing blood flow and halting inflammation. "You want some inflammation. You want the body to heal itself," he explains. "I only advise icing for pain control." If you have significant pain, you can apply an ice pack wrapped in a thin towel for fifteen minutes every two to three hours for the first two to three days.

Immediately following a ligament injury, your recovery reflex creates inflammation to initiate the healing process. The redness, heat, pain, and swelling are signs that your blood vessels are dilating, bringing in armaments to manage the injury, remove damaged tissue cells, and stimulate the proliferation of healthy cells.[4] While it may feel soothing, prolonged icing delays these cellular healing actions. A meta-analysis found no evidence that icing improves clinical outcomes.[5] Even Dr. Gabe Mirkin,[6] who coined the term RICE back in 1978, no longer advocates icing for sprained ankles. "It's perfectly fine to ice if you want, but realize it's delaying healing," he admitted a few years ago.[7]

The newly recommended approach to treating injured ligaments is the PEACE and LOVE method, which stands for: *Protect, Elevate, Avoid* anti-inflammatories, Compress, Educate, and Load, Optimism, Vascularization, and Exercise.[8] This method avoids ice, NSAIDs, and other anti-inflammatories, while emphasizing the importance of early and controlled use of your injured limb to activate your recovery reflex and accelerate healing. Here is how to get started:

Protect: Immediately following any ankle sprain (even a mild one), it is important to prevent further injury by protecting the ankle from excessive movement for one to three days. This can be accomplished with an elastic bandage, tight trainer or sneaker, air cast, or walking cast. When compared to longer immobilization, early weight-bearing with support improves the range of motion, accelerates the return to sports and work, reduces swelling, and improves patient satisfaction.[9] For more severe sprains, crutches can be used for the first several days or longer, if directed by a doctor.

Elevate: Keep your injured ankle elevated above the level of the heart to promote drainage of swelling and blood circulation. When sleeping or sitting, keep your ankle propped up on a stack of pillows.

Avoid Anti-Inflammatories: Do your best to avoid taking anti-inflammatory medications (such as ibuprofen) and applying ice. Remember that inflammation is a natural and necessary part of the healing process and will speed your recovery.

Compression: Compression can help minimize swelling while providing support to the injured ankle. You can purchase an elastic bandage wrap or an ankle compression "sleeve" at any pharmacy. If you notice joint instability, taping your ankle can also provide functional support. Ask your physiotherapist or sports medicine doctor to show you the proper technique.

Educate: Understand that your recovery reflex needs time to activate. Give your body a sufficient healing window to avoid exacerbating the injury.

Load: Instead of resting the ankle for long periods of time, begin early supported movement. For mild to moderate sprains, this could include walking around the house. If that is too painful, you can draw the alphabet with your toes (see "Exercise," following). Early ankle loading promotes healing by stimulating tissue repair and maintaining strength and flexibility. Avoid activities that cause outright pain, but a little discomfort is okay. Once healed, wear a high-top trainer or hiking boot that provides plenty of ankle support to prevent reinjuring the joint.

Optimism: Maintain a positive mindset and stay confident in the healing process. A positive outlook can impact physical recovery.

Vascularization: Choose pain-free, non-weight-bearing activities that promote blood flow to the injured joint, such as cycling on a stationary bike with minimal resistance, walking in water to offload your weight, or gentle range-of-motion exercises in the pool. For more severe sprains, ask your physiotherapist or sports and exercise medicine specialist for a longer list of rehab exercises.

Exercise: This includes progressive rehabilitation activities aimed at restoring your strength, flexibility, proprioception, and function. Initiate gentle range-of-motion exercises (a strategy I often recommend is to draw the letters of the alphabet with your foot and ankle) and gradually increase the intensity as the pain and swelling decrease. I recommend walking if your ankle can support your weight. Resistance-band exercises, in which you dorsiflex, plantarflex, invert, and evert the ankle are useful to strengthen the joint. Once your healing is well progressed, you can add balancing on one leg and hopping to prepare for higher-impact activities.

Plantar Fasciitis

Plantar fasciitis (PF) is a common musculoskeletal condition that causes pain in the heel of the foot.[10] My patients who have it usually tell me, "My first step onto the floor in the morning just *kills* me!" Subsequent steps are easier unless they are inactive for a period, and then the stabbing pain returns.

The underlying cause of PF is thought to be degenerative changes to the plantar fascia, the tough band of tissue running across the bottom of the foot that connects the heel bone to the toes. This tissue supports the arch of the foot and helps absorb shock. Over time, repeated stress or excessive strain can cause micro-tears in the tissue, leading to irritation, inflammation, and thickening of the plantar fascia, leading to pain. As many as one in ten people develop PF in their lifetime,[11] though it's more common among people who are overweight or have diabetes, pregnant women, runners, and those who practice step aerobics.

You may find some relief with icing and occasional NSAIDs. I recommend purchasing special compression socks, which apply gentle, graduated pressure to the foot and ankle to improve blood circulation. They are available over the counter at pharmacies, and they will make mornings more comfortable, when PF pain is often at its worst.[12] Look for compression socks that also provide arch support.

Another strategy for easing PF is to massage the fascia on your foot with a tennis ball. Place it under the ball of your foot and roll it from side to side. Repeat the massage under the arch and then finally the heel. You can also roll forward, using the tennis ball to apply pressure from the ball of your foot all the way back to the heel. When you begin, you might be surprised by how tight or painful this feels. Trust that it gets much easier with daily repetition.

Another option, extracorporeal shock wave therapy (ESWT), is often effective in people who continue to have symptoms despite conservative treatment. During ESWT, a device applies acoustic shock waves to the area of injury or pain. These waves pass through the skin and soft tissues to reach the targeted area, creating micro-damage in the tissue, which jump-starts the body's recovery reflex.

Seven prospective randomized controlled trials included 294 participants in a ESWT group and 369 participants in a placebo group;[13] the former had significantly less pain twelve weeks after treatment. Typical ESWT treatment occurs weekly for four to six weeks. A recent study revealed the value of also using ESWT to treat trigger points, which are painful knots in your muscles that are sensitive to touch.[14] People with PF who had calf trigger points treated in addition to their heels had further improvement in pain, function, and quality of life than those treated in the heel alone—a reminder that pain can be referred from distant locations!

Other effective treatments include Botox injections, platelet-rich plasma injections (more about this later), percutaneous electrolysis, dry needling, and electroacupuncture—all of which show similar and sometimes better results than the older treatment of corticosteroid injections (which can have more side effects).[15] My patient Maria, meanwhile, swears by reflexology, which uses deep pressure on specific points along the feet to relieve symptoms of PF. While it can be painful, she said it was the most effective treatment of all, allowing her to get back on the golf course—which she walks!

Muscle and Tendon Strains

My thirty-four-year-old patient Rusty loved to garden on the weekends. After forty hours in the office, gardening was his way of relieving stress. One day, while carrying a heavy brick, he turned and instantly felt a bolt of pain in his back that radiated into his buttocks and thigh. He rested, applied heat to his back, and took ibuprofen; after a few days, he felt better. But from then on, every time he crouched in his garden, the crippling pain returned.

To prevent these painful recurrences, Rusty gradually put together a set of yoga stretches he practiced at least three times a week to keep his back muscles loose and his stress levels low, allowing him to enjoy gardening pain free. Downward dog, cobra, and pigeon were the most helpful poses for Rusty owing to tightness in his hamstrings, but you may find success with a different routine.

While the information in this section is useful for all sorts of muscle strains, I am going to focus on lower-back pain, which 80 percent of people experience at some point in their lives. In fact, a recent study in *The Lancet* found that lower-back pain is the leading cause of disability worldwide.[16]

For most people, lower-back pain is considered "nonspecific," meaning it comes from neuromuscular dysfunction of muscle, ligaments, facet joints, fascia, nerve roots, or the vertebral disk. Much of it is "mechanical" in origin, meaning it is a result of abnormal forces or mechanics—at times due to misalignment—occurring in the tissue. Encouragingly, if a position, movement, or activity caused the issue, it is likely that improving your posture, strengthening your core muscles, and stretching tight hamstrings will activate your recovery reflex and help resolve the pain.

A sudden movement—like the twist that injured Rusty—can overstretch the ligaments or tendons or strain the muscles. Poor posture, which is a result of being out of alignment, can create excess tension, making you more susceptible to muscle strain. A weak core can place you at risk, as well. Ligament damage can also occur from repetitive movements and overuse. Years ago, when the videogame Tetris was released in the United States, I played it so often that I developed swelling and aching pain at the base of my thumb. Today this condition is better known as "texter's thumb," and it is a form of repetitive strain injury. Similarly, I occasionally treat patients with wrist pain because of prolonged hours typing at their computers without a break. Of course, the best way to address this is to stop the offending activity. If it cannot be avoided, see if you can alter your movement, improve your alignment, use ergonomic equipment, or take frequent breaks so your recovery reflex has time to heal the injury.

The following integrative-medicine recommendations can quickly activate your recovery reflex for muscle and tendon strains.

Again, Minimize Bedrest

Just as with ankle sprains, large-scale studies have shown that bedrest actually lengthens your recovery period from muscle strains.[17] Prolonged inactivity can lead to muscle weakness and even atrophy; it can also lead to stiffer joints, reduced blood flow, and loss of flexibility.

While intermittent rest can feel good, limit the time you spend lying down. Two to four days after injury, do your best to avoid bedrest altogether. Functional activities enhance blood circulation, delivering essential nutrients and oxygen to the injured area and facilitating the removal of waste products. In 90 percent of cases,[18] lower-back pain will get better on its own, and returning to your normal activity expedites this process.

In one clinical trial,[19] people in Helsinki, Finland, with lower-back pain were randomized into three groups: strict bed rest for two days, back-mobilizing exercises, or the continuation of ordinary activities as tolerated. After both three and twelve weeks, the study found that continuing ordinary activities led "to more rapid recovery" compared to the other groups. Of course, do use your judgment, and if you are in extreme pain, see your doctor for an evaluation.

Note that if you have back pain, you may have trouble finding a comfortable sleeping position. One way to reduce discomfort is to place a pillow under your knees when lying on your back, or between your knees when lying on your side.[20]

Exercises for Pain Relief

As we saw earlier with the Olympian Hannes Daube, when your body is aligned correctly, your muscles, ligaments, and joints work more efficiently. Poor posture may strain or overwork some muscles and weaken others, leading to misalignment.

There are many specific exercises to strengthen your back and improve your flexibility and posture (and therefore your alignment). I frequently recommend the McKenzie Method, which emphasizes extension exercises. (To get started, visit uk.mckenzieinstitute.org or do an online search for your area.) Another approach designed to decrease back pain by improving posture and body mechanics is the Gokhale Method, which I discuss in the "Deactivating Pain Signals" chapter.

Stuart McGill, PhD, is a professor emeritus at the University of Waterloo in Ontario, Canada, and a renowned lecturer in spine function, injury prevention, and rehabilitation. He emphasizes building core stability for both treating and preventing back pain. He recommends his "Big Three" exercises to increase strength and protect your back: curl-ups, side planks, and bird dogs. You can find detailed videos on how to perform them on YouTube.

Tools for Healing

In addition to the above exercises, I recommend the following strategies for enhancing your recovery reflex and helping you realign, gain flexibility, and build strength.

Foam Rollers: These are popular tools used to help alleviate muscle pain, increase flexibility, and stimulate recovery.[21] They apply direct pressure to the muscles and the connective tissue surrounding them, enhancing range of motion and reducing both acute and delayed onset muscle soreness.[22] Here's the side benefit: Rolling out the hamstrings also relieves longstanding back pain, a reminder that the origin of pain is not always the same as the location it is experienced.[23] Foam rollers come in various densities and contours, and you can even use tennis or lacrosse balls for smaller knots or aches. I usually recommend the softer rollers to start, but denser rollers can be helpful for larger or stronger muscles. Begin by rolling each muscle for 30 to 120 seconds, one to three times. Roll at a slow, controlled pace (about two to four seconds per roll in one direction).[24]

Acupuncture: Acupuncture can be an effective treatment to ease muscle strain.[25] It is believed to work by reducing excessive inflammation, improving circulation, and reducing muscle tension. Clinical studies reveal that acupuncture may be just as effective as medication for acute back pain.[26]

Pilates: Pilates focuses on strengthening muscles, improving flexibility, and enhancing overall body awareness. It was invented by Joseph Pilates, a German-born émigré to Britain who experimented during World War I with attaching springs to hospital beds so soldiers could tone their muscles while bed-bound.[27] His experiments resulted in a device known as the "reformer machine," which consists of a bedlike frame connected with springs to a flat, movable platform that rolls back and forth on wheels. The springs can be adjusted to provide different levels of resistance.

Pilates exercises engage your whole body to improve muscle tone, strength, and alignment, thereby improving posture. They especially strengthen your core, including the abs, pelvic floor, and muscles around your spine. The exercises are repeated in sets and target specific muscles.[28] Many Pilates exercises are carried out while lying down, so the back muscles do not engage as you strengthen your core. Pilates has been shown to improve muscle endurance and flexibility,[29] with wonderful side benefits that include less chronic pain,[30] anxiety, and depression.[31]

Chiropractic: Chiropractors use their hands or specialized tools to apply controlled, sudden force to joints, particularly those in the spine. This process aims to improve spinal alignment and joint mobility. The evidence supporting the effectiveness of chiropractic goes back thirty years, with inclusion in the Agency for Health Care Policy and Research's Clinical Practice Guidelines for acute low back pain in 1994.[32] A recent study found that patients with acute back injuries who immediately sought out chiropractic care had shorter pain episodes overall.[33]

Heat Therapy: Applying heat to injured or sore muscles can alleviate pain and promote healing. It may sound like a simple approach, and in some ways it is, but heat has been found to have multiple effects that support your recovery reflex.[34] It activates temperature-signaling nerves, thereby blocking the pain signals from using those pathways, and it improves circulation, which helps relax tight muscles and reduce spasms. The increase in tissue temperature also reduces fascia stiffness, which restores normal gliding and helps normalize pain sensing in those tissues. Finally, heat therapy increases metabolism and vasodilation, accelerating the healing processes. One clinical trial followed people aged twenty to fifty with acute low back pain.[35] Twice-daily application of heat in the form of a hot water bag for twenty minutes (in addition to NSAIDs) was significantly more effective at treating lower-back pain after five days compared to NSAIDs alone.

Medication and Supplements

After a muscle strain, you might be tempted to take an NSAID such as ibuprofen or naproxen. While NSAIDs can suppress pain, there is evidence they may also inhibit your recovery reflex by suppressing inflammation.

Of even greater concern, the regular use of NSAIDs for acute back pain increases the risk of developing *chronic* back pain. Data from the UK Biobank found that people with acute back pain who took NSAIDs had almost double the chance of developing chronic back pain, compared to those not taking NSAIDs.[36] This was not a randomized controlled trial, so it is not definitive, but other evidence supports the concept that NSAIDs interfere with healing. For instance, one study evaluated biological markers in nearly one hundred people when they first reported acute back pain, and then again three months later.[37] Those whose pain resolved had rapid and intense inflammation, which diminished by three months. Those who did not mount an inflammatory response had persistent pain.

Rather than taking an NSAID, consider what has worked well for you in the past. Perhaps that is heat, massage, or PT, or you might also wish to experiment with use of a transcutaneous electrical nerve stimulation (TENS) unit, acupuncture, and stretching. Together, these interventions will do more to support your healing response and restore homeostasis.[38]

There is evidence of effectiveness for several supplements in treating back and neck pain. Here is what I recommend:

Capsicum: The genus name for a wide variety of sweet and hot peppers, some capsicums contain an active compound called *capsaicin*, which is found in hot peppers and is responsible for their characteristic heat. Capsaicin binds to TRPV1 receptors on sensory nerve endings. This binding initially causes a sensation of heat and pain that desensitizes the nerve endings, reducing their ability to transmit pain signals. Capsaicin effectively subverts the pain-carrying nerve signal by sending a tingling sensation instead. Studies indicate that capsaicin is an effective treatment for muscle pain.[39] Apply a small amount of capsaicin cream or gel to the affected area up to four times daily. Be sure to wash your hands thoroughly afterwards to avoid transferring capsaicin to sensitive areas like the eyes or mucous membranes. (An effective over-the-counter alternative to capsaicin is a lidocaine patch, an anesthetic that stops nerves from sending pain signals to the brain.[40])

Liniments: Another set of topical products are liniments, also known as *salves*. These have been around for a long time! An herbalist in Rangoon developed and brought Tiger Balm to market in the 1870s. It contains menthol and oil of wintergreen. (Wintergreen oil is a source of methyl salicylate, a key component in Bengay heat rub, which was developed in 1898.) The ingredients in liniments can cool, numb, or send tingling sensations along the nerve pathway, blocking the pain signal from reaching the brain. In addition to these ingredients, doTERRA's Deep Blue is a soothing massage cream that contains the botanicals peppermint, ylang ylang, helichrysum, blue tansy, blue chamomile, and osmanthus. The usual directions for liniments are to apply two to three times daily. Avoid products with methyl salicylate if you have an allergy to aspirin, and be aware that excessive use can lead to dermatitis or increased internal absorption (potential symptoms are nausea, vomiting, and dizziness).[41]

Platelet-Rich Plasma

Platelet-rich plasma (PRP) therapy is a treatment in which a concentrated amount of your own platelets (the tiny cells in your blood that form clots to stop bleeding) is injected to promote healing of injured tissues. Your doctor draws a small amount of blood and places it in a centrifuge, where it's spun at high speed to isolate the plasma from the rest of the blood components. The PRP is then injected directly into the injured area. PRP is rich in several growth factors that promote tissue repair and regeneration. It has been shown to be effective for a wide variety of musculoskeletal injuries, including rotator-cuff injuries, muscle strains, Achilles ruptures, and patella damage. Dr. Rao, mentioned earlier, even successfully uses PRP in the damaged big toes of ballet dancers. Orthopedic specialists, sports-medicine doctors, dermatologists, and pain-management specialists are often trained to administer PRP. Note that PRP is usually considered a "second-line" therapy and has limited availability.

One study followed thirty professional athletes who received either PRP or standard treatment for various musculoskeletal injuries.[42] After fourteen days, 80 percent of the PRP group showed significant improvement in the regenerative healing process compared to just 20 percent for the control group. After three weeks, these figures were 100 percent and 73 percent, respectively. Dr. Rao notes that while PRP is effective, he suggests athletes wait until the off-season, owing to the recommended six-week recovery period after a PRP injection.

But PRP is not just for athletes! A sixty-year-old colleague of mine, Andrea, tripped and fell, resulting in terrible hip pain that lingered for months despite regular chiropractic adjustments. The pain was so bad she could barely walk, sleep, or perform her physiotherapy exercises. Finally, an ultrasound and MRI revealed torn muscles in her hamstring, gluteus medias, and gluteus minimus. Andrea was thrilled when her doctor suggested PRP. She had three injections spaced two weeks apart. She felt some relief after the first shot, and by the third her pain was 90 percent gone. Her doctor raved, "PRP has literally cleared out our physical rehab program. People are finally getting better!" Success rates of PRP vary depending on the condition being treated and its severity. For instance, one study of osteoarthritis of the knee found that about 60 percent of people with mild or moderate arthritis saw greater improvement compared to those with severe arthritis.[43]

Broken Bones

Sometimes it can be difficult to tell the difference between a bad sprain or bruise and a broken bone. A history of a direct blow, a fall from a height, or hearing a snap with sudden, severe pain is a potential indicator of a fracture; usually an X-ray will confirm. The treatment varies depending on the specific bone broken and how extensive the fracture is.

Fractures can be open (the bone pierces the skin) or closed (the skin is intact). Sometimes the bone is in perfect alignment and the fracture does not initially show up on an X-ray. Other times, bone fragments are not aligned, or the bone is broken into many pieces, and you may require surgery.

Most broken bones are placed in a splint, sling, brace, or cast to immobilize them. The healing of a bone fracture is another beautiful example of your recovery reflex in action. Your body knows exactly what to do and deploys overlapping stages to fully heal: Blood clots form around the injury to stabilize the area; a soft substance called *callus* forms to bridge the fracture; and specialized cells called *osteoblasts* begin remodeling the callus into mature bone.

My colleague Dr. Patricia Lebensohn was in a bicycle accident that injured her right foot a few weeks before leaving for a hiking trip in Europe. She immediately suspected a broken bone and went to a clinic, where an X-ray showed swelling and inflammation of the soft tissues but did not confirm a fracture. Patricia wrapped her foot, iced it, and took ibuprofen.

She flew to Europe with two pals and proceeded to hike 640 kilometres (400 miles) with intermittent pain. Upon arriving home, her doctor ordered an MRI, which indeed revealed a non-displaced fracture of the calcaneus (the large heel bone). This time, she ceased all strenuous activity and allowed the bone to heal for six weeks.

Earlier in this chapter I explained that too much rest can inhibit the healing process for ligament damage and muscle strains. A broken bone requires exactly the opposite: immobilization and rest. These two steps reduce the likelihood of complications, such as the bone shifting out of alignment or a nonunion (failure of the bone ends to grow together). Resting allows the body to form callus at the fracture site. You can engage in activities that don't put direct pressure on your healing bone. For instance, Patricia was able to ride a bike and swim even as she stopped hiking.

Become a Successful Weekend Warrior

Many years ago, my friend Nadine came over to my house with her kids. After watching them jump on the trampoline in my yard for an hour, she said: "I just *have* to jump, too!" She had been a gymnast back in high school, and though she was two decades removed from competition, she couldn't resist the urge to do a backflip. You can probably see where this is going: after a few bounces, Nadine summersaulted in the air, landed the flip, and then groaned in pain. She had thrown out her back.

You may have a story—or know someone who has a story—like Nadine's. Musculoskeletal injuries are common, particularly when you ramp up your activity levels after a long break. It is never a good idea to suddenly move from a state of rest to explosive movement. This is especially true as we get older. "It's a very bad idea to go zero to sixty without any sort of warm-up," explains Dr. Rao, who always leaves space open on his Monday morning calendar for weekend-warrior walk-ins. Preparing your body for activity can make all the difference between a pain-free weekend or one spent lying on the couch! Here is what I recommend.

Practice Dynamic Stretches

Back in middle-school gym class, you probably learned how to stretch before running. From hamstring stretches to quadricep stretches and shoulder stretches, they all likely had one thing in common: You were not moving. These "static" stretches involve extending a muscle to its farthest point and holding. However, as Dr. Rao notes, this can lead to a decrease in muscle temperature and blood flow, which may not adequately prepare the muscle for intense activity. "I've stopped recommending static stretches because they've never been proven in studies to decrease injury rates," he explains.

Instead, he recommends dynamic stretches, which put your muscles through a full range of motion to increase blood flow, muscle temperature, and neuromuscular readiness. Dynamic stretches include continuous movement, better preparing the muscles for the movements they will perform during your workout. There are many popular dynamic stretches you can look up on YouTube, but Dr. Rao's favorite are "Frankensteins," which target the hamstrings, hip flexors, and lower back. This stretch mimics the stiff-legged walk of Frankenstein's monster, hence the name. It is an excellent addition to a warm-up routine before activities such as running, jumping, or playing sports.

Here is a short primer: Stand tall with your feet hip-width apart and your arms extended parallel to the ground. Kick your right leg straight in front of you, keeping the knee locked. As you lift your leg, try to touch your right foot with your left hand. (You are unlikely to reach, so just aim to get as close as you comfortably can.) Lower your right leg back to the ground and then repeat the exercise with your left leg. As you walk forward slowly, repeating the exercise ten to fifteen times, be sure to keep your spine upright.

Remember that cool-down exercises can be just as important as warm-ups, and they are often neglected. A cool-down period after intense exercise will help your heart gradually return to its resting rate; it also reduces delayed onset muscle soreness.[44] To cool down, I recommend slow-paced walking and using a foam roller to stretch any muscles that may have tightened.

Hydrate

I have a patient, Samira, who loves to backpack on the weekends but frequently develops cramps, which are sudden, involuntary contractions or spasms of one or more muscles. It turns out that to lighten her load she scrimps on carrying water, which of course is quite heavy. After encouraging her to pre-hydrate with water and electrolytes (more on these in a bit), her cramping resolved.

Proper hydration is essential for maintaining the synovial fluid that lubricates the joints, while hydrated tissues, including muscles and cartilage, provide better shock absorption. As Samira discovered, dehydration can cause electrolyte imbalances, particularly of sodium, potassium, magnesium, and calcium, which aid muscle contraction and relaxation.

As you sweat during a workout, you're not only losing fluids but in addition you're losing critical electrolytes. These are the minerals in your body that maintain fluid balance, transmit nerve impulses, and support muscle function. Drinking enough water so your urine is pale yellow helps ensure hydration, but it doesn't tell you about your electrolyte status. Unfortunately, short of blood testing, which is not commonly available outside of a lab, you will not know what your electrolyte levels are; instead, you will learn over time to read your body's signals. Higher intensity and longer exercise and hotter temperatures all require more fluids and electrolytes. I recommend adding electrolyte powders to your water bottle. Note that sugars in electrolyte formulas may be useful if you are exercising for longer periods of time.

Stretch to Relieve Cramps

Stretches are the best way—better than pickle juice or other salty brines—to relieve exercise-induced muscle cramps.[45] For calf cramps, sit on the floor, keeping your leg straight while pulling the top of your foot toward your body. (You can use a strap or a towel looped around your foot if it feels too far to reach.) Alternatively, stand up and put your weight on the affected leg, then gently bend your knee and lift your toes repeatedly. For a hamstring cramp, sit on the floor with your back straight and your legs extended. Reach forward with both hands toward your toes and hold for thirty seconds. Additionally, foam rollers can stretch and help stimulate blood flow to the cramping area, encouraging it to release knots or trigger points.

Photo-Biomodulation Therapy

A truly remarkable innovation in medicine is the use of photo-biomodulation therapy (PBMT) to enhance athletic performance and recovery from exercise.[46] During PBMT, or red light therapy, light at specific wavelengths penetrates the skin and is absorbed by cells, stimulating healing, reducing pain and inflammation, and promoting tissue regeneration.

PBMT is now recommended by the International Olympics Committee to improve acute muscular recovery. The directions are to use PBMT for thirty seconds at least five minutes before and after the strength-training activity. Ideally, treat all the muscle groups engaged in the activity. This is one of many areas, including hair growth and migraine relief, where light is beginning to be used as a medical tool to support your recovery reflex. PBMT is generally available privately and for certain treatments on the NHS, and personal devices are now sold online.

Your Rapid Recovery Prescription for Mending Musculoskeletal Pain

Musculoskeletal injuries are common occurrences, and your recovery reflex is designed to kick in as you heal from sprains, strains, cramps, and broken bones. With an integrative approach you can quickly return to an active lifestyle.

Ligament Injuries
- Use the PEACE and LOVE method for mild to moderate sprains. Strive to return to normal activities as soon as possible.

Plantar fasciitis
- Treat by rolling on a tennis ball, icing, wearing compression socks, taking NSAIDs, and with massage. For stubborn cases, ESWT is a good option.

Back Pain (and Other Muscle or Tendon Strains)
1. Minimize rest and return to functional movement as soon as possible. If you have trouble sleeping with back pain, place a pillow under your knees when lying on your back, or between your knees when lying on your side.
2. The McKenzie and Gokhale methods can improve posture and decrease pain. To strengthen your core and prevent back pain, practice Stuart McGill's "Big Three" exercises: curl-ups, side planks, and bird dogs.
3. Foam rollers, acupuncture, Pilates, chiropractic, and heat therapy can enhance your recovery reflex.
4. Capsaicin and liniments are safe and effective alternatives to NSAIDs.

For more severe ligament and muscle injuries, PRP injections can help jump-start your recovery reflex.

Broken Bones
- Broken bones—usually diagnosed with a hospital visit and an X-ray—require immobilization and rest.

Finally, for weekend warriors, remember to practice dynamic warm-up stretches, stay hydrated, and use stretches to relieve cramps.

6

Supporting Healthy Skin and Hair

Your skin is a magnificent part of your body. It serves as your first line of defense against the world, acting as a barrier to protect you from pathogens, harmful chemicals, and physical injuries. It is also your largest organ, covering about 2 square metres (22 sq. ft.) and weighing 3.6 kilograms (8 lb).[1]

Skin is made up of three layers: the epidermis, which is the outermost layer; the middle dermis layer, which contains collagen and elastin fibers, blood vessels, nerve endings, sweat and oil glands, and hair follicles; and the hypodermis, the protective innermost layer made up of fat and connective tissue.

Roughly every month, the epidermis completely renews itself, shedding dead skin cells and replacing them with new ones.[2] We have surprising control over how our skin looks and feels during this process. Variables from the content of your diet (lots of fruits and vegetables), the amount of sun exposure (minimize, and use zinc or titanium sunscreen), and the products you use on your skin (more on these following) can help keep it more supple, smooth, and firm. Though it ages over time, your skin beautifully showcases the body's recovery reflex. As soon as the skin is cut, blood clotting commences to stop the bleeding and create a temporary barrier against pathogens. Your immune response then creates puffy inflammation as the skin heals, a scab forms, and healthy pink tissue forms underneath.

As impressive as our skin's healing abilities are, however, there are conditions that can prevent us from feeling and looking our best. Fortunately, integrative medicine can help.

Acne

Acne can make people feel unattractive, embarrassed, and in the case of young adults, so self-conscious that they avoid social activities.[3] More than a simple nuisance, blemishes are closely linked with self-confidence and mental health, and large-scale studies reveal that acne can increase suicide risk.[4] And acne is not limited to youth alone; while it affects 85 percent of people aged twelve to twenty-four, research shows that approximately 50 percent of women in their twenties, 33 percent of women in their thirties, and 25 percent of women (and 12 percent of men) in their forties suffer from it, too.[5]

Acne is linked to hormones called *androgens*, which, among other things, increase the production of sebum, an oily substance produced by the sebaceous glands that lubricates your hair and skin. Sometimes, hair follicles become clogged with dead skin cells and sebum. This is what causes acne to form. The bacterium *Cutibacterium acnes* (*C. Acnes*) multiplies inside the clogged follicles, leading to inflammation, redness, and pus-filled pimples.

For many years, antibiotics—primarily doxycycline and minocycline—were the primary treatments for acne. While they were effective, doctors and scientists are increasingly aware that antibiotics can disrupt the delicate balance of microbiota in the gut.[6] Similarly, birth control pills, which are often used to treat acne as they can reduce androgen levels, can have a variety of unwanted side effects. These two therapies, which doctors still prescribe despite their adverse consequences, may ultimately go the way of radiotherapy—which was once an actual treatment for acne, too![7]

Fortunately, we now have safer methods that support your recovery reflex as it kicks into gear to fight off acne-causing bacteria. Here are my favorite integrative strategies.

Eat the Rainbow

My nineteen-year-old patient Ashley was struggling with acne flare-ups. While she had had a few pimples in high school, the canteen food at her college seemed to make it much worse. My advice was simple: "Eat the rainbow!" This meant loading up her plate with as much color as possible, including green beans, squash, carrots, tomatoes, oranges, chard, blueberries, and a smaller amount of grains and protein. I also recommended avoiding dairy and adding a dietary supplement of zinc and topical green tea solution (more about these later). Ashley's acne cleared up, and she shared her methods with all her friends.

Colorful fruits and vegetables contain phytonutrients, compounds that give plants their color and help protect them from disease. They protect humans from disease, too, and they help with acne by reducing inflammation. Vitamin A, found in orange and yellow vegetables, helps regulate skin-cell production and reduce the risk of clogged pores, while vitamin C, present in citrus fruits, strawberries, and bell peppers (capsicums), supports collagen production and helps repair damaged skin.[8]

Certain foods can exacerbate acne. Dairy, particularly cow's milk, has long been linked to outbreaks. Cow's milk contains insulin-like growth factor 1 (IGF-1),[9] which can stimulate oil glands in the skin and increase sebum production. It also contains the hormones estrogen, progesterone, and androgen precursors. Lower-fat milks may be particularly problematic, with skim milk conveying the highest risk of acne breakouts.[10]

Foods with a high glycemic index (GI), such as baguettes, pastries, and sugary cereals, cause rapid spikes in blood sugar levels, and the resulting inflammation may trigger the body to produce more sebum. Following a low-glycemic diet can help prevent outbreaks. In one study of more than two thousand two hundred Americans placed on a low-glycemic diet, 87 percent reported having less acne, and 91 percent said they needed less medication.[11] (See the "Reversing Type 2 Diabetes" chapter for more information about high- and low-GI foods.) Generally speaking, population-wide studies show that people who avoid the standard American diet (with the appropriate acronym SAD), which is rich in saturated fats and refined carbohydrates, are much less acne prone.[12]

Consider the Kitavan Islanders of Papua New Guinea, who don't eat any refined foods. In one study of one thousand two hundred islanders,[13] *zero* were found to have acne!

Use a Gentle Cleanser

As we have become more knowledgeable about our skin microbiome, we have discovered that soap can disrupt its homeostasis owing to its high pH (usually 9 to 10). Your skin naturally has a slightly acidic pH level, and overly alkaline cleansers can contribute to bacterial growth and acne breakouts.[14] Indeed, one study of 120 young adults with acne found that those who used cleansers with a pH between 5.5 and 7 had less acne and less irritation.[15]

There are a number of products available with lower pH levels that may be gentler on the skin. One product that meets the standard with a pH of 5.5 is Cetaphil Cleansing and Moisturizing Syndet Bar (or Gentle Cleansing Bar).[16] Another product shown to be effective at significantly reducing acne is Effaclar Cleansing Gel,[17] made by La Roche-Posay. Also look for body wash products that generally include certain ingredients such as include salicylic acid, lactic acid, glycolic acid, and botanicals to exfoliate skin and unblock pores.[18] CeraVe Hydrating Facial Cleanser has not been in a clinical study, but it has a pH no greater than 5.5, and some of its ingredients—namely, ceramides and hyaluronic acid—have been proven to help restore the skin barrier and improve skin hydration. Finally, a set of seven herbal products made by Shaant—a cleanser, oil-control cream, exfoliator, toner, spot treatment, clay mask, and body scrub—were studied on both the face and body and shown to reduce acne and inflammation, improve skin hydration, and even improve mood.[19]

Mind–Body Practices

The link between psychological stress and acne is well established. During tense situations, the brain releases stress hormones including cortisol, which can increase the production of sebum in the skin.[20] And just as high stress levels can slow wound healing, they also make existing acne breakouts linger.[21] (I encourage you to read the "Unwinding Anxiety" chapter, where I discuss strategies for dealing with anxiety.)

There are many ways to reduce stress and soothe your skin, and strong evidence exists for hypnosis, meditation, and biofeedback.[22] Biofeedback teaches you to control physiological processes that are normally involuntary, such as heart rate, muscle tension, and body temperature, using techniques like deep breathing, progressive muscle relaxation, visualization, and mindfulness meditation. In a study of thirty people,[23] one group underwent twelve biofeedback sessions and the other was given traditional attention therapy sessions focusing on happiness. After six weeks, the biofeedback group saw a significant reduction in acne severity compared to the control group. Guided imagery can also be helpful. Here is my recommendation: Before going to bed, in your mind's eye, take a few moments to imagine your face with clear, vibrant, and healthy skin.

Treating Breakouts

The occasional breakout happens to many of us, no matter how hard we try to avoid them. Happily, there are safe and effective products you can use to help your skin recover quickly. Here are the topical remedies and oral supplements that I recommend.

> **Tea Tree Oil:** Tea tree oil is an essential oil derived from the leaves of the *Melaleuca alternifolia* tree, which is native to Australia. It contains compounds such as terpinen-4-ol, which have strong antibacterial and antifungal properties.[24] I usually recommend using a 5 percent tea tree oil solution. To apply, first add 7 to 10 drops of tea tree oil to 1 tablespoon of witch hazel extract. Apply it topically with a cotton bud to the spot or with a cotton wool ball all over your face (or other acne location) while avoiding your eyes. Tea tree oil has been shown to be effective in treating mild to moderate acne, and has also been compared to benzoyl peroxide. In a study of 124 people, the two products were equally effective, and while the tea tree oil took a bit longer to work, it had fewer side effects.[25]
>
> **Green Tea:** Green tea is high in polyphenols, which are plant compounds that contain powerful antioxidants that reduce inflammation. Studies

prove that green tea is an effective treatment for reducing acne lesions.[26] I recommend topically applying a lotion containing 2 to 3 percent green tea extract. Or, a simple DIY home remedy can be made by infusing a green tea bag in hot water for 10 minutes, allowing it to cool, and then applying the bag to the outbreak area or smoothing it all over your face.

Nicotinamide: Also known as vitamin B3, nicotinamide has potent anti-inflammatory effects and reduces sebum production. In one study, a 4 percent nicotinamide gel used for eight weeks was found to reduce sebum levels, and thirty of the thirty-eight participants were moderately to highly satisfied with their treatment results.[27] The same gel was also compared to 1 percent clindamycin gel (an antibiotic) in a randomized trial of seventy-six people.[28] After eight weeks, the two products were found to be comparable and effective. Given the worry about resistant microorganisms from antibiotics, I believe nicotinamide is the safer choice. And as a side benefit, nicotinamide reduces wrinkles![29]

Lactobacillus plantarum: This species of bacteria is commonly found in fermented foods and is known for its beneficial effects on gut health. Recent studies suggest that a *Lactobacillus plantarum* extract can reduce the number of skin lesions among people with acne due to its antimicrobial properties.[30] I recommend applying a 5 percent lotion daily.

Zinc: Zinc is a mineral with antibacterial and anti-inflammatory properties that has the novel effect of increasing the effectiveness of antibiotics when treating antibiotic-resistant strains of *C. acnes*.[31] Zinc can be used topically (and is included in many cleansers) or taken orally.[32] While not as effective as antibiotics, it is much safer. In one study involving 332 participants,[33] one group received 30 mg of zinc gluconate and the other received 100 mg of minocycline. At the end of the study, 63 percent of the antibiotic group saw a significant reduction in inflammatory lesions compared to 31 percent of the zinc users. For topical use, I recommend a lotion with 5 percent zinc sulfate.

Oral Probiotics: Probiotics can act in multiple ways to reduce acne:[34] They can inhibit *C. acnes*,[35] decrease inflammation, and improve the skin barrier function. Oral *Bifidobacterium bifidum* and *Lactobacillus acidophilus* have both been successfully used at a dose of 10 to 20 CFUs per day.[36] In one study, *Saccharomyces cerevisiae* (a yeast) dosed at 250 mg three times daily led to improvements in acne when compared to a placebo over a five-month period.[37]

Omega-3 Fatty Acids: Omega-3 fatty acids, particularly EPA and DHA, have strong anti-inflammatory properties. They can help reduce the systemic inflammation that contributes to acne, leading to fewer and less severe breakouts. A study found that patients with acne who adhered to a Mediterranean diet (which is rich in omega-3 foods) while taking a DHA/EPA supplement (600 mg DHA and 300 mg EPA in weeks one through eight, increasing to 800 mg DHA and 400 mg EPA in weeks eight through sixteen) saw their acne lesions improve significantly.[38] (Notably, 98 percent of the participants were deficient in omega-3s at the onset of the study!) In another study, forty-five participants with mild to moderate acne were treated with a daily dose of 1,000 mg EPA plus 1,000 mg DHA plus 400 mg of borage oil and were found to have significant improvements compared to a control group.[39]

NicAzel: This is a prescription dietary supplement available in the U.S.A. consisting of vitamins and minerals. While costly, my patient Debra loved this product and has been taking it regularly for several years. When I asked about her acne, she told me that she "went from a full-blown breakout every month in the week before her period to just an occasional zit." In one trial, 235 people with acne added NicAzel to their daily regimen.[40] After eight weeks, 88 percent of them saw an improvement, and three-quarters thought NicAzel was as effective as oral antibiotics. Speak to your healthcare provider to ask about similar products available in your area.

Conventional Acne Treatments

If you walk into your local pharmacy, you may find an entire section devoted to acne products. Treating acne is big business, with the U.S. market alone valued at more than $5 billion.[41] But do the most popular commercial products actually work? Let's review them.

Salicylic Acid and Benzoyl Peroxide: One of the most popular remedies on store shelves is salicylic acid, which is typically found in scrubs and cleansers. While there are few studies supporting its effectiveness, salicylic acid has been shown to reduce inflammatory lesions and comedones,[42] which are small, flesh-colored acne "bumps" or papules. However, my patients have much better results with benzoyl peroxide (BP), an organic compound that acts as an antibacterial agent and exfoliant. When applied directly to acne, BP can effectively kill the bacteria responsible for acne development.[43] Note that some people do not tolerate BP and have side effects, including redness, peeling, dryness, sensitivity to sun, and itching.

Retinoids: Retinoids are a vitamin A–derived class of compounds commonly used to treat acne and prevent or minimize wrinkles, and they are highly effective.[44] Retinoids accelerate the turnover of skin cells, which helps prevent the formation of clogged pores, and they treat existing acne by reducing redness and swelling. Start with a lower concentration, as retinoids can dry out your skin. You can gradually increase the potency as your skin adjusts. Begin by applying a pea-size amount at night. Be sure to use sun protection during the day, as retinoids increase UV light sensitivity.

Spironolactone: A diuretic that is sometimes used to treat high blood pressure and PCOS (polycystic ovary syndrome), spironolactone has an anti-androgen effect. A recent trial divided 133 women with moderate acne into two groups.[45] The first group received doxycycline and BP for three months, followed by a three-month treatment with a placebo and BP, while the second group received spironolactone and BP for six months. While the onset was slower, spironolactone was almost three times more effective than doxycycline at the sixth month. Women described spironolactone as easy to tolerate and reported they had better quality of life than when taking the antibiotic.

Dermatitis

When *itis* is added to a word, it signals inflammation. *Tendonitis* means inflammation of a tendon, *colitis* is inflammation of the colon, and *dermatitis* is inflammation of the derma (skin). Dermatitis is characterized by a range of symptoms that include redness, swelling, itching, and scaling. There are three common forms: Atopic dermatitis (eczema) is a condition characterized by dry, itchy, and inflamed skin that affects nearly ten million children and more than sixteen million adults in the United States.[46] Contact dermatitis occurs when skin comes into contact with an irritant or allergen and causes similar symptoms. Finally, seborrheic dermatitis causes scaly patches, redness, and dandruff, often affecting oily areas of the body (like the scalp and face) and is thought to be caused by an overgrowth of yeast on the skin. There are many integrative tools at your disposal that can dramatically reduce the symptoms and recurrences of all three types.

Stress and Eczema

My forty-two-year-old patient Sarah had a severe onset of seborrheic dermatitis. We tried a few integrative treatments with mixed results, including omega-3 fatty acids, topical chapparal brewed as tea and applied as a poultice on her scalp, and an oral dietary supplement called quercetin. When her symptoms still didn't resolve fully, instead of turning to more powerful medication, we looked within. Sarah's mother had recently died, and Sarah was grieving. We began a program of simple guided imagery that called for Sarah to relax and then visualize a healthy, comfortable scalp covered with beautiful thick hair. After practicing this technique for a few weeks, her eczema cleared up entirely.

See the chapter "Unwinding Anxiety" for more information about integrating ways to de-stress into your daily routine.

Topicals

Eczema leaves your skin dry, inflamed, or extremely itchy. One key to minimizing discomfort and preventing flares is maintaining proper hydration. Moisturizers help to restore the skin barrier by providing essential lipids and forming a protective layer on the skin's surface. While you'll find pharmacy shelves devoted to moisturizers specifically formulated for eczema, one effective product is in your supermarket.

Coconut Oil: Coconut oil is a natural oil extracted from the meat of mature coconuts. It is an effective moisturizer that helps to hydrate dry, flaky skin by forming a protective barrier on its surface. Coconut oil contains lauric acid, which has anti-inflammatory properties that reduce redness, swelling, and itching. Lauric acid also has antimicrobial properties, which can reduce the risk of infections on compromised skin.[47] I recommend using cold-pressed or virgin organic coconut oil, which does not contain solvents that may further irritate your skin. Unlike most oils, coconut oil is solid at room temperature, so you'll want to lather it in your hands to liquefy it. I recommend applying it immediately after bathing, while your skin is still damp and well hydrated; this will "trap" the moisture in your skin. You can apply coconut oil directly to an area that has eczema, but I also recommend you use it (or one of the following moisturizers) all over your skin to prevent outbreaks.[48]

Other Moisturizers: There are many additional products on the marketplace that hydrate the skin, relieve itching, and improve skin barrier function. It is important to find one that feels good, is affordable, and leaves out fragrance and irritants. Once you find a product you like, use it once or twice a day. Moisturizers that have been researched and that I recommend include those made by CeraVe, Aveeno, and Eucerin.[49] CeraVe, which contains ceramides and hyaluronic acid, has been studied and shown to help hydrate the skin and restore its natural barrier.[50] Aveeno Eczema Therapy Moisturizing Cream was studied in fifty patients ages twelve to sixty over an eight-week period.[51] Dermatologists noticed improvement after just two weeks of twice-daily use. Participants described less discomfort, improved skin texture, and an overall improvement in the look and feel of their skin. Look at the ingredients list for oats, urea, ceramides, and hyaluronic acid. Avoid anything with fragrance and parabens.

Licorice Gel: Derived from the root of the licorice plant (*Glycyrrhiza glabra*), licorice gel is a topical product noted for its anti-inflammatory, soothing, and healing properties, and has been shown to be an effective treatment for eczema.[52] Apply a thin layer of gel to eczema-affected areas after cleansing. It can be used once or twice daily, depending on the severity of your symptoms.

Black Tea Compress: Black tea contains tannins, which have anti-inflammatory, antibacterial, and astringent properties. It is effective for eczema when used as a compress. Here is how to make one: Soak a clean cloth or cotton pad in brewed black tea and apply it directly to the skin. In one study, people who used black tea compresses saw a dramatic reduction in facial eczema severity within three days.[53] Apple Bodemer, MD, a dermatologist who completed our Integrative Medicine Fellowship and now serves on the faculty at our Center, recommends infusing the compress in tea for 5 to 10 minutes and letting it cool until lukewarm. (Green, black, and white teas will all work, as they originate from the same plant.) As an alternative to a cloth compress, she recommends using rice paper, as it is highly absorbent and gentle on the skin. Apply the compress to the affected area and leave it on for 10 to 15 minutes. This process can be repeated several times a day, depending on the severity of the eczema. If the tannins dry out your skin, apply your moisturizer immediately afterwards.

Environmental Factors

My forty-seven-year-old patient Samir suddenly developed blotches of eczema on both his arms. Nothing had changed about his daily routine, and he had no family history of eczema. He saw multiple dermatologists, and while steroids helped, when he went off them, the rash reappeared. Flummoxed, Samir came to see me. After deconstructing his routine, we figured out the cause: a university-themed coffee mug given to him by his former college roommate. It was his favorite mug, and he drank coffee from it every morning. One day, Samir looked down and noticed bits of plastic floating in his coffee. After many years of use, the plastic had become brittle. When Samir switched to a new ceramic mug, his eczema disappeared entirely.

Environmental factors besides plastics can trigger or exacerbate eczema symptoms. Cold and dry climates can sap the skin of moisture, while excessive heat and humidity can increase sweating, which may irritate the skin especially in its folds and areas prone to friction. Certain foods can also be a trigger; see the "Your Rapid Recovery Toolkit" (appendix 1) for information on how to begin an elimination diet that can pinpoint potential dietary culprits.

Skincare products may also cause flare-ups. I had one patient, Jessica, with severe eczema on her face. The skin around her eyes, nose, cheeks, and chin was red, hot, and incredibly itchy; she hated the way her face looked and went to one dermatologist after another looking for help. They were all stumped. We eventually figured out the offender was her moisturizer, which contained a variety of allergenic chemicals. I switched her to a simple regimen of a thin layer of coconut oil before bedtime, and her eczema cleared up for good.

When bathing, take care to avoid harsh soaps that can irritate eczema. I recommend the "soak and seal" method:[54] Take a short (5 to 10 minutes) bath or shower while avoiding scrubbing affected skin; pat (don't rub) yourself dry with a towel, leaving your skin slightly damp; immediately apply moisturizers before your skin has a chance to dry out.

Clothing, too, can contribute to eczema outbreaks. Fabrics with rough or abrasive textures can create friction against the skin, leading to irritation. Wool in particular is known to be irritating for people with sensitive skin. If you are prone to eczema, avoid synthetic materials, including fabrics containing polyester, nylon, and acrylic, which can trap heat and moisture. Choose soft, breathable fabrics like cotton or silk, which are gentle on the skin and allow for air circulation. It's also a good idea to wash new clothing before wearing it to remove excess dyes and chemicals. Speaking of laundry, note that many detergents contain fragrances and other chemicals that can irritate sensitive skin. And don't get me started on fabric softeners! (I recommend you use wool dryer balls instead.) Unfortunately, shopping the "clean" product line at the store is not sufficient. Several brands available in stores' "green section" actually score quite poorly when it comes to hazardous chemicals. Detergents labeled "fragrance-free" or "unscented" often score better. It's best to scan the bar code with one of the apps mentioned below before purchasing.

If you are wondering about your own products, I highly recommend you download one of the apps that allow you to check what's in your products such as the Yuka app developed in France, which contains information on three hundred thousand cosmetic products. Scan the barcode of your favorite products and you will discover whether they contain allergens, reproductive toxicants, or carcinogens. Look for online sites that also have lists of verified products that are free of hazardous chemicals.

Probiotics

Finally, taking probiotics can also help clear up eczema. A meta-analysis of six randomized trials found a significant reduction in eczema symptoms when probiotics were used.[55] In a separate clinical trial focused on treating dry skin and wrinkles,[56] 110 participants between the ages of forty-one and fifty-nine were randomized to receive either oral probiotics or placebo. Granted, dry skin and wrinkles are not the same as eczema, but I include this study because after twelve weeks, the probiotic group not only experienced significantly improved skin hydration (an important issue for eczema) but they also had fewer wrinkles!

I recommend purchasing probiotics that contain *Lactobacillus plantarum*, *L. acidophilus*, or *L. rhamnoses*, all of which have been studied and found to reduce dryness and improve skin barrier functions.[57]

Medication

Eczema is conventionally treated using topical corticosteroids, which reduce redness, swelling, and itching by suppressing the inflammatory response in the skin and reducing blood flow to the inflamed area. They are effective,[58] and I do prescribe them for the occasional flare-up. You can purchase relatively weak over-the-counter products containing 0.5 or 1 percent hydrocortisone cream or ointment. It is best to avoid prolonged use of potent (or fluorinated) topical steroids, which can lead to thinning of the skin, making it more fragile and susceptible to bruising, tearing, and stretch marks (striae).[59]

Dermatologists have developed a safer alternative to steroids: topical calcineurin inhibitors (TCIs), a class of medications that work by modulating the immune response and reducing inflammation. TCIs usually come in two strengths: pimecrolimus cream for mild to moderate eczema,[60] and tacrolimus ointment for moderate to severe eczema. Unlike topical steroids, TCIs do not cause skin atrophy, making them suitable for long-term use on delicate skin areas, including the face, genital area, and armpits.[61] You can use TCIs for long-term maintenance or intermittently to treat flare-ups, but ideally you will want to detect the underlying cause of the eczema and eliminate it.

Hair Loss

We wash, brush, and comb our hair each morning, yet we rarely pause to consider how impressive the human scalp is! Hair is a filament that grows from a follicle in your skin and consists primarily of tightly packed cells filled with a fibrous protein called *keratin*. Your individual hairs may not seem strong, but the average strand can support roughly 100 grams (3½ oz) of weight.[62]

Hair growth has three distinct phases:[63] anagen, catagen, and telogen. The anagen, or active growth, phase lasts two to seven years, during which hair grows nearly 2 centimetres (½ in) per month. Nearly 90 percent of your hair is usually in the anagen phase. During the catagen phase, which lasts about two to three weeks, the hair follicle shrinks and detaches from the dermal papilla, the structure at the base of the hair follicle that supplies nutrients to growing hair. Finally, during the telogen phase, which lasts about three to four months, hair stops growing altogether and falls out. At any moment, some of your hair is in the telogen phase, and it is perfectly normal to lose fifty to one hundred hairs daily.[64]

Hair loss beyond this norm, also known as alopecia, is the gradual or sudden loss of hair from the scalp or other parts of the body where hair naturally grows. It can occur in both men and women and can be temporary or permanent, depending on the underlying cause. Sometimes hair loss is genetic, and sometimes it's caused by a stressor. The most common forms of alopecia is androgenic alopecia, which is the hereditary type that affects roughly 50 percent of men and many women over the age of forty.[65]

To be clear, many men wear their baldness or shaved head from androgenic alopecia with pride!

Other forms of hair loss include alopecia areata, an autoimmune disease that can cause hair loss just on the head or across the body; and telogen effluvium, which involves rapid hair loss after a stressful event or sudden hormonal changes (such as childbirth). I experienced telogen effluvium after each of my three children were born; I initially noticed very short hairs growing in at my hairline like a fringe (bangs), and my first thought was: *Who cut my fringe so short?*

Your recovery reflex is effective at regrowing hair—provided you act before scar tissue has formed. The strategies that follow can help dramatically slow down hair loss—and in many situations, help you to grow new hair.

Diet

Can the food you eat—or, as we'll see, what you drink—impact hair loss? The results from a large-scale study involving more than one thousand men suggest *yes*. After studying the habits of eighteen- to forty-five-year-old men, researchers from China's Tsinghua University concluded that men who consume sugary beverages such as juice, energy drinks, or sweet tea more than seven times per week were about 3.4 times more likely to have male-pattern hair loss compared to those who did not consume sugary beverages.[66] More concerning, the high sugar consumption was linked to a 25 percent higher rate of depression.

Diets that emphasize vegetables, fruits, and omega-3 fatty acids—all of which are naturally anti-inflammatory—may help stimulate hair growth.[67] Research suggests that a Mediterranean-style diet is especially effective. In one study that controlled for age, education, body-mass index, and family history,[68] men who ate three or more servings of raw vegetables and three or more servings of fresh herbs each week reduced their risk of male-pattern hair loss.

Topicals

Should you start noticing excessive hair loss, I recommend you speak to your physician and have lab work done, including iron, total iron-binding capacity, ferritin, thyroid-stimulating hormone, and vitamin D. This is because hair loss can be a sign of another health issue, such as hypothyroidism, or a nutritional deficiency of iron, zinc, vitamin D, or protein. It is important to diagnose and begin treating your scalp to address any issues before fatty infiltration or scarring occurs. Here are some integrative recommendations I recommend you begin immediately.

> **Pumpkin Seed Oil:** One clinical trial showed that massaging pumpkin seed oil or 5 percent minoxidil foam into the scalp daily for three months were both equally effective.[69] For maximum effectiveness, massage 1 teaspoon into the scalp, rather than your hair, one to three times a week. As you apply the pumpkin seed oil, focus on areas you want to stimulate growth. Massage gently for 5 to 10 minutes to improve blood circulation, then leave it on for at least 30 minutes. For deeper penetration, wrap your hair with a warm towel or shower cap and leave pumpkin seed oil on your scalp overnight. Like other topicals for hair growth, pumpkin seed oil is messy. You may prefer to use the oral supplement at a dose of 400 to 500 mg daily. One study of seventy-six patients compared 400 mg of oral pumpkin seed oil to placebo and found a 40 percent increase in hair count among the pumpkin-seed-oil users.[70]
>
> **Saw Palmetto Oil:** Like pumpkin seed oil, saw palmetto oil inhibits the action of 5-alpha reductase. In one study, eighty healthy men and women aged eighteen to fifty received either 400 mg of oral saw palmetto oil, 5 cc of a topical formulation containing 20 percent saw palmetto, or a placebo.[71] At the end of the study, both the oral and topical saw palmetto formulations were found to reduce hair loss by 29 percent and 22 percent, respectively, compared to the placebo. There were no serious side effects. Note that in my experience, saw palmetto usually takes six to twelve months to show an effect, so be patient!
>
> **Essential Oils:** A number of essential oils have been shown to promote hair growth. One study followed eighty-six people with alopecia areata who were randomized into two groups.[72] The essential-oils group massaged carrier oils (jojoba and grapeseed) infused with a mixture of thyme, rosemary, lavender, and cedarwood into their scalp daily. The control group massaged only the carrier oils. In the active group, 44 percent showed

significant improvement in hair growth compared to 15 percent of the control group. Other studies have found that rosemary oil alone is effective. In one trial, one hundred men with androgenic alopecia were treated with either rosemary essential oil or minoxidil.[73] After six months, both groups saw significant increases in hair count.

Laser Therapy

An exciting new treatment approach in medicine is the use of light therapy, or photo-biomodulation, which can promote anti-inflammatory effects.[74] These laser devices are available in hair salons or for home use as bonnets, helmets, or handheld combs. HairMax LaserComb is available to use at home for reversing thinning hair. A meta-analysis of laser hair loss devices found a significant increase in hair density,[75] with equal effectiveness found across the different types of devices and therapy duration.

Conventional Treatment for Hair Loss

For many years, the only sanctioned medicine for hair loss was minoxidil, which you may recognize under several different brand names. It is an over-the-counter treatment available in spray, liquid or foam formulations. Minoxidil is a vasodilator, meaning it expands blood vessels. When applied to the scalp, it can boost blood flow to hair follicles, providing them with more nutrients and oxygen, while extending the anagen phase of the hair cycle. The shampoo forms of minoxidil are effective, and usually come in strengths of 2 percent and 5 percent.

Minoxidil is also effective when taken orally in tiny doses.[76] In one study, 105 men and women with androgenic alopecia and telogen effluvium were given oral minoxidil at a dose of 0.6 to 2.5 mg.[77] After one year, 52 percent of the patients demonstrated clinical improvement and 43 percent demonstrated stabilization. This is a genuine breakthrough! One of my twenty-six-year-old patients, Cyndi, developed classic alopecia areata on her scalp when her parents went through a divorce. She was distraught about the oval bald patches, and while she could cover it up with careful blow-drying, she wanted to do all she could to heal. In addition to following my advice about lifestyle measures—including using a meditation app for relaxation, prioritizing eight hours of restful sleep, and eating a Mediterranean diet—Cyndi took oral minoxidil. She did well and within a couple of months had new hair growth. The dose is substantially lower than the 5 to 40 mg used for high blood pressure (the original indication for minoxidil) and is usually quite well tolerated. I usually begin with a dose of 0.25 mg for women and 0.5 mg for men.

Other oral prescription medications, some of which are available only privately, for hair loss include finasteride and spironolactone, both of which inhibit the 5-alpha-reductase enzyme and prevent conversion of testosterone to dihydrotestosterone. Your dermatologist may also inject an area on your scalp with steroids. Some newer biologic medications called *JAK inhibitors* usually prescribed by a dermatologist, are now approved for hair loss.[78] I see them as exciting especially for severe alopecia, but they must be used with great caution owing to potential side effects, including immune suppression and acne. While effective, hair loss resumes for most users when the medication is discontinued,[79] supporting the case for all the integrative strategies that activate your innate healing response.

Your Rapid Recovery Prescription for Supporting Healthy Skin and Hair

Everyone wants to feel good and confident in their own skin. The following integrative strategies for skin conditions and hair loss can help you look and feel yourself again:

Acne
1. Eat the rainbow by filling your plate with colorful fruits, vegetables, and a smaller amount of grains and proteins. Avoid dairy products and high-GI foods.
2. Use a cleanser with a pH between 5.5 and 7 to minimize bacteria and maximize skin health. Benzoyl peroxide can be used as well.

3. Mind–body techniques including hypnosis, meditation, and biofeedback can reduce overall stress levels, which affect sebum production in the skin.
4. Treat occasional breakouts with one or more of the following: tea tree oil, green tea, nicotinamide, *Lactobacillus plantarum* lotion, zinc, oral probiotics, and omega-3 fatty acids.
5. If you need additional treatment, speak with your doctor about the safest medications with the fewest side effects. This includes retinoids, spironolactone, and the prescribed supplement NicAzel, where available.

Dermatitis
1. Keep your skin hydrated with coconut oil or moisturizers like CeraVe, Aveeno, or Eucerin. Look on the ingredients list of products for oats, urea, ceramides, and hyaluronic acid. Avoid anything with fragrance and parabens.
2. Treat eczema breakouts with licorice gel and a black tea compress.
3. Stay away from harsh soaps and plastics. Avoid environmental irritants and allergens in skincare products and laundry detergents by scanning products with an app.
4. Taking probiotics can also help clear up eczema. I recommend products that contain *Lactobacillus plantarum*, *L. acidophilus*, or *L. rhamnoses*.
5. Low-dose corticosteroids (0.5 or 1 percent hydrocortisone) are available over the counter. Alternatively, ask your doctor for stronger prescribed topical steroids for occasional flare-ups.
6. If you need to use medication for a prolonged period, I recommend a trial of TCIs, which have few side effects.

Hair Loss
1. Avoid sugary beverages such as juice, energy drinks, and sweet teas. A Mediterranean-style diet can lower your risk of hair loss.
2. Should you notice excessive hair loss, request the following tests from your doctor: iron, total iron-binding capacity, ferritin, thyroid-stimulating hormone, and vitamin D. It is important to diagnose and

begin treating your scalp to address any issues before fatty infiltration or permanent scarring occurs. Women have long been underrepresented in clinical research.

3. Treat patchy hair loss or thinning hair with pumpkin seed oil, saw palmetto oil, essential oils, or with red-light therapy.
4. Topical minoxidil is effective and widely available in shampoo form.
5. Ask your doctor about medications for hair loss, such as oral minoxidil, finasteride, or spironolactone.

7

Preventing PMS and Upholding Urogenital Health

In 2022, researchers from Brigham and Women's Hospital in Boston, Massachusetts, released the results of a study analyzing more than 1,400 clinical trials involving three hundred thousand participants.[1] The conclusion affirmed what many had been pointing to for decades: Women are underrepresented in medical research. Despite constituting 50.8 percent of the U.S. population, women make up only 41.2 percent of trial participants. Fifty-one percent of people with cancer are female, yet they only make up 41 percent of cancer-trial participants. The figures are similar for heart disease: 49 percent and 41.9 percent, respectively. The discrepancies are even worse among mental-health trials: 60 percent of people with psychiatric disorders are female, but women constitute only 42 percent of participants in psychiatric drug trials.

Before U.S. Congress passed a law in 1993 mandating that women be included in clinical research, these statistics were far, far worse.[2] Researchers have long been flummoxed by the challenge of studying women, in part because fluctuating hormonal cycles could potentially impact the outcomes of a trial. Many researchers even avoid using female lab mice owing to concerns about hormones, as well as perceived greater costs.[3] For decades, the male body was simply treated as the "default" in medical research, leading to trials of male participants alone and findings that were generalized to women without evidence of equivalent efficacy or safety.[4] One serious result of this underrepresentation is that women experience adverse side effects from medication at twice the rate of men.[5]

Simply put, we have much to learn about women's bodies and we need a lot of research to catch up. While I am eager to help everyone recover faster, I felt it vital to devote three chapters of this book to women's health issues. (In the next chapter I will cover menopause, and in Part Three, I will discuss breast cancer and its surgery.)

Premenstrual syndrome

Arti, a twenty-seven-year-old woman, came to see me complaining of terrible premenstrual syndrome (PMS) symptoms, including cramping, breast tenderness, and mood swings. "It's now to the point where I don't go to work and I snarl at my family!" she exclaimed. Her doctor recommended she take antidepressants or birth control pills,[6] both of which can help mitigate symptoms, but Arti did not want to take medication for a condition that affected her only a few days per month. She remembered as a little girl how her grandmother would give her teas and herbs when she didn't feel well. "Aren't there any herbal medicines for PMS?" she asked me.

"Yes!" I said, letting her know about the research supporting chasteberry, saffron, and curcumin. I also suggested she take calcium, vitamin B6, and magnesium. She altered her diet by cutting down on animal products and limiting simple carbohydrates. When combined with 4-7-8 breathing (see "Your Rapid Recovery Toolkit," appendix 1) and daily thirty-minute walks, Arti was able to dramatically reduce her PMS symptoms, and for the first time in a long time, she felt in better control of her body.

Premenstrual syndrome refers to a group of physical and emotional symptoms that many women experience in the days or weeks leading up to their menstrual period, such as bloating, breast tenderness, headaches, fatigue, changes in appetite, cramps, mood swings, anxiety, depression, difficulty concentrating, and sleep trouble. PMS occurs during the luteal phase of the menstrual cycle, which is the time between ovulation and the onset of menstruation.

The exact cause of PMS is not known, but changes in neurotransmitter levels (which affect mood and behavioral symptoms) and tiny immune-modulating molecules called *prostaglandins* (which affect physical symptoms) play a major role.[7] Hormonal fluctuations during the menstrual cycle are also believed to have an impact,[8] as are genetics and nutritional deficiencies, particularly magnesium, calcium, and B vitamins. All told, as many as three in four women will experience PMS symptoms at some point in their reproductive life.[9]

Here are the integrative-medicine strategies I recommend for reducing PMS.

Supplements

As discussed earlier, micronutrient deficiencies may be a major contributor to PMS. Before proceeding to botanicals or medications, I advise seeing whether a three-month period of supplementation will correct these deficiencies, support your recovery reflex, and lead to either a significant improvement or complete resolution of symptoms. Here is where to start.

> **Calcium:** An essential mineral, calcium has a well-documented ability to stabilize mood and reduce irritability, depression, and anxiety symptoms associated with PMS. It is estimated that nearly half the world's population has inadequate access to dietary calcium.[10] One randomized trial treated nearly five hundred women with PMS with either 1,200 mg calcium carbonate per day or a placebo for three menstrual cycles.[11] The calcium group saw a 48 percent reduction of symptoms by the third month. A more recent randomized trial of sixty-four university students found that taking calcium supplements at a dose of 500 mg per day effectively reduced psychological and physical symptoms, including feeling anxious, depressed, water retention, breast tenderness, abdominal bloating, leg swelling, feeling cold, nausea, frequent urination, back pain, headaches, and muscle pain.[12] Side benefits of calcium supplementation include maximizing bone growth during adolescence and young adulthood, thereby reducing the risk of osteoporosis in the post-menopausal period. Additional potential side benefits include reducing the risk of high blood pressure, polycystic ovary syndrome (PCOS), multiple sclerosis, and breast cancer.[13] I recommend beginning with 500 mg of calcium citrate daily.

Vitamin B6: This vitamin plays an essential role in the synthesis of neurotransmitters such as serotonin and dopamine. When taken as a supplement, vitamin B6 has been found to reduce physical symptoms of PMS, including bloating and water retention, as well as alleviate mood swings and irritability.[14] I recommend a daily dose of 50 mg of vitamin B6, either alone or as part of a multivitamin-multimineral supplement.

Magnesium: Magnesium is an essential mineral involved in numerous physiological processes, particularly muscle relaxation and nerve function. Taking a magnesium supplement has been found to help relieve both the physical and psychological symptoms of PMS, especially cramping and irritability.[15] I recommend a dose of 400 mg daily and increasing to 600 mg as needed. Magnesium may be even more potent when combined with a vitamin B6 supplement.[16] Side benefits of magnesium include reduced constipation and improved sleep.

Zinc: Zinc is effective at relieving PMS symptoms, including cramps, breast tenderness, and depression. Notably, zinc levels are frequently lower in women with PMS.[17] One study randomly assigned sixty women with PMS aged eighteen to thirty to receive 30 mg of zinc gluconate or a placebo for twelve weeks.[18] The women who received zinc had significant improvement in physical and psychological symptoms. I recommend zinc gluconate at daily a dose of 25 to 30 mg.

Botanical Medicines

Botanical medicines, also known as herbal medicines, are therapeutic products derived from plants. The following can help with PMS symptoms:

Chasteberry: Known botanically as *Vitex agnus-castus*, chasteberry is a medicinal herb native to the Mediterranean region that has long been used to treat a variety of women's issues. Its popular name stems from folklore that it reduces sexual desire; monks during the Middle Ages planted it in their gardens and reportedly consumed it regularly.[19] While there is little science to support chasteberry's effect on libido, studies are much clearer about its usefulness for PMS. Chasteberry reduces levels of the hormone prolactin (which can be associated with PMS[20]), while it stimulates dopamine (a reward neurotransmitter) and opioid (painkilling) activity—all of which reduce PMS symptoms.[21] Studies show that chasteberry can reduce PMS symptoms by as much as 50 percent.[22] It is recommended for PMS by the German Commission E, a national scientific advisory board that evaluates the efficacy of herbal medicines. I recommend taking 40 mg every morning of dry chasteberry extract.[23] It can take a full three months to show an effect and is considered safe for long-term use.

Saffron: Saffron, a spice derived from the flower of *Crocus sativus*, can help alleviate mood swings, irritability, and depression associated with PMS. One study found that women aged eighteen to thirty-five who took saffron at a dose of 30 mg once per day had a significant reduction in fatigue, headaches, bloating, irritability, and depression compared to those who took a placebo.[24] Another study of 120 women compared saffron, the antidepressant fluoxetine, and placebo;[25] saffron was just as effective as fluoxetine, but had far fewer side effects. I recommend taking 15 mg twice daily during the luteal phase.

Curcumin: By reducing inflammation in the body, curcumin can help alleviate menstrual cramps, breast tenderness, and general discomfort.[26] Another way curcumin works is by altering levels of neurotransmitters, including serotonin, dopamine, and norepinephrine, exerting an antidepressant effect. One randomized trial showed that curcumin is effective at a dose of 100 mg taken twice daily for ten days, beginning a week before you expect your period and continuing for three days after it begins.[27] Side benefits of curcumin that support your recovery reflex include less metabolic syndrome, arthritis, anxiety, depression, and lower cholesterol;[28] it can also reduce muscle soreness after exercising.

Nutrition

You're not alone if you crave chocolate and other sweets before your period.[29] (Before the onset of your period, blood sugar levels can drop, sometimes leading to cravings.) However, sugary foods can increase inflammation in the body, which is correlated with PMS symptoms.[30] I recommend cutting back on chocolate and other sweets.

In addition to cutting out sugar, the American College of Obstetricians and Gynecologists also recommends increasing fiber-rich complex carbohydrates to improve PMS symptoms.[31] Fiber helps to regulate your body's hormones, especially estrogen, excess levels of which can contribute to PMS symptoms.[32] Fiber binds to estrogen in your gut and removes it through your bowel movements. In general, diets rich in fiber augment your recovery system, and as a side benefit, it will reduce constipation and contribute to a healthy microbiome!

I also recommend drinking raspberry leaf tea. Traditionally known as the "women's herb," raspberry leaf tea contains fragarine, a compound thought to help tone and relax the muscles of the uterus. This can reduce the menstrual cramps associated with PMS. The tea can also soothe the digestive system and reduce bloating and cramping. Raspberry leaf tea is yummy and can be consumed hot or iced. You can sweeten it modestly with 1 teaspoon of sugar or honey, if desired. I recommend drinking a cup daily for ninety days, then assessing its impact on your PMS symptoms.

Finally, recent studies have doubled down on the importance of avoiding alcohol if it worsens your PMS. One meta-analysis found that the risk for PMS was 45 percent higher among moderate drinkers and 79 percent higher among heavy drinkers (more than one drink per day).[33]

Medication

Taking medication can benefit women with significant PMS symptoms. The following meds can help.

> **Ibuprofen:** My thirty-two-year-old patient Hailey was suffering from terrible menstrual cramping after she stopped taking birth control pills. I recommended she use ibuprofen, which has been found to reduce PMS symptoms by inhibiting the production of prostaglandins.[34] She found that taking two tablets (200 mg each) at the first hint of cramping worked like a charm. (Hailey also found that the ibuprofen worked extremely well in conjunction with a heating pad over her low abdomen and pelvis.)

I also recommended a trial of calcium, magnesium, and vitamin B6 to help prevent those cramps in the first place.

Birth Control Pills: The first oral contraception was approved in the 1960s, an incredible advance that gave women control over their reproductive health for the first time in human history. Birth control pills are often chosen by young women not only for their ability to prevent unwanted pregnancy but also to regulate irregular cycles, reduce PMS, and clear up acne. These are all positive outcomes, and I believe that birth control pills can be a good choice for young women with more difficult to manage PMS. Yet, I have some concerns. In some women, birth control pills can cause weight gain, perhaps because the hormones in birth control pills are synthetic and not bioidentical. They may also increase the risk of depression and anxiety and lower libido. As women age pass thirty-five, the risk of blood clots rises (especially among women who smoke). A more subtle worry is that taking birth control pills can mask underlying health issues that deserve attention, such as PCOS or endometriosis, leading to a late discovery that may impair fertility.[35] (I write about this in my previous book, *Be Fruitful: The Essential Guide to Maximizing Fertility and Giving Birth to a Healthy Child*.)

SSRIs: Selective serotonin reuptake inhibitors (SSRIs) are a class of antidepressant medications that increase levels of serotonin (for more information, see the "Defeating Depression" chapter) and have been proven effective for women with severe PMS. Interestingly, research shows it may not be necessary to take an SSRI every day.[36] If you have stubborn emotional PMS symptoms, you may want to discuss with your doctor a daily dose of 10 to 20 mg of fluoxetine for ten to fourteen days, taken only during the luteal phase.

I don't want to minimize the pain and emotional distress that PMS can cause. At the same time, I want to acknowledge and suggest you explore the positive aspects of the cyclical nature that is the bedrock of all women of reproductive age. Throughout this book I write about our circadian clock, but other biological cycles are less well known; for instance, evidence supports circalunar rhythms as well.[37] The menstrual cycle's hormonal fluctuations are even thought to inspire creativity.[38] As women, we can choose to mindfully tune into our cycle, track mood and energy during different phases, and treat ourselves with kindness.

Urinary-Tract Infections

Urinary-tract infections (UTIs) are infections of the lower urinary system, which includes the bladder and urethra. Yes, men get UTIs too, and more so as they age, but UTIs are far more common in women; 12 percent of men will have one in their lifetime, compared to 50 to 60 percent of women.[39] Typical symptoms include pain or a burning sensation while urinating, feeling the urge to go to the toilet despite having little urine in the bladder, experiencing pressure or cramping in the lower abdomen, finding occasional blood in the urine, and in more than 80 percent of premenopausal women with UTIs, suffering dyspareunia (pain during intercourse).[40]

The likelihood of developing a UTI increases with age. Menopause leads to an abrupt decline in estrogen, which maintains the health of the urethra and vulvar tissues. (For more information about menopause, see the "Mastering Menopause" chapter.) As estrogen levels decrease, over time, urogenital tissues become thinner and drier, making them more susceptible to irritation and infection.

Drink Fluids

Drinking plenty of fluids supports your recovery reflex by flushing bacteria from the urinary tract. A well-hydrated urinary system creates a less favorable environment for bacteria, and frequent urination helps keep bacteria from adhering to the walls of the bladder and urethra. A study of 140 women with an average age of thirty-six and a history of recurrent UTIs revealed that drinking 1.5 liters (6+ glasses) of water a day dropped the likelihood of developing a UTI by 50 percent.[41] (This amount of water may not sound like much, but a study of more than sixteen thousand women and men across thirteen countries found that fewer than 50 percent of women get an adequate intake![42]) Being fully hydrated has side benefits, including better muscular performance, fewer headaches, and less constipation.[43]

The type of fluids you drink also matter. While water is best for flushing out bacteria and staying hydrated, cranberry juice is a potent adversary for UTIs.[44] Cranberries contains proanthocyanidins, which are compounds that naturally inhibit bacteria, particularly *E. coli,* from adhering to the walls of the bladder. (*E. coli* is the organism that most commonly leads to UTIs.) Cranberry juice has been proven in multiple studies to help prevent UTI recurrences among women who are prone to them.[45]

Probiotics

As discussed earlier in this book, probiotics are the healthy bacteria (and sometimes yeast) that support your gut microbiome.[46] It may seem odd that consuming more bacteria can help prevent bacterial infections such as recurrent UTIs, but probiotics, particularly *Lactobacillus,* produce compounds that inhibit the growth of pathogens.[47] *Lactobacilli* also produce lactic acid and hydrogen peroxide, creating an acidic environment that is less favorable for the growth of *E. coli.* Look for products that contain *L. rhamnosus* GR-1 and *L. reuteri* RC-14.[48] In a randomized trial, these two strains at an oral dose of 109 CFUs twice daily for one year was as effective at preventing UTI recurrence as daily ingestion of an antibiotic.[49] And as a side benefit, there was less antibiotic resistance in the women who took lactobacilli.

You can also add probiotic-rich foods to your diet. I recommend yogurt, kefir (a fermented milk drink rich in probiotics), kombucha, sauerkraut, kimchi, pickles, miso, and tempeh.

Estrogen Creams

My sixty-seven-year-old patient Sally was prescribed an antibiotic to take after sexual intercourse because of frequent UTIs. She was not happy about using antibiotics regularly, but she hated the sensation of burning and painful urination from the UTIs that followed lovemaking. When I examined her, I found a different reason for the infections: atrophy, or thinning of the tissues around the urethra. She achieved a full and rapid recovery of her vulvar tissue by spreading an estrogen cream around her urethra and inside her vagina for three months. Sally happily reported she no longer gets urinary infections when she makes love with her husband and she was able to discontinue the antibiotics altogether.

Topical estrogen creams are applied directly to the vulva and urethral area and they improve the health of these tissues by rejuvenating mucosal cells.[50] Typically, these creams are used for a condition called *vaginal atrophy*, which presents as vaginal dryness, itching, burning, and discomfort during sex. (It's an awful name, I know, and the new name, *genitourinary syndrome of menopause*, is not much better!)

Vaginal estrogen creams can prevent recurrent UTIs by restoring the thickness and elasticity to the vaginal lining.[51] Menopause isn't the only thing that lowers estrogen levels, though; breastfeeding can, too. I recommend a bioidentical estrogen cream, meaning its hormones are chemically identical to the ones your body produces. (You will need to ask your doctor for a prescription.)

What About Antibiotics?

Antibiotics are the primary treatment for UTIs, but we are increasingly aware of how they disrupt the microbiome and contribute to the development of antibiotic-resistant bacteria.[52] To minimize these outcomes, whenever possible, I recommend "narrow-spectrum antibiotics," which are active only against a select group of bacterial types;[53] oral nitrofurantoin for five days is the usual first choice. Fosfomycin is also used as an antibiotic for treating UTIs, but it is "broad spectrum," meaning it kills off a wide variety of bacteria, including beneficial kinds.[54] Your doctor can also order a urine culture to ascertain the sensitivity of the bacteria to various antibiotics.

Vaginitis

Vulvovaginitis, or vaginitis for short, can occur due to an infection (yeast, bacterial, or protozoan) or have a non-infectious cause such as irritation, allergy, dermatitis, or atrophic vaginitis.[55] Typical symptoms include redness, itching, swelling, and vaginal discharge. The healthy vagina has a microbiome dominated by *Lactobacillus* and contains traces of yeast and anaerobic bacteria. Most of the time your recovery reflex keeps this complex ecosystem in homeostasis, but sometimes unhealthy bacteria can overpower the healthy bacteria and lead to a condition called *bacterial vaginosis* (BV). Symptoms include a thin, grayish-white discharge with a fishy odor; itching; and burning during urination.

Healthy vaginas also contain a fungus genus called *Candida*. Normally, these fungi are part of the healthy microbiome of the vagina and don't cause any trouble; under certain circumstances (such as taking an antibiotic) they can multiply out of control, causing a yeast infection. Symptoms include itching and irritation in the vagina and vulva; a burning sensation while urinating or during sexual intercourse; and a white, odorless discharge with a cottage-cheese appearance. It is these two forms of vaginitis—yeast infections and BV—that I will focus on in this section.

Vaginitis may not get spoken about much, yet it is common: Three in four women will have a yeast infection and around 35 percent of women will get BV in their lifetime.[56] Here's how to quickly recover from both.

Yeast Infections

One major cause of yeast infections are antibiotics, which can kill off bacteria, leading to an overgrowth of yeast. Women with higher estrogen levels, pregnant women, or those on high-dose estrogen birth control pills are at an increased risk as well.[57]

Another major risk factor for vaginitis is douching, which is the practice of cleansing the vagina with vinegar, bicarbonate of (baking) soda, iodine, antiseptics, or other fragranced products. While rinsing the vulva (external genitalia) is important, the vagina is considered a "self-cleaning oven." I find the phrase funny and accurate! The cervix produces mucus, which traps and helps expel bacteria, dead cells, and other debris from the vaginal canal. The vagina also maintains a slightly acidic balance of flora, which inhibits the growth of yeast. The cleaning chemicals in douching products strip away these beneficial bacteria. They also compromise the protective mucus that acts as the vagina's first line of defense against infection.

Equally concerning, studies have shown links between douching and other adverse health outcomes, including pelvic inflammatory disease, cervical cancer, low birth weight, ectopic pregnancy, and increased risk of sexually transmitted infections.[58]

In addition to avoiding douching, I recommend forgoing products that contain perfumes, parabens, chlorhexidine, citric acid, and polyquaternium. It will come as no surprise that I strongly recommend against the recent vaginal steaming fad, sometimes called *yoni*, or V-steaming. Popularized by the actress Gwyneth Paltrow and her lifestyle brand Goop, vaginal steaming involves "cleaning" the vagina with hot water infused with various herbs. To put it simply, the vagina is not meant to be steam-cleaned! No credible studies have shown a benefit to steaming, while the dangers—from disrupting the natural pH balance to second-degree burns—are well documented.[59]

I recommend cleansing the external genital area with mild soap and water, or even better, products specifically manufactured to have a slightly acidic pH designed to support the vagina's naturally acidic environment. Please avoid using harsh soaps, scented products, or antiseptics on the vaginal area.

A diet rich in sugars and refined carbohydrates can also cause trouble, as *Candida* thrive on sugar; this also leads people with uncontrolled diabetes to be more susceptible to yeast infections.[60] Western diets high in fat and sugar, and low in vegetable fiber, alter the gut microbiota, leading to an imbalance of microbes—sometimes called *dysbiosis*—and an overgrowth of *Candida*. Following a *"Candida* diet" may be helpful. While it has not been scientifically studied yet, this diet has been around for decades, and many women swear by its effectiveness. Here are the basics:

- Consume lean proteins; nonstarchy vegetables (avoid potatoes and enjoy rocket/arugula, courgettes/zucchini, broccoli, and cauliflower); and a limited amount of complex carbohydrates (such as quinoa and brown rice) and fat (think avocados).
- Avoid all refined carbohydrates, including added sugars, corn syrup, dextrose, and fructose, as well as any refined or processed foods.

- Avoid starchy vegetables such as potatoes, corn, and peas.
- Avoid beans.
- Avoid fruit and milk for three full weeks. Attempt to add them back into your diet after that interval and see if they trigger any recurrent symptoms.
- Avoid all yeast and mold-containing foods for three weeks or longer. (Yeast-containing foods are not the same as *Candida*. However, it's important to avoid them because they may spur the growth of *Candida*.)

The *Candida* diet is a healthy one rich in vegetable fiber, omega-3 polyunsaturated fatty acids, and vitamins D and E. It also contains many micronutrients that improve microbiome diversity and short-chain fatty-acid production, while reducing fungal species in the gut.[61] Other foods shown to have antifungal properties include garlic, cinnamon, lemongrass, coconut oil, ginger, seaweed, thyme, olive oil, fermented vegetables, apple cider vinegar, and yogurt.[62]

If you come down with a yeast infection, rest assured they are usually quite treatable at home with antifungal medications, which work by destroying the membranes of fungal cells.[63] There are many creams, ointments, and pessaries are depending on local availability, such as Miconazole, Clotrimazole, and Ticonazole. There are also stronger antifungal medications available by prescription as vaginal or oral medications. Miconazole is effective 80 to 90 percent of the time when used for the specified duration (usually one to seven days, depending on the product).[64]

For a single yeast infection, such as one triggered by an antibiotic or a wet bathing suit, it is perfectly reasonable to use an over-the-counter antifungal product. Around 6 percent of women will develop recurrent yeast infections,[65] which is defined as four or more vaginal infections per year. Worldwide, this is estimated to affect some 370 million women over their lifetime,[66] leading to considerable suffering. The following are integrative strategies that can dramatically help to reduce recurrences.

Probiotics: I recommend that you take *Lactobacillus*, as it supports your recovery reflex by producing lactic acid and hydrogen peroxide, which respectively acidify the vagina and have antibacterial properties. As a side benefit, it also helps prevent UTIs by adhering to the epithelium, making it harder for *E. coli* to attach to the bladder wall.[67] Probiotics are especially useful when treating recurrent yeast infections. Note that they can take two to six months to fully recolonize the healthy bacteria in your vagina.[68] I recommend a dose of eight billion CFU of *Lactobacilli* daily.

Boric Acid: Boric acid is a compound with antifungal and antiseptic properties that can be used to treat yeast infections, as well as bacterial vaginosis (see later). It works by directly killing *Candida* cells and helping to maintain the vagina's acidity.[69] Boric acid is available over the counter in some products in the form of vaginal capsules or pessaries. The typical dosage is a pessary once daily for seven days. A meta-analysis reviewing women with recurrent vulvovaginal candidiasis found that using boric acid resulted in a cure rate of 40 to 100 percent.[70]

Zinc: Research suggests that zinc can prevent recurrent *Candida* vaginitis.[71] If you have recurrent yeast infections, I recommend using a zinc-containing hydrogel nightly for two weeks, and then twice per week ongoing.

Bacterial Vaginosis

My patient Gena had frequent bouts of bacterial vaginosis (BV). She could not pinpoint what caused them, but they made sexual intercourse with her husband painful. Most of the triggers seemed random, although she noticed episodes after wearing a wet bathing suit and a stressful cross-country trip for a friend's law school graduation. Hoping to avoid antibiotics, I offered Gena an alternative—boric acid vaginal pessaries—which effectively treated the infection. She used them nightly and her discharge resolved. With regular courses of probiotics and a gentle vulvar wash, both of which support homeostasis, Gena was finally able to prevent relapses.

Unlike yeast infections, which are caused by the overgrowth of yeast, BV is caused by an overgrowth of harmful bacteria (vaginal dysbiosis) that overpowers the healthy acid-producing bacteria, primarily *Lactobacillus*. As the volume of healthy bacteria decreases, the vagina becomes less acidic, making it easier for harmful bacteria to proliferate. Symptoms include pain, irritation, discharge, odor, and itching. Risk factors include having multiple sex partners or a new sex partner, having unprotected sex, and as with yeast infections, douching.[72]

Your doctor will test for BV by performing a pelvic exam and then examining a swab sample under a microscope for "clue cells," which are vaginal epithelial cells covered with bacteria; these are considered a key indicator of BV. If you have BV, you will usually be prescribed an antibiotic, such as metronidazole or clindamycin, which can be administered orally or as a vaginal cream or gel. (I recommend vaginal antibiotics, as they are less likely to disrupt your gut microbiome.)

A course of antibiotics will usually clear the BV symptoms in a week, but there is a 50 percent risk of BV reoccurrence within twelve months.[73] Activate your recovery reflex to ward off another infection by supporting your vaginal microbiome. I recommend newer vulvar-cleansing products that can help moisturize dry tissue, restore healthy pH levels, and deliver beneficial *Lactobacillus* to prevent bacterial overgrowth. One clinical trial showed that women using one such product had reduced frequency of pain, itching, and irritation, and had zero recurrences of BV over a twelve-month period.[74] Another botanical vulvar product is made of burdock (*Arctium majus*), chamomile (*Chamomilla recutita*), and aloe (*Aloe barbadensis*). A study comprising 137 women found that when it was used either alone or with antibiotics, it resulted in significant improvements in redness, itching, and vaginal discharge.[75]

Probiotics can also help prevent recurrence of BV. A trial of 544 women revealed that those taking oral probiotics containing *Lactobacillus rhamnosus* GR-1 and *Lactobacillus reuteri* RC-14 for six weeks had a roughly 62 percent restoration of the normal vaginal microbiome compared to about 27 percent for the placebo.[76] Another meta-analysis involving about two thousand participants found that adding a probiotic to an antibiotic regimen led to a 73 percent cure rate of BV.[77] I recommend visiting the free resource at www.probioticguide.uk for help in choosing which brand to buy; there is an entire section on vaginal health that details the evidence for various products.

Boric acid pessaries also have been shown to prevent recurrence of BV.[78] In one study, 105 women with extremely challenging recurrent BV used a combination regimen of oral nitroimidazole (500 mg twice daily for seven days) simultaneously with vaginal boric acid (600 mg daily for thirty days), followed by a vaginal metronidazole gel (the same antibiotic in vaginal form) twice a week for five months. Six months after this treatment, 69 percent of the participants were cured.

Your Rapid Recovery Prescription for Preventing PMS and Upholding Urogenital Health

Science has a lot of catching up to do when it comes to understanding women's bodies, so I am pleased to provide you with strategies to address PMS, UTIs, and vaginitis. Here is how you can activate your rapid recovery reflex to resolve these health challenges and prevent recurrences.

For PMS
1. Reduce sugar intake, eat more fiber-rich complex carbohydrates, drink raspberry leaf tea, and avoid alcohol.
2. The following supplements can significantly improve or fully resolve symptoms of PMS: calcium, B vitamins, magnesium, and zinc.
3. Botanical medicines that have been proven to reduce the severity of PMS include chasteberry, saffron, and curcumin.
4. If you have significant PMS symptoms, taking ibuprofen for symptom control or SSRIs in the luteal phase of your cycle can help.

For UTIs
1. Drink at least of 1.5 liters (6+ glasses) of water per day.
2. Take a *Lactobacillus* probiotic supplement or add probiotic-rich foods to your diet, such as yogurt, kefir, kombucha, sauerkraut, kimchi, miso, and tempeh.

3. For women with atrophic changes to their urogenital tissues, topical estrogen creams applied to the vulva can resolve thinning of tissue and reduce UTI recurrences.
4. For UTIs that require antibiotics, ask your doctor to treat you with a narrow-spectrum antibiotic to reduce disruption of the microbiome.

For Vaginitis
1. Treat yeast infections by using over-the-counter antifungal creams.
2. Avoid douching to prevent recurrences. Cleanse the vulva with mild soap and water or a specialty product.
3. Consider a trial of the *Candida* diet.
4. For recurrent yeast infections, use probiotics, boric acid, and zinc.
5. Treat BV with boric acid or antibiotics, ideally using a vaginal cream or gel.
6. You can reduce the risk of BV recurrences by using a specialty intimate moisturizing product, taking probiotics and boric-acid supplements, not douching, and avoiding products that contain perfumes, parabens, chlorhexidine, citric acid, and polyquaternium.

8

Mastering Menopause

Several years ago, a fifty-two-year-old woman named Catherine came to see me about severe sleep disturbances. Although she'd had mild—and in her mind, insignificant—sleep problems for a few years, in the weeks before she saw me, she'd suddenly started experiencing intense night sweats and hot flushes. They had progressed to the point she was barely getting five hours of sleep each night. Her work as a high-powered CEO was suffering. She needed a solution—fast.

Catherine's symptoms, as you probably guessed, were due to menopause, a normal life passage that marks the end of a woman's menstrual cycle. Curiously, menopause is defined in hindsight after a woman has not had a period for a full year. While the average age of menopause onset is fifty-one, there is a significant range among women, typically between forty-five and fifty-five.[1] The transition into menopause, known as perimenopause, lasts around seven years on average, but can be significantly shorter or longer. While it is neither a disease nor a disorder, menopause causes some women to experience symptoms that can be quite severe and debilitating.

The hot flushes and night sweats that Catherine experienced, also known as *vasomotor symptoms*, are common, as are mood swings, vaginal dryness, and cognitive issues. Hot flushes are often accompanied by sweating, heart palpitations, dizziness, fatigue, and anxiety, and they can last anywhere from thirty seconds to five minutes. When they happen at night, they disrupt sleep. They can be intrusive and greatly impact work and relationships. The overall result is to make women feel depleted—even those who are intricately aware of the workings of their bodies. A survey of female doctors by the British Medical Association found that "a significant number have reduced their hours, left management roles or intend to leave medicine altogether, despite enjoying their careers, because of the difficulties they faced when going through menopause."[2] I find the results of this survey—that professional women at the height of their success are stalled or derailed by these treatable symptoms—incredibly disturbing.

For Catherine, reducing her hours and lightening her workload were simply not options. After discussing various strategies, we decided the best course forward was a treatment called *hormone replacement therapy* (HRT). I prescribed an estradiol patch together with oral micronized progesterone. (I'll talk more about treatments options later in this chapter.) Within a week, her hot flushes subsided, the night sweats dissipated, and her sleep returned to normal. Five weeks later she exclaimed, "You saved my life!" I hadn't, but hormone therapy had; I was simply the doctor writing the prescription.

The resolution for Catherine's symptoms—hormonal medication—might sound surprising in a book about integrative medicine. While it's true I often emphasize nonpharmaceutical interventions, a hallmark of integrative medicine is tailoring treatments to the individual, and modern HRT can be customized based on a woman's symptoms, preferences, and risk factors. As we'll see in this chapter, HRT is often a wise and safe strategy for women who have menopausal symptoms, as well as to prevent several common health challenges. Nevertheless, HRT is not for everyone, so I will also explore how dietary supplements, acupuncture, diet, and avoiding environmental triggers can provide symptom relief.

Hormone Replacement Therapy

During the menopausal transition, the ovaries decrease production of sex hormones, including estrogen and progesterone. One function of estrogen is to act like a thermostat in the brain's thermoregulatory region. When estrogen levels drop, this thermostat becomes more sensitive to changes in body temperature.[3] If the body gets even slightly warmer, the brain thinks it's overheating, triggering hot flushes and sweating. HRT replaces estrogen and progesterone, thereby relieving symptoms of hot flushes, night sweats, and vaginal dryness. It also reduces the risk of osteoporosis (a disease that causes bones to become weaker), colon cancer, and potentially heart disease, and restores women's sense of well-being.

There are many misconceptions about HRT, especially about its long-term risks. When I was beginning my practice in the late 1980s, it was common to prescribe HRT preventively to every woman going through menopause. Research showed it could protect against osteoporosis and was associated with a reduced risk of heart disease. Bestselling books framed menopause as a "hormone deficiency disease, curable and totally preventable"[4] by taking estrogen. No woman, it seemed, had to experience uncomfortable menopause symptoms ever again. There was just one problem: Only a few randomized controlled trials had compared the benefits of HRT with its potential long-term risks.

This all changed in the early 2000s, when researchers began publishing data from the Women's Health Initiative (WHI), a major research program established by the U.S. National Institutes of Health to prevent disease in post-menopausal women. The WHI enrolled about twenty-seven thousand post-menopausal women aged fifty to seventy-nine to assess the effects of HRT on preventing heart disease, fractures, and colorectal cancer, as well as to investigate its effect on risk of breast cancer and embolisms. The trial was halted early when it was found that the women who were prescribed a combination of equine (horse) estrogen and a synthetic version of progesterone had an increased risk of breast cancer, heart attacks, strokes, and blood clots. (Mostly ignored in the negative news reports was that HRT also resulted in a reduced risk of colorectal cancer and fractures.) Meanwhile, women who had undergone a hysterectomy were prescribed estrogen alone; their trial was also halted early owing to an increased risk of strokes and blood clots. (This trial also revealed a reduced risk of fracture.[5])

When the findings from the WHI were made public, women discontinued HRT en masse, and doctors almost immediately stopped prescribing it, even for women who had terrible menopausal symptoms. One study showed the use of systemic hormone replacement therapy plummeted by as much as

80 percent.[6] The risk of cancer and stroke, it seemed, was too significant. As an integrative doctor, I was constantly fielding calls from women whose hot flushes, night sweats, and sleep problems had returned with a vengeance because they had quit HRT cold turkey.

Today, our understanding of HRT has evolved significantly. It now seems that women who start HRT shortly after experiencing menopause symptoms in fact have a *lower* risk of death compared to those who do not begin HRT. Why the about-face? One major shortcoming of the WHI has been labeled the "timing hypothesis." The average age of participants was sixty-three, and almost a fourth of the women enrolled were in their seventies. While this made logical sense at the time—the researchers wanted to see if HRT prevented heart disease, which most often occurs at a more advanced age—women usually start taking HRT in their late forties and fifties, when menopausal symptoms begin. Subsequent analyses have found that starting HRT close to the onset of menopause symptoms *does not carry the same cardiovascular risk*. In fact, an eighteen-year follow-up study of the participants in the WHI found that HRT use (either estrogen-only or estrogen-plus-progestin) for five to seven years during the menopause transition "was not associated with risk of all-cause, cardiovascular, or cancer mortality."[7] All in all, the research found that women who started HRT in early menopause actually tended to live longer than women who did not take hormones. Another pooled statistical analysis of thirty subsequent randomized controlled trials found that women who began HRT before age sixty had a 39 percent reduced risk of death compared to women who did not take HRT.[8]

It appears that the health effects of estrogen replacement differ depending on how quickly a woman begins HRT after the onset of menopausal symptoms. For instance, animal studies have shown that when estrogen is given immediately following surgical removal of the ovaries—which triggers the immediate onset of menopause—it produces anti-inflammatory and heart-protective effects.[9] However, if estrogen is given only after a long delay, these beneficial effects do not appear. In other words, for effective heart protection, it is best to begin HRT at the onset of menopausal symptoms.

Preliminary evidence indicates that acting during this critical window of time may also benefit the brain. In its 2022 position statement, the North American Menopause Society concluded that HRT may be beneficial to cognition in women if initiated within five years of the last menstrual period or immediately after hysterectomy with oophorectomy (removal of ovaries).[10] On the other hand, the data are mixed about the benefits and harms of HRT to memory and cognition when initiated in women aged sixty-five or older.

HRT also plays a crucial role in maintaining bone density by regulating a process called *remodeling*,[11] wherein old bone is removed and replaced by new bone. When you produce less estrogen, the body begins breaking down bone faster than it can build new bone, leading to a reduction in bone density. (For more information about bone health, see the "Building Stronger Bones" chapter.) Because HRT increases the estrogen levels in the body, it considerably reduces the risk of osteoporosis.[12] This alone can be a reason to consider HRT. For instance, when I entered menopause, my symptoms were generally mild and manageable. But because of a history of osteoporosis among the women in my family and heart disease in my father, I began HRT immediately.

Today, HRT is considered an excellent option for symptom management for many women—with certain caveats. Here are the general criteria that might make you a good candidate:

1. **You have bothersome menopausal symptoms:** These may include hot flushes, night sweats, sleep disturbances, mood swings, cognitive changes, vaginal dryness, or discomfort during intercourse.
2. **You recently entered perimenopause:** HRT is most effective, and the long-term risks are lowest, when you initiate it soon after symptoms begin. Studies also show that women who enter menopause early (before age forty) due to surgery (hysterectomy with oophorectomy) or premature ovarian failure are also good candidates for HRT, at least until they reach the natural age of menopause (early fifties).[13]
3. **You have a higher risk of osteoporosis:** HRT replaces estrogen, which regulates bone density and can substantially lower the risk of osteoporosis later in life.
4. **You have an absence of contraindications:** Women with a personal or

family history of hormonally driven cancers (breast, ovarian, or endometrial); a history of stroke or deep-vein thrombosis; liver disease; or heart disease are not good candidates for HRT.

The Benefits of Bioidentical Hormone Therapy

Should you decide to begin hormone replacement therapy, I highly recommend bioidentical estrogen and progesterone to my patients. Bioidentical hormones are customized to have the exact same molecular structure as the hormones are customized to naturally produced by your body. I always prescribe bioidentical hormones, and I recommend that you request them from a reputable private clinic or specialist pharmacy. In the U.K., bioidentical hormones, in oral, transdermal or vaginal form, are available on the NHS. Of note, there is some confusion about product terminology and origin; the NHS prefers that bioidentical hormones are obtained from regulated pharmaceutical companies rather than purchasing compounded bioidentical hormones.

There are numerous delivery mechanisms for HRT, each with a different application and different considerations. Here are the most common ones, along with my recommendations:

- **Oral:** In this form of HRT, estrogen or combined estrogen-progestin pills (progestin is a synthetic version of progesterone) are taken daily. I do not recommend oral estrogen because it requires larger doses, has to be metabolized in your liver (which comes with an unintended side effect of creating unhealthy lipids), and increases the risk of blood clots and pulmonary embolism.[14] It's also important to note that the troubling WHI findings were associated with oral, non-bioidentical HRT. But I do recommend and prescribe oral micronized progesterone, a bioidentical form with a better safety profile than synthetic progestins.[15] *Micronized* means that the drug particles are reduced to a tiny size (microns), making them much easier to absorb into the body.

- **Transdermal:** Transdermal HRT is administered via adhesive patches placed on the skin, usually on the lower abdomen or buttocks, which release estrogen (and sometimes progesterone) steadily into the bloodstream. Transdermal HRT generally requires just one-twentieth the dose of oral HRT. The negative impacts on blood pressure, lipids, or blood clotting are also considerably lower than for oral HRT. For these reasons, it is my preferred delivery mechanism, and I recommend it to most of the women I see. (I do not prescribe the combined patches with estrogen and progesterone, as they contain a synthetic progesterone.)
- **Vaginal:** When my fifty-five-year-old patient Stacey began menopause, she avoided hormone replacement therapy because of her family history of breast cancer. But she hesitated when I asked whether she'd had any sexual problems in the past twelve months, such as lack of interest, pain, dryness, or difficulty with orgasm. Then she tearfully described that she was having increasing issues with vaginal dryness and pain during intercourse. Married for almost thirty years, she and her husband had always had a satisfying sexual relationship. A four-week course of vaginal estrogen put an end to her symptoms and brought back her love life. Vaginal estrogen is a localized treatment designed primarily to address vaginal and urinary symptoms of menopause, including painful intercourse, dryness, burning, and frequent urinary-tract infections. It is unlikely to have systemic effects and is a good option if you don't suffer from more general menopausal symptoms, such as sleep disturbances, hot flushes, night sweats, or mood changes. If your doctor does not ask about your sex life, be brave and bring it up yourself. Many effective strategies can address the range of sexual issues for women and men. Products containing vaginal estrogen require a prescription and come as a cream, ring, or as tablets inserted into the vagina. (For more information, see page 371.)
- **Pellets:** Available in the U.S., these are tiny implants, usually injected every three to four months into muscles in the buttocks, that release estrogen steadily over several months.[16] Pellets are less commonly used than other methods. While they are effective, I do not recommend pellets to my patients because they require a small procedure,

initially release high levels of hormones, and cannot easily be removed in the event of complications.

Note that unless you've had a hysterectomy, you should expect to be prescribed the hormone progesterone alongside estrogen as part of your HRT regimen. This is because estrogen stimulates growth of the uterine lining, called the *endometrium*. Before menopause, this thickening prepares a woman's body for a potential pregnancy; if pregnancy does not occur, the lining is discarded in the form of a menstrual period. Unopposed estrogen—that is, HRT that uses estrogen without progesterone—taken during menopause can lead to endometrial overgrowth,[17] increasing the risk of endometrial cancer. Taking progesterone counterbalances estrogen's effects, causing the uterine lining to shed just like it would with a period. (Later in life you will likely be prescribed continuous progesterone, which will suppress the build-up and shedding of the uterine lining.) If you have had a hysterectomy, you will not need to take progesterone, as you no longer have an endometrium.

Finally, you might be wondering how long you should be on HRT. At this time, there is no simple answer to this question. The duration of HRT is individualized based on your symptoms and risk factors. Generally speaking, I recommend HRT at the lowest effective dose needed to relieve menopausal symptoms for as long as they last. The duration and intensity of symptoms in women varies from no symptoms at all—when I ask these women about the date of their last period, they sometimes give me a blank stare and then marvel that they haven't noticed its absence!—to truly difficult and lasting ten years or longer.[18]

Most studies show that the risk of breast cancer increases after five years of HRT,[19] but some show an increase after as little as one year.[20] This can feel scary and may lead you to avoid HRT completely. However, it is important to put the risk into context with the severity of your symptoms right now and the potential long-term health benefits of HRT. While women understandably fear breast cancer—which over a lifetime occurs in one in eight women[21]—the most common cause of death in women is heart disease, which we now understand is lessened by HRT. There is even evidence that both estrogen-alone and estrogen-plus-progesterone HRT reduce the risk of another serious condition, diabetes (by 26 percent when estrogen is taken alone and by 11 percent when taken together with progesterone).[22]

I and many other doctors often contemplate whether there is a dose of bioidentical HRT that, if prescribed at menopause, would protect women's bones and heart, relieve menopausal symptoms, but not increase the risk of breast cancer. Unfortunately, finding out would require a study on the scale of the WHI, which could cost in the range of $250 million to carry out. It's unlikely to happen anytime soon. Until such research is available, I recommend periodically discussing with your doctor what your lowest effective dose would be. As your symptoms improve, you can re-evaluate the benefits and risks of continuing HRT and when it is appropriate to taper or stop.

Supplements

While HRT is the most effective method for addressing symptoms of menopause, it is certainly not the only option. If you have a personal or family history of hormonally driven cancers (breast, ovarian, or endometrial), liver disease, stroke, deep-vein thrombosis, or heart disease, then HRT may not be a good option. Additionally, if your symptoms are generally mild, or if you simply prefer to approach menopause without pharmaceutical medications, there are a host of treatment options that can help. Supplements are an option but they are regulated as food so the requirements are less stringent compared to medications, which can makes choosing products more challenging. (See "How to Choose a Supplement," appendix 2, for tips choosing high-quality products.) Here are my favorite supplements.

> **Black Cohosh:** My patient Sandra had bothersome hot flushes. Her night sweats were so bad she sometimes required a change of pajamas, and she often had to remake her bed in the middle of the night after soaking her bedsheets. This was wreaking havoc on her career and her sleep, and therefore on her well-being. She did not want to use hormone replacement therapy, so I recommended a botanical called *black cohosh*. A perennial plant native to North America, black cohosh (*Actaea racemosa*) has long been used

by Native Americans for many ailments, including menstrual cramps, childbirth, and menopausal symptoms.[23] Why does it work? Research points to phytochemicals in black cohosh that impact the temperature regulation centers in the brain, thereby reducing hot flushes.[24] It has been studied in women with breast cancer taking the drug tamoxifen (which can worsen hot flushes), and was found to be safe and effective.[25] In my own practice, I've seen black cohosh help patients with night sweats and sleep disturbances. It's my first choice of botanical for menopausal symptoms; I recommend 40 to 160 mg per day, taken in two divided doses. Sandra took 80 mg twice a day and found that her hot flushes resolved completely. Her restful sleep was restored, and she felt "like herself" again!

St. John's Wort: Known by the scientific name *Hypericum perforatum*, St. John's wort is a plant that has been used for centuries in herbal medicine to treat melancholia and pain. When it comes to menopause, St. John's wort is particularly lauded for its mood-regulating properties,[26] but randomized control trials have shown it can also help reduce hot flushes.[27] St. John's wort can be taken alone, but studies indicate it may be particularly effective when combined with black cohosh.[28] The usual dose is 300 mg three times a day (of a 0.3 percent hypericin product). It's important to note that St. John's wort revs up the metabolism of drugs by the liver and can interact with many medications, so be sure to consult with your doctor or pharmacist before beginning if you are taking any prescription medications.

Valerian: Valerian can be useful for easing a variety of menopause symptoms. For instance, one randomized placebo-controlled trial concluded that "Valerian improves the quality of sleep in women with menopause who are experiencing insomnia."[29] Other controlled trials have seen success treating hot flushes with valerian, whose phytoestrogenic (plant estrogen) components appear to mimic the effects of estrogen in the body.[30] I recommend buying the capsules rather than an extract or tea, as valerian has a strong and, to most people, unappealing odor. You can take valerian just at bedtime if sleep is your main concern but I often recommend taking up to 250 to 300 mg three times a day to help manage hot flushes and anxiety symptoms.

Hops: While hops (*Humulus lupulus*) are famous for their role in brewing beer, they also have phytoestrogenic (plant estrogen) properties that may reduce symptoms of hot flushes, sleep disturbances, and mood swings.[31] Randomized controlled trials indicate that hops can effectively reduce early menopausal symptoms,[32] but you're likely to see results only with dietary supplements, not pilsner—sorry, beer lovers! To match the results seen in the studies,[33] I recommend taking a standardized extract in capsule form once per day. (Look for a phrase such as: "100 mcg of 8-prenylnaringenin per 300 mg dose" on product labels.)

> ### Traditional Chinese Medicine and Menopause
>
> Getting stuck with needles might seem like a surprising way to manage hot flushes and night sweats, but many randomized controlled trials have shown that acupuncture is effective. For instance, a 2015 meta-analysis concluded that acupuncture treatments could improve the frequency and severity of menopause symptoms with effects lasting up to three months.[34]
>
> While the exact physiological mechanism of acupuncture is debated, many Western scientists believe it modulates hot flushes through its effect on endorphins, which affect the thermoregulatory center in the brain.[35] One randomized controlled trial found acupuncture to be as effective as the antidepressant medication Effexor, which is sometimes prescribed to treat hot flushes, in women with hormone receptor positive breast cancer.[36] In addition to acupuncture, Chinese herbal medicine can be used to treat menopausal symptoms. It is best to consult a knowledgeable herbalist to select the best remedy from the large number of herbs and mixtures available.

Exercise

Maintaining an exercise routine is valuable for decreasing some menopause symptoms—namely, anxiety, weight gain, altered sleep, an increased risk of heart disease, and bone loss—in the short and long term.

As discussed earlier, the decrease in estrogen production associated with menopause can lead to an increased risk of osteoporosis, so you'll want to do exercises for bone health. (For more information about the best exercises for bone health, see the "Building Stronger Bones" chapter.) After menopause, women also face an increased risk of cardiovascular disease.[37] Regular aerobic exercise, such as cycling, swimming, or brisk walking for thirty minutes on most days of the week, can help improve heart health, reduce blood pressure, and maintain healthy cholesterol levels. Here's more reason to exercise: Hormonal changes during menopause can cause weight gain,[38] particularly a redistribution of fat from the buttocks and thighs to the abdomen,[39] which is another risk factor for cardiovascular disease. (Note that HRT may help prevent this weight gain.) Regular exercise boosts metabolism and will help you maintain a healthy body weight.

While exercise has been proven to reduce your long-term risk of osteoporosis and cardiovascular disease, does it mitigate other symptoms of menopause? Exercise has not been shown to help hot flushes or night sweats, but many studies do show a huge benefit for mental health, sleep, and overall well-being. For instance, in one clinical trial, researchers investigated the efficacy of a twelve-week training program—including walking, stretching, and resistance band workouts—on quality of life for menopausal women between the ages of forty and sixty-five. The results: Exercise was highly correlated with improved vitality and mental health.[40]

Diet

Can the food we eat have a direct effect on symptoms of menopause? Yes! A study of more than six thousand women revealed that both the Mediterranean diet and a high-fruit diet were associated with 20 percent fewer vasomotor symptoms compared to a dietary pattern with high sugar and fat, which was associated with increased hot flushes and night sweats.[41] For more information about the Mediterranean diet, see "Your Rapid Recovery Toolkit," appendix 1.

I also recommend eating soy foods, which contain compounds called *isoflavones*, a type of phytoestrogen that has a structure similar to human estrogen. A twelve-week study from 2021 demonstrated that eating a diet rich in soy foods can reduce severe hot flushes.[42] The study, sponsored by the Physicians Committee for Responsible Medicine and known as the Women's Study for the Alleviation of Vasomotor Symptoms (WAVS) trial, assigned women reporting two or more hot flushes daily to one of two groups: an intervention group that incorporated a low-fat, plant-based diet including 90 grams (3 oz) of cooked soybeans daily, and a control group that made no dietary changes. The conclusion: "Total hot flushes decreased by 79 percent and moderate-to-severe hot flushes decreased by 84 percent in the intervention group. At the study's conclusion, 59 percent of intervention-group participants reported becoming free of moderate and severe hot flushes. There was no change . . . in the control group."[43]

When you are adding soy foods to your diet, I highly recommend products that are minimally processed, such as edamame, tofu, tempeh, soy milk, and miso; avoid soy-based imitation meats and ultraprocessed soy cheeses. I also recommend choosing organic or non-GMO (genetically modified organism) varieties. Organic products are not allowed to be sprayed with the herbicide glyphosate, which was declared "probably carcinogenic to humans" by the International Agency for Research on Cancer.[44]

How about foods to avoid when it comes to menopause symptoms? Spicy foods, highly processed foods, caffeine, and alcohol have been found to trigger hot flushes in some women.[45] Data from a large online nutrition study known as the ZOE trial concluded, "Eating a healthy, varied diet, rich in fiber, complex carbohydrates, healthy fats, and healthy proteins—and saving sweets and desserts for an occasional treat—may therefore lessen the impact of these effects of menopause on women's bodies."[46]

Environmental Triggers

Vivian was only forty-three when she came to see me after experiencing extremely uncomfortable symptoms that included hot flushes, heavy bleeding, and swollen nodules (erythema nodosum) on the front of her shins. She is frequent public speaker, and her symptoms were not only making her miserable physically but they were also affecting her confidence onstage. After taking a full history (including her diet) and ordering lab tests and a pelvic ultrasound, I asked her to make a list of products she used daily, such as household cleaners, laundry detergents, shampoo, conditioner, soap, plastic containers—anything she touched or ate with.

I explained to her that environmental factors can play a big role in the severity of menopausal symptoms. Sometimes the trigger can be obvious, such as smoking, which is strongly linked to hot flushes and night sweats.[47] But even innocuous-seeming items we use every day can cause issues. Here is what I recommend investigating:

- **Environmental chemicals:** Minimize exposure to plastics, phthalates (common chemicals in personal-care products such as soaps, shampoo, and hair spray, as well as in flooring and plastic tubing), pesticides, DDE (a breakdown product of the pesticide DDT), furans (a byproduct created when trash is burned or pesticides manufactured),[48] PCBs (polychlorinated biphenyls often used as an insulator),[49] and β-hexachlorocyclohexane (an insecticide).[50] These may contain xenoestrogens, which have a molecular structure similar to estrogen. By binding to estrogen receptors, xenoestrogens can disrupt the normal functioning of the endocrine system, leading to a hormone imbalance and potentially causing menopausal symptoms.[51] If "fragrance" is on the label of a product, it likely contains phthalates. Pure essential oils are unlikely to contain phthalates, making them a better fragrance choice, although they are not completely free of risk for allergic reactions, irritation, or other issues. (Note that companies are not required to disclose the ingredients contained in fragrances.)
- **Temperature:** Hot environments or sudden temperature swings can trigger hot flushes. I recommend keeping your bedroom between 15.5°C and 20°C (60–68°F) for the best night's sleep.[52] Experiment in this range to find the ideal temperature for you. Wearing breathable clothing while sleeping can also be helpful.
- **Stress:** Chronic anxiety or sudden stressful events can exacerbate mood swings, irritability, insomnia, and even hot flushes. Stress can even cause falls in estrogen levels, potentially exacerbating hormonal

imbalances associated with menopause.[53] (See the "Unwinding Anxiety" chapter for more information about stress-reduction techniques.)

Because Vivian had a sudden onset of menopausal symptoms, I advised her to take a close look at any recent changes in her home or workplace. Two weeks after our consult, I called her with the results of her blood work. Before I could get three words out, she exclaimed: "I figured it out!" Apparently, just before her symptoms began, she'd hired a new employee who began using a plastic coffee pot. Vivian switched to a glass cafetiere, and her symptoms resolved entirely. Sure enough, a few months later, I came across a study revealing that substances in plastics known as endocrine-disrupting chemicals (EDCs) can mimic, block, or interfere with the body's hormones, leading to an earlier onset of menopausal symptoms.[54] When I sent the study to Vivian, she let me know that she was still using the cafetiere—and her symptoms had not returned.

Cooling off Hot Flushes

A breakthrough treatment for moderate to severe hot flushes is available in the U.K. privately and as of 2025 is being reviewed by the NHS. The oral medication, fezolinetant, is a new class of drug designed to target the neurons in the brain's hypothalamus that are responsible for triggering hot flushes. Although I have not yet prescribed it, I anticipate it will be especially useful for women with hot flushes who cannot take hormone replacement therapy.[55]

There are other products available that can help with hot flushes. Two small studies were conducted, one testing a cooling mattress pad and the other a device that cools the forehead. While both study groups were quite small—fifteen to twenty women—the results were impressive. The mattress pad reduced hot flushes (both during the day and night) by more than half at eight weeks, while also reducing sleep disturbances.[56] The forehead cooling device improved sleep onset: Women fell asleep 39 percent faster and had about half the number of nighttime awakenings. Most notably, the device cut hot flush severity in half.[57]

Your Rapid Recovery Prescription for Mastering Menopause

Integrative medicine provides many strategies to effectively manage the symptoms of menopause. Decide what is best for you depending on your preferences, symptom intensity, and personal and family history. Here is what I recommend:

1. If you decide to take HRT after talking with your doctor, begin within ten years of menopause. Consider transdermal, bioidentical estrogen, and be sure to take oral micronized progesterone if your uterus is intact. For symptoms that are more localized (vaginal and/or urethral), vaginal estrogen is a great option.
2. If you prefer to avoid HRT, or are not a good candidate, dietary supplements can help manage symptoms. Black cohosh, St. John's wort, valerian, or hops can be used depending on the symptoms that bother you most.
3. Traditional Chinese medicine, particularly acupuncture, is another option that can effectively treat menopausal symptoms.
4. Exercising for 150 minutes per week reduces the risk of osteoporosis and heart disease; it also improves mood and minimizes the weight gain that can be associated with menopause.
5. Eating a Mediterranean-style diet and adding soy foods daily to your diet can decrease hot flushes and strengthen bones.
6. Pay close attention to environmental triggers that increase menopausal symptoms, including toxic chemicals, temperature, and stress levels.

Part Two

Recovery from Longstanding Conditions

9

Healing Heart Disease

My fifty-year-old patient Steve considered himself healthy. He'd never had a serious illness—that is, until he began experiencing chest tightness after a particularly stressful day at work. Steve's doctor quickly referred him to a cardiologist, who conducted a stress test and then scheduled him for an angiogram. This scan, which shows how well blood flows through the arteries, revealed that Steve had a significant blockage, so his cardiologist inserted a stent—a small mesh tube designed to hold arteries open. Steve took this as a warning sign. Both his parents had died young of heart disease, and he knew it was time to make major changes in his life. He came to see me to discuss how to prevent any further heart trouble.

During our visit, Steve explained that he had worked hard his entire life at a large accounting firm, and the stress had taken its toll. We talked about his career successes and the good family life he had been able to create, but he understood it was time to cut back on his travel and focus on mentoring younger colleagues. Steve also had abdominal obesity. For years he had tried diet after diet, only for all of them to fail. When I brought up a concept called *time-restricted eating* (TRE), he was intrigued and excited. ("You mean I can still eat all the foods I like?" he exclaimed.) Steve embraced TRE and lost nearly 9 kilograms (20 lb) in six months by limiting his eating window to ten hours a day. With the freedom he gained from cutting out travel for work, Steve revived his passion for trail running and began exercising six to eight hours per week. At a one-year follow-up appointment with his cardiologist, Steve's blood pressure and cholesterol levels were normal and he aced his stress test. Today, Steve jokes that when he sees his cardiologist, he is the healthiest person in the waiting room.

Steve is one of millions of adults living with some form of heart disease,[1] a condition that arises when the coronary arteries supplying oxygen-rich blood to the heart become narrowed by the buildup of a waxy substance called *plaque*, which is a combination of fat, cholesterol, cells, and cellular waste products. The heart is forced to work harder owing to diminished blood flow, causing the muscles to thicken and become weaker over time. If a chunk of plaque breaks off, the resulting clot can completely block the flow of blood, causing a heart attack.

At the dawn of the twentieth century, heart disease was an uncommon cause of death. Within a few short decades, however, it became our leading killer in the United States, the U.K. and elsewhere.[2] How is that possible? Human DNA did not change significantly in that time, but our lifestyles did, impairing the function of our recovery reflex. We became increasingly sedentary and adopted a diet rich in sodium, sugar, saturated fat, and refined grains. We were exposed to new environmental toxins and experienced high levels of stress at work.

Thanks to blood-pressure and cholesterol-lowering medications, as well as a reduction in smoking, hospitalizations from heart attacks have dropped by nearly 40 percent since the mid-1990s.[3] Still, heart disease remains one of the leading causes of death in the U.K. and other countries. But experts believe that close to 80 percent of these cases are *completely preventable*.[4] Cholesterol and blood-pressure-lowering medications are effective preventive measures, but they do not address all the root causes of heart disease. Lowering your risk involves making the kind of lifestyle modifications Steve had.

In this chapter, we will see that while heart disease is the world's number-one cause of death, it may also be the world's most preventable form of death.

Testing for Heart Disease

To assess whether you have heart disease, your doctor will begin by taking your blood pressure, which is the force exerted by the circulating blood against the walls of your arteries. It's reported as two numbers: systolic (the pressure when the heart beats) and diastolic (the pressure when the heart is at rest between beats). The ideal blood pressure is below 120/80 mm Hg; as those numbers get higher, the risk of heart disease increases. Additionally, your doctor may order a number of blood tests. Let's take a closer look at what these labs test for and how to interpret the results:

- **Cholesterol Level:** Cholesterol is a waxy, fat-like substance essential for building cells and producing certain hormones. Your total cholesterol level is composed of HDL (high-density lipoprotein) cholesterol, known as "good" cholesterol, which helps remove more dangerous forms of cholesterol from the bloodstream; LDL (low-density lipoprotein) cholesterol, known as "bad" cholesterol, which contributes to plaque buildup in arteries; and triglycerides, which are a type of fat. Generally speaking, targeted cholesterol numbers for optimal heart health are as follows: total cholesterol under 5.0 mmol/L (193 mg/dL), fasting triglycerides under 1.7 mmol/L (150 mg/dL) or non-fasting triglycerides below 2.0 mmol/L (177 mb/dL), LDL cholesterol under 3.0 mmol/L (116 mg/dL); plus HDL cholesterol higher than 1.0 mmol/L (39 mg/dL) for men and higher than 1.2 mmol/L (46 mg/dL) for women.
- **High-Sensitivity C-Reactive Protein (hs-CRP):** This test measures inflammation levels, which can indicate a higher risk of atherosclerosis (hardening of the arteries from plaque buildup).
- **Hemoglobin A1C and Fasting Blood Sugar:** These tests assess the presence of prediabetes or diabetes.

If your LDL cholesterol is elevated, I highly recommend you get the following advanced cardiac tests, but some may not be available on the NHS. They can provide a fuller picture of your risk for heart disease:

- **Lipoprotein(a), or Lp(a):** Lp(a) is a cholesterol particle whose level is mostly determined by genetics. About one in five Americans have an elevated Lp(a), which increases the risk of cardiovascular disease. If you are at risk, your doctor can refer you to a specialist lipid clinic to have an Lp(a) genetic test, which helps identify individuals who may be at increased risk even if other cholesterol levels are normal. I recommend that everyone have this test once in adulthood. A normal level is less than 50 mg/dl. While there is no specific treatment for elevated Lp(a) as of this writing, it is an additional factor in determining your risk of heart disease and the merit of taking medication. Note: There are drugs in trial that show promise in reducing Lp(a).

- **Apolipoproteins A-I and B:** This test provides detailed information about cholesterol particles in your blood. For instance, LDL particles can be big and fluffy or small and dense; the latter are much more dangerous.[5] A regular LDL test does not distinguish between these forms.
- **Homocysteine:** Homocysteine is an amino acid that, when elevated, can damage the lining of your blood vessels (endothelium), leading to inflammation and atherosclerosis.
- **Omega-3 Index:** This test reflects the omega-3 status of your body for the past four months. It measures the amount of EPA (eicosapentanoic acid) and DHA (docosahexaenoic acid) in your red blood cell membranes.
- **Coronary Artery Calcium Score:** A coronary calcium test is an ultrafast CT scan that assesses your risk of coronary artery disease by measuring the amount of calcified plaque in the walls of the arteries. A calcium score of 0 is ideal and means there is very little risk for a cardiovascular event. A score of 100 to 300 signifies moderate plaque deposits, and a score greater than 300 means there is a high heart-attack risk.[6] I recommend men and women get this test by age forty and fifty, respectively, if other risk assessments put them in a "moderate" risk category. In my view, a calcium score test is not necessary if your heart disease risk is determined to be very low, or if you already know you have heart disease.

Your doctor may also order a stress test, which involves walking (or running) on a treadmill while wearing an electrocardiogram (ECG) monitor to record your heart's activity. Finally, if you have predictive symptoms of heart disease, you may need a coronary angiography. This can reveal blockages or narrowing of your arteries from plaque buildup. Research shows that among people with existing heart disease,[7] if their plaque continues to accumulate, they have a 15 to 20 percent increased risk of having further cardiac events within the next twelve months, when compared to people whose plaque does not progress. Conversely, a meta-analysis involving more than seven thousand patients with heart disease found that even a 1 percent decrease in plaque can lower your odds of a major cardiovascular event like a heart attack or stroke by 25 percent.[8]

What Increases Your Risk of Heart Disease?

Unlike many longstanding conditions I cover in this book, heart disease presents with few initial symptoms, even as it silently begins damaging the layer of cells lining your blood vessels. How do you know if you are at risk? The Interheart study was a fifty-two-country analysis of the risk factors for heart attack involving nearly thirty thousand individuals.[9] Here are the most important modifiable factors the researchers discovered:

1. **Smoking:** According to the study, smoking was the single biggest risk factor for a heart attack. Even just one cigarette per day increases the risk of heart attack by 5 percent, compared to not smoking at all.
2. **Abnormal Lipids:** High levels of bad cholesterol (LDL) and low levels of good cholesterol (HDL) contribute to heart disease.
3. **Hypertension:** Also known as high blood pressure, hypertension forces the heart to work harder, leading to damage in the heart's arteries. A blood pressure over 120/80 is considered elevated, while a reading over 130/80 is stage 1 hypertension.
4. **Diabetes:** As discussed in the "Reversing Type 2 Diabetes" chapter, having diabetes increases the amount of sugar in your blood, which can damage the heart over time.
5. **Abdominal Obesity:** The fat that develops around your belly, known as visceral fat, is different from the fat on your thighs or buttocks. Visceral fat releases substances that lead to insulin resistance, elevated LDL cholesterol, and inflammation, which can increase high blood pressure. Men with a waist circumference over 101.6 centimetres (40 in), and women with a waist over 89 centimetres (35 in), are at the highest risk.

6. **Stress:** Chronic stress increases your risk of heart disease. Stress hormones like cortisol raise your blood pressure and increase the levels of glucose and fat in the blood, contributing to plaque buildup.
7. **Diet:** The Interheart study noted that individuals who ate the fewest vegetables and fruits had a much higher risk of heart disease.
8. **Physical Activity:** People who engaged in regular physical activity had a lower risk of experiencing a heart attack compared to those who were inactive.

Here is the bottom line: By minimizing your modifiable risk factors, you can enhance your recovery reflex and significantly decrease your risk of heart disease. In 2010, a team of researchers led by the epidemiologist Dr. Donald Lloyd-Jones and his team published the ideal risk factor profile for avoiding heart disease:[10] not smoking, keeping your body-mass index (BMI) under 25, getting 150 minutes of moderate exercise per week, eating a healthy diet, keeping your total cholesterol under 5.0 mmol/L (193 mg d/L), keeping your blood pressure under 120/80 mm HG, and keeping your fasting blood sugar under 100 mg/dL. Unfortunately, the team found only 5 percent of Americans manage to hit all seven. (An eighth metric, optimal sleep, was added in 2022.)

Do not panic if you don't, either! The rest of this chapter will discuss strategies to address these risk factors (as well as a few others not considered in these trials). I'll begin with the most common treatment of all: cholesterol-lowering medications, and how to think about whether they might be a good option for you.

Cholesterol-Lowering Medications

Cholesterol-lowering medications, known as statins, are among the most prescribed drugs worldwide, with some forty million Americans taking them daily.[11] They work by blocking HMG-CoA reductase, an enzyme in the liver that controls LDL cholesterol production. And, indeed, statins work well, often lowering LDL cholesterol by as much as 30 to 50 percent.[12] Statins also have two additional heart-protective benefits: They reduce inflammation and they stabilize plaque in the arteries. With these three effects, statins lower the risk of death from cardiovascular disease by 25 percent or more,[13] prevent plaque buildup from worsening, and are a major reason why the rate of death from heart attacks fell from about eighty-seven deaths per one hundred thousand people in 1999 to about thirty-eight deaths per one hundred thousand people in 2020.[14]

So, you might be thinking, *If statins are that effective, why shouldn't everyone take them?* Despite their obvious benefits, statins can have side effects. The most common is muscle pain, which can range from mild soreness to aches serious enough to limit your daily activities. In very rare cases, statins can cause life-threatening muscle damage called *rhabdomyolysis*, which can lead to liver damage or kidney failure. Some studies show that statins interfere with insulin production in your liver, raising glucose levels and increasing the risk of type 2 diabetes.[15]

Statins have a number needed to treat (NNT) of 400 for people without a personal history of heart disease; this means 400 patients need to be treated before preventing a non-fatal heart attack in one person, and a NNT as low as 25 for patients at the highest risk of heart disease.[16] Conversely, they have a number needed to harm (NNH) of 50 for diabetes, meaning for every fifty people (with or without existing heart disease) taking a statin, one developed diabetes. The NNH for muscle damage is just 10. In individuals with existing heart disease, the NNT for fatal heart attacks is 83, and the NNT for non-fatal heart attacks is 39. Thus, for people who already have heart disease, the benefits of taking a statin usually outweigh the risks.

So, should *you* take a statin? Doctors have access to a risk estimator tool known as "QRISK3" that can calculate your risk and help you determine if you might benefit and it is available online. After you enter your risk factors, it assesses your odds of having a cardiovascular event in the next ten years. I generally recommend against taking a statin if your risk is less than 5 percent. If your risk is in the gray zone—between 5 and 15 percent—you may ask your doctor about getting a coronary calcium score that can help you decide.

Consult with your doctor about whether a statin is the best course of action. If so, the next question is: Which one do you take? Among the two most prescribed are atorvastatin and rosuvastatin. I generally recommend starting with rosuvastatin, as atorvastatin can cross the blood-brain barrier and sometimes has the highly unwanted side effect of cognitive impairment.[17] Rosuvastatin, on the other hand, has a very limited ability to cross the blood-brain barrier.[18] If you experience muscle aches, discuss taking a lower dose or switching to a different statin with your health team.

What if you don't tolerate statins because of significant muscle pain, or if a high dose of statin medication does not get you to your target LDL?[19] Dr. Vivian Kominos, a cardiologist and fellowship graduate from our Integrative Medicine Center, usually recommends adding a second LDL-lowering medication, ezetimibe, a drug that reduces cholesterol absorption in the gut. The Improve-It trial,[20] which followed eighteen thousand patients who had suffered a cardiac event like a heart attack or unstable angina, revealed that adding ezetimibe lowered LDL by nearly one-fourth. More important, it further decreased the occurrence of cardiovascular events by 2 percent.

Once again, remember that an elevated LDL cholesterol is just one of many risk factors for heart disease. Even if you begin a statin, to fully activate your recovery reflex you will need to also address your stress, exercise, weight, abdominal obesity, and any other modifiable risk factors!

Supplements and Medications to Consider

If you have a borderline risk for heart disease, are reluctant to take medication with an NNT of 400, or are experiencing uncomfortable side effects from statins, there are other ways to lower your cholesterol, including dietary supplements, other medications, and lifestyle modifications. Talk to your doctor about these strategies:

Supplements
- **Red Yeast Rice:** The product of rice fermented with *Monascus purpureus* yeast, red yeast rice has been repeatedly studied and found to lower cholesterol. Interestingly, it contains small amounts of monacolin K, a compound that is identical to the pharmaceutical

lovastatin. It is available online in the U.K. as a supplement. I recommend a starting dose of 600 mg twice daily. If you decide to try a supplement, be sure to check any product you're considering with your pharmacist or doctor, as red yeast rice's potency varies and some products contain a toxin called *citrinin*. See "How to Choose a Supplement" (appendix 2) for more information.

- **Garlic Extract:** The active compounds in garlic are believed to have lipid-lowering properties. Studies have shown that garlic supplements may be able to lower total cholesterol by 7 percent and LDL cholesterol by 10 percent,[21] although the results vary. Garlic (and garlic extract) may also offer another cardiovascular benefit: blood pressure reduction.[22]

- **CoQ10:** Coenzyme Q10 is an antioxidant that improves heart function and blood flow. It also helps protect LDL cholesterol from oxidation, potentially reducing atherosclerosis risk. One study found that patients who were given CoQ10 within three days of having a heart attack were less likely to have a recurrent event compared to those who did not receive the supplement.[23] Taking CoQ10 when a statin has been prescribed is especially important, as statins reduce the levels of CoQ10 in the body. I recommend starting with a dose of 100 mg daily.

- **Vitamin D:** Low levels of vitamin D are associated with an increased risk of heart disease and hypertension,[24] though we're not exactly sure why. It may be the case that vitamin D affects heart health through its role in regulating blood pressure, inflammation, and glucose metabolism. Studies also show that people with normal vitamin D levels don't benefit from supplements.[25] I recommend checking your vitamin D level to determine whether to add a supplement. (See "How to Choose a Supplement," appendix 2, for more information.)

- **Magnesium:** Magnesium helps maintain normal heart rhythm, regulates blood pressure, and is involved in energy production in heart cells. Approximately 50 percent of Americans don't get the daily recommended intake of magnesium in their diet.[26] This is important because magnesium deficiency is linked to an increased risk of cardiovascular problems.[27] While food sources include green leafy vegetables, avocados, dark chocolate, nuts, and seeds, I also commonly recommend daily magnesium citrate supplements at a dose of 400 mg in the evening.

Other Medications

- **Ezetimibe:** As discussed earlier, ezetimibe is a medication that can be taken with a statin if taking one alone does not get you to the desired LDL level. It can also be taken in place of a statin that is causing intolerable side effects.[28]
- **Colchicine:** Colchicine is an older medication primarily used to treat gout, but recent studies have shown it can also significantly reduce plaque volume, thanks to its anti-inflammatory properties.[29]
- **Prescription Fish Oil:** Rich in omega-3 fatty acids, fish oil can lower cholesterol by reducing triglycerides. It can also help improve overall heart health by reducing inflammation and the risk of blood clots. Icosapent ethyl is a prescription form of fish oil. A major trial found that icosapent ethyl led to plaque regression,[30] but critics point out that the control oil chosen—mineral oil—can *increase* inflammation and may increase your risk of bleeding,[31] which may have skewed the results in the fish oil's favor.

The Gum–Heart Connection

It might seem odd that the plaque on your teeth can lead to a completely different form of plaque in your arteries, but research increasingly points to a connection. The sticky film, known as dental plaque, that builds on your teeth is primarily composed of bacteria and forms an acidic substance that harms tooth enamel and your gums. While the exact mechanism is not fully understood, it appears these bacteria also enter your bloodstream, causing inflammation and fatty plaque buildup in your arteries.

Research shows that people with periodontal (gum) disease have as much as three times the risk of heart attack, stroke, or other serious cardiac events.[32] Brushing, flossing, and seeing your dentist regularly for cleanings and check-ups will not only keep your teeth and gums happy and healthy, but your heart will benefit, too!

Heart Disease Reversal Diet

Statins and other drugs can be a lifesaving tool for reversing the buildup of atherosclerotic plaque in your arteries, but they do not address the unhealthy behaviors that contribute to plaque buildup in the first place. To fully support your recovery reflex, you need to alter the food you eat.

The Lifestyle Heart Trial was first published back in 1990.[33] The study was led by Dr. Dean Ornish, who recruited forty-eight people with advanced coronary artery disease and divided them into two groups. The first group followed the usual care by their doctors—statin and blood-pressure medications, smoking cessation, and in some cases, surgery—while the other group adopted four specific lifestyle changes: (1) They consumed a less-than-10-percent-fat vegetarian diet, (2) they participated in small emotional-support groups, (3) they practiced yoga, and (4) they followed a modest exercise routine. Remarkably, the study revealed that participants in the lifestyle intervention group were able to reverse coronary artery blockage after just one year, while the control group showed a progression of the disease. A five-year follow-up study found that the lifestyle group had further reversal of their coronary artery blockages[34]—another example of an activated recovery reflex leading to a healthier heart![35]

Meanwhile, other dietary studies have continued to clarify the link between diet and heart health. The Predimed study, a large trial carried out in Spain and published in 2018 in the *New England Journal of Medicine*,[36] randomly divided nearly seven thousand five hundred participants with a high risk of heart disease into two groups following variations on a Mediterranean diet: one supplemented with extra-virgin olive oil, the other with mixed nuts. A third control group consumed a diet of low-fat foods. This study represented the largest-ever examination of the efficacy of the Mediterranean diet on cardiovascular disease. The conclusion was: "The incidence of major cardiovascular events was lower among those assigned to a Mediterranean diet supplemented with extra-virgin olive oil or mixed nuts than among those assigned to a reduced-fat diet."[37]

An earlier trial, the Lyon Heart Study, similarly randomly grouped participants with heart disease into a group that followed a Mediterranean-style diet and another group that solely cut down on fat consumption.[38] After nearly four years, the participants assigned to the Mediterranean diet had a "50 to 70 percent lower risk of recurrent heart disease," including cardiac death, nonfatal heart attacks, and unstable angina, compared to the control group. For more information about how to begin a Mediterranean diet, see "Your Rapid Recovery Toolkit" (appendix 1).

Another effective diet is the Dietary Approaches to Stop Hypertension (DASH) plan, which was developed by a team of researchers sponsored by the U.S. National Institutes of Health. The DASH diet is similar to a Mediterranean-style diet in its emphasis on vegetables and fruits, whole grains, nuts, and seeds, but it allows more lean, animal-based protein, such as poultry. Many studies have shown that the DASH diet can effectively lower blood pressure and reduce the risk of heart attack and stroke.[39]

Another heart-protection strategy is to follow a vegan diet, meaning no animal products whatsoever. A study published in 2023, by Stanford University researcher Christopher Gardner, PhD, compared twenty-two pairs of identical twins to see how a vegan diet compared to an omnivore diet.[40] Both diets were minimally processed, excluded sugars and refined starches, and were heavy on vegetables, fruits, pulses (legumes), and whole grains. The omnivore diet also included chicken, fish, eggs, cheese, dairy, and other animal products. Four weeks later, "The participants with a vegan diet had significantly lower low-density lipoprotein cholesterol (LDL-C) levels, insulin and body weight—all of which are associated with improved cardiovascular health—than the omnivore participants."[41]

Impressively, the vegan group's LDL cholesterol dropped on average from a high 2.86 mmol/L (110.7 mg/dL) to a normal 2.47 mmol/L (95.5 mg/dL).

The evidence is less strong for Atkins or keto diets which emphasize more animal fats and little to no carbohydrates. Dr. Kominos, mentioned earlier, explains that she's "not a fan of long-term keto diets because we just don't have the evidence." The data are in fact fairly clear that eating more meat is associated with worse cardiovascular health. In a 2023 *European Heart Journal* article, researchers reviewed forty-three trials of more than four million people and concluded that eating red meat significantly increased the risk of cardiovascular disease.[42] Oxford University researchers have even narrowed down the specific amounts: Every 50 grams (1¾ oz) per day higher intake of unprocessed red meat (such as beef, lamb, or pork) increases the risk of coronary heart disease by 9 percent.[43] If you need a visual, consider that 50 grams (1¾ oz) of meat is about 2½ slices of ham or a cut of meat the size of your palm.

Here are the most important takeaways from the studies on diet and heart disease: First, eating more vegetables, fruits, and whole grains is protective against heart disease and can help reverse it among people with a history of heart attack. Second, eating processed meats dramatically increases the risk of heart disease. In a decade-long study, researchers examined the eating habits of 135,000 people across twenty-one countries, concluding in *The American Journal of Clinical Nutrition* that eating approximately 140 grams (5 oz) of processed meats per week increased the risk of cardiovascular disease by 46 percent and the risk of death by 50 percent compared to eating no processed meats at all.[44] (For context, 140 grams (5 oz) equates to five rashers of bacon, five slices of deli meat, or fewer than two hotdogs.) Additionally, when you eat meat, the bacteria that inhabit your gut—the microbiome at work again!—create trimethylamine, which your liver oxidizes into trimethylamine N-oxide (TMAO). High levels of TMAO are associated with an increased risk of atherosclerosis.[45]

When cooking, you can reduce the amount of oxidized LDL, which is significantly more likely to cause atherosclerotic plaque buildup, by avoiding dry, hot cooking (over 200°C/180°C Fan/400° F/Gas Mark 6). High temperatures increase the formation of advanced glycolic end products (AGEs), which are harmful compounds formed when proteins or fats combine with sugars. You can mitigate the risk of an occasional barbeque by first marinating your food in vinegar or lemon, which reduces the formation of AGEs.[46]

Finally, consuming too much sugar is also associated with an increased risk of heart disease. Sugar increases inflammation in the body, which contributes to the buildup of atherosclerotic plaque, even if you are not overweight. In one study,[47] participants who consumed 25 percent or more of their calories from sugar were more than twice as likely to die from heart disease, compared to people who derived less than 10 percent from sugar. Perhaps 25 percent sounds impossibly high, but consider that the average American adolescent gets 17.3 percent of their calories from sugar, the average American adult is not far behind at 13.5 percent and other high-income countries are fast catching up. Unfortunately, artificial sweeteners are no better; they are associated with as much as a 9 percent increased risk of heart disease and an 18 percent increased risk of stroke.[48]

Time-Restricted Eating

As we saw at the beginning of this chapter, my patient Steve reversed his heart disease in part by restricting his eating to a ten-hour window. Time-restricted eating (TRE) is an eating pattern that focuses on *when* you eat, rather than *what* or how much you eat. It confines your food intake to a specific number of hours each day and prescribes fasting for the rest of the time.

Many of my patients have successfully integrated TRE into weight loss and diabetes reversal, and studies show it is also valuable for reversing heart disease.[49] For instance, eating within a ten-hour window has been shown to "significantly reduce" blood pressure, blood sugar, and cholesterol levels among shift workers with erratic eating schedules.[50] It is uncommon to have side effects when following TRE, and when they do occur, they are usually mild and transient—such as fatigue or dizziness—and are easily resolved with a snack.[51]

Exercise

Here is another effective way to prevent, arrest, or even reverse heart disease: exercise at a moderate intensity for 150 minutes per week. Exercise improves the efficiency of the cardiovascular system, dilates blood vessels, and reduces arterial stiffness, ultimately lowering blood pressure by an average of 5 to 7 mm/Hg among those with high blood pressure. This translates to a 20 to 30 percent reduced risk of heart disease![52] Additionally, exercise improves lipids by increasing HDL cholesterol and lowering LDL cholesterol and triglycerides.[53]

It can be challenging to fit 150 minutes of moderate exercise into your average week, especially if you have a house full of kids, a long commute, or any of the other stresses and obligations that prevent 72 percent of Americans from meeting the recommended physical activity guidelines.[54] The good news is that even the smallest amounts of exercise make a difference! Getting *any* activity has a huge benefit over being sedentary. Studies have shown that people who walk seven thousand steps per day have a 50 to 70 percent lower risk of death,[55] and dramatically more plaque regression,[56] compared to those who walk fewer steps. But don't be dissuaded if you can't hit that benchmark immediately. Every step counts! Many people find it helpful to use a smartphone, Apple Watch, Fitbit, Oura ring, or other device to track their steps.

Data from a trial following more than one hundred thousand participants for thirty years found that 300 minutes or more per week of moderate exercise can bring as much as a 19 to 25 percent lower risk of cardiovascular mortality.[57] If you are pressed for time, keep in mind that as little as 75 minutes per week of vigorous exercise can afford similar heart protection.[58]

So, what counts as moderate exercise? Begin by subtracting your age from 220, which gives you a rough sense of your maximum heart rate. For moderate exercise, you should aim to exercise between 64 and 76 percent of your maximum. (Seventy-seven percent to 85 percent of your max counts as vigorous.) For example, if you are fifty years old, your maximum heart rate will be about 170 beats per minute. So, a moderate workout might be a bike ride or jog that elevates your heart rate to somewhere between 109 and 129 beats per minute. A simpler way to measure this is use the talk test: During moderate exercise, you should be able hold a conversation but not sing. If you have difficulty speaking, the exercise is considered vigorous.

De-Stressing

Revving up your heart isn't the only way to improve your cardiovascular health. Yoga can reduce stress, lower blood pressure, improve cholesterol levels, and enhance overall physical fitness. One review of clinical research found that compared to people who remained sedentary, those who began a yoga practice lowered their total cholesterol by 0.5 mmol/L (18 mg/dL), triglycerides by 0.28 mml/L (25 mg/dL), and both systolic and diastolic blood pressure by roughly 5 mm/Hg.[59] In another study, participants with metabolic syndrome—defined as having a waistline over 101.6 centimetres (40 in) in men or 89 centimetres (35 in) in women, high blood pressure, high blood sugar, high triglycerides, and low HDL cholesterol—were randomized into two groups.[60] The first received dietary interventions designed to help them lose weight, while the other began a yoga program. After twelve weeks, 45 percent of those in the yoga group recovered from their metabolic syndrome compared to 32 percent of the diet group.

Various forms of meditation, including mindfulness-based stress reduction, mantra meditation, and transcendental meditation, have also been found to lower blood pressure and reduce stress and anxiety.[61] These practices may also reduce other heart disease risk factors, including type 2 diabetes and high cholesterol.

The Interheart study mentioned earlier revealed that four types of psychological stress accounted for up to 32 percent of the attributable risk of heart attack; those four sources were stresses at work, at home, concern with finances, and major life events in the past year. The good news is that research studies have consistently shown that relaxation techniques can reduce recurrent cardiovascular events by 29 percent and reduce mortality by 34 percent; as side benefits, they also improve blood pressure, cholesterol, and body weight.

Environmental Toxins

When my patient John came in with high blood pressure, I was surprised: he was thirty-seven years old, ate a healthy diet, didn't smoke, exercised daily, and had no family history of hypertension. As I sat across from him, I kept thinking, *Could there be something else affecting his heart?* I inquired about his daily routine, and he mentioned that he drank five or six cans of unsweetened iced tea every day. As an experiment, I asked him to make his own iced tea instead. Sure enough, when I saw him next, his blood pressure was normal. The iced-tea cans had likely contained bisphenol A (BPA), a chemical used in the linings of food and drink cans, jar lids, and bottle caps that can significantly raise blood pressure.[62] BPA is an endocrine disruptor, meaning it interferes with your body's hormones. The good news is that BPA is excreted by your kidneys, so ceasing exposure—typically from plastics, can liners, and thermal receipt paper—will lead to a rapid drop in your body burden of this chemical. Another bit of good news: Manufacturers are eliminating BPA from can liners.

The larger takeaway from John's story is that your heart health isn't just affected by the food and beverages you consume; it's also affected by environmental toxins, potentially including those in the air you breathe. Alarmingly, the European Environmental Agency reports that "Around 8.8 percent of Ischemic Heart Disease (IHD) deaths are due to air pollution, as are 9.3 percent of stroke deaths."[63] Air pollution exposes us to particulate matter and ozone,[64] which increase the risk of heart disease and respiratory problems, including asthma. Airborne pollution can be hard to avoid, depending on where you live and work; fortunately, HEPA (high-efficiency particulate air) filters can help create a clean air sanctuary in your home.

Additionally, heavy metals can have detrimental effects on heart health. Exposure to lead—often from old paint, contaminated water, or industrial pollution—can cause high blood pressure and arteriosclerosis.[65] Another damaging heavy metal, mercury, is most commonly encountered by eating contaminated seafood. Mercury can cause damage to the endothelial cells lining the blood vessels, leading to increased risk of arteriosclerosis.

It can also disrupt the oxidation of fats, leading to increased levels of LDL cholesterol.[66] Note that health officials recommends eating low-mercury fish for the healthy nutrients they contain, including iodine, choline, iron, and omega-3s.[67] The fishes to avoid eating include shark, swordfish, king mackerel, marlin, orange roughy, bigeye tuna, and tilefish, as they tend to have high levels of mercury.

Your Prescription for Healing Heart Disease

Heart disease is largely preventable. There are many steps you can take to improve your heart health—and at the same time yield side benefits as these lifestyle changes also prevent cancer, diabetes, and depression.

1. Address any modifiable risk factors for heart disease, include smoking, abnormal lipids, hypertension, abdominal obesity, stress, an unhealthy diet, and lack of physical activity.
2. Adopt a diet rich in vegetables, fruits, and whole grains. Eating processed meats and added sugars increases your risk. I recommend following the Mediterranean diet, the DASH diet, a vegan diet, or practicing time-restricted eating.
3. Exercise at a moderate intensity for at least 150 minutes per week.
4. Practice relaxation techniques, such as yoga and meditation.
5. Use the QRISK3 risk estimator tool to assess your odds of a cardiovascular event.
6. If you have abnormal cholesterol levels, ask your doctor to order advanced cardiac tests for a better understanding of your risks.
7. If your risk of heart disease is borderline, or if you have serious side effects from statins, a variety of supplements can help, including red yeast rice, fish oil, garlic extract, CoQ10, vitamin D, and magnesium.
8. To the best of your ability, limit your exposure to environmental toxins and air pollutants, which can have detrimental effects on your heart.

10

Deactivating Pain Signals

Two curious stories provide fascinating insights into how the body experiences acute pain.[1] The first involves a twenty-nine-year-old construction worker who, in 1995, accidentally jumped onto a seven-inch nail. When he saw the nail sticking through the top of his boot, he screamed in pain and was rushed to the hospital. Doctors quickly sedated him and cut off the boot. To their astonishment, the nail had passed between his toes without piercing skin. The injury was imaginary, it turns out, though the pain was nevertheless very real.

About a decade later, another construction worker was using a nail gun when it unexpectedly discharged near his face. He felt a twinge, but assumed the nail had glanced off his jaw, leaving him only with a minor toothache and some bruising. Six uneventful days later, he visited a dentist. To his shock, the X-rays revealed a four-inch nail embedded in his head. Because the construction worker firmly believed the nail had missed him, his brain simply did not detect the injury.

So what do these two stories tell us? Pain is real; at the same time, it is not fully correlated with physical damage—or lack thereof. Rather, it correlates with your brain's best guess of how much protection your body needs. Usually this system works well, such as when you burn your hand on a hot pot and immediately pull it away. But at other times the system fails, as with the construction worker who didn't feel the nail in his head. More commonly, the body's pain system fails in the opposite direction and leads to chronic pain, in which pain signals get stuck "On" despite the physical injury having healed. This process, in which acute pain becomes chronic pain, may prevent you from returning to homeostasis, and to recover requires an entirely different approach that involves addressing the story our mind tells us about pain, one that is entangled with our fear and arousal.

The brain's very neuroplasticity, or ability to change—which is incredibly helpful most of the time—can pose a challenge when it comes to pain. Chronic pain seems to deepen the grooves in the brain that react to discomfort, such that increasingly weak stimuli—in some cases, even a cool breeze—can cause a spasm of pain. The underlying mechanisms of longstanding pain include changes in the brain networks, in neurotransmitters, and in some cases in sympathetic nervous system tone.[2] This process, which creates a heightened sense of pain, is called *central sensitization* (CS).

In this chapter I will examine several common pain syndromes, including chronic back pain, headaches (migraines and tension), nerve pain, and osteo- and rheumatoid arthritis. Recovery is possible, and the recommendations that follow can help.

Your Pain Is Real. It's in Your Body—and in Your Brain

Accumulating evidence suggests that one aspect of longstanding pain results from our fear of the pain itself. If you have longstanding pain, this may not be what you want to hear. It is normal to crave simple answers to health problems. How can such intense pain—such *specific* pain—not have a physical cause?

As Dr. Howard Schubiner, director of the Mind Body Medicine Center at Ascension Providence Hospital in Southfield, Michigan, explains, "Whether pain is triggered by stress or physical injury, the brain generates the sensations. And—this is a mind-blowing concept—it's not just reflecting what it feels, it's deciding whether to turn pain on or off."[3] Dr. Schubiner is the protégé of Dr. John Sarno, whose famous 1991 bestseller, *Healing Back Pain,* theorized that the brain sometimes creates pain to distract us from repressed anxiety and anger. Dr. Sarno believed that this could manifest in the back, but also as migraines, nerve pain, fibromyalgia, or gastrointestinal upset. He correctly postulated that the psychological stress of repressed emotions, coupled with forcing yourself to meet standards set by other people, causes physical symptoms. When we feel stress, our brain creates pain by inhibiting blood flow to nerves, tissues, and muscles.

No one wants to be told that the pain is "all in your head." It makes us feel discounted or even downright offended. So, it's critical to understand that pain is *real*, no matter its source. Dr. Sarno named this brain-generated pain "tension myositis"; it was later renamed *neural circuit pain* by Dr. Schubiner. Neural circuit pain is caused by neural pathways in the brain rather than structural damage in the body. One of the clearest examples of neural circuit pain is "phantom limb syndrome." Up to 64 percent of amputees feel excruciating pain in an arm or leg that has been amputated from their body.[4]

The first step toward relieving neural circuit pain is accepting that while your pain is real, your physical body may be fine. I recommend creating a mantra for yourself to repeat when you have flare-ups. If you have back pain, for instance, you can use this mantra developed by Dr. Sarno: "Your pain is a result of a process initiated by the brain to protect you from feelings that you have inside that the brain considers to be too painful, too sad, or too threatening. The same brain that brings this on can make it go away."

The second step is to work on accepting there is likely a psychological component influencing your pain. Through journaling exercises, guided meditation, or counseling, see if you can discern the stressors that aggravate your pain. (See the "Unwinding Anxiety" chapter for more information.) Make a list of the things that are weighing on your mind, as they are likely weighing on your ailing body part. Simply acknowledging the presence of psychological stressors will sometimes reduce pain.

The good news is that the brain's neuroplasticity—a part of your recovery reflex—can help turn down your heightened pain sensitivity. For instance, in one study, patients with chronic musculoskeletal pain and central sensitization who received one-on-one neuroscience education ended up with less pain, disability, and psychosocial distress.[5]

Let's now take a closer look at some of the most common forms of longstanding pain syndromes, starting with back pain.

Back Pain

Nearly ten years ago, I became one of the sixteen million Americans who experience persistent back pain. It began shortly after my father died. I had been at his bedside with my sisters, my father's partner, his doctor, and a hospice nurse. It was a gentle and peaceful passing. Three weeks later, my first book was published, and a New York City friend threw a bash for me at her Manhattan apartment. Just as I stood up to make a speech, I felt intense spasms in my mid-back. I managed to deliver my remarks, but the pain didn't subside. At times it would keep me from sleeping, and I spent countless nights lying on the floor, seeking respite from the pain. When my first grandchild was born, I was afraid that holding him would make my back pain worse and that I would not be able to have the relationship I longed for. I would run my fingers over my mid-back, pressing as hard as I could on the muscle spasm and struggling to understand the physical processes that were to blame.

I am someone who prefers a "less is more" approach to medical care, and I never considered back surgery. I sought treatment from chiropractors, osteopaths, physiotherapists, massage therapists, and energy-work providers. I learned posture exercises and used guided imagery, shamanic healing, trauma-releasing exercises, and Pilates. Some of these integrative approaches helped, others did not. Regardless, nothing fixed the pain completely. It wasn't until I stopped searching for a singular cause of my pain and instead accepted I had developed central sensitization that I began to improve.

I studied my triggers—which included sitting for more than five minutes in a chair that lacked back support, as well as emotional stressors. I learned the principles of the Alexander and Gokhale techniques (more on these later), gradually retaught myself to sit, and attended to how I stand and walk. I added low-dose naltrexone (more on this later) and repeated Dr. Sarno's mantra nightly before I went to sleep. Gradually, my pain dissipated. Now, when my back pain flares (about once every two or three months), I see it as a sign I need to realign my body for better posture or deal with something that is upsetting me.

If you also suffer from back pain, you are far from alone. It's among the most common reasons people visit their doctor. For some, back pain presents as a dull, constant ache. Others—like me—experience intense spasms. Sometimes back pain is the result of an accident; other times it just seems to show up.

As we will see in the "Recovery from Orthopedic Surgery" chapter, back surgery is sometimes the correct course of treatment. But if you are like me and the tens of millions of people whose back pain comes and goes with little apparent reason, there is an excellent chance you can heal yourself. And, surprisingly, as just noted, it begins by accepting there may not be anything physically wrong with you. This can be a challenging thing to do, but the evidence is compelling.

Consider, for instance, the power of mindfulness exercises. In 2016, researchers from the University of Washington published a landmark study[6] in *The Journal of the American Medical Association* in which 342 adults with back pain were randomly assigned to either conventional medical care; mindfulness-based stress reduction (MBSR), such as meditation, yoga, and body awareness exercises; or cognitive behavioral therapy (CBT), which involves education about chronic pain, sleep hygiene, guided imagery, and other relaxation skills. Those who received MBSR and CBT experienced greater improvement in their pain compared to the group that received conventional care, and the results persisted for a full year.

Ask yourself: How is your back currently feeling? If there is pain, can you observe it with compassion and curiosity? Notice if sending breath to the area softens the discomfort. Mindfulness helps you see that the pain is not static, that there is an ebb and flow to its intensity, and that it can be influenced. In addition to MBSR and CBT, other useful options include breath work, guided imagery, biofeedback, progressive muscle relaxation, and hypnotherapy. Find the one that best resonates for you and make it a daily practice.

A Simple Scan to Relieve Back Pain

While there are many effective mindfulness exercises for back pain, one of my favorites is the "Body Scan,"[7] courtesy of Dr. Jon Kabat-Zinn, a pioneering mindfulness teacher and researcher. I recommend that you practice it every day for twenty minutes.

1. Lie on your back in a comfortable place, close your eyes, and focus on how your belly rises and falls while breathing.
2. Focus on your left foot. Be aware of every sensation, including pain, for a few minutes. When your mind wanders, calmly bring your attention back to your foot.
3. If you notice pain anywhere in your body, acknowledge it and gently breathe through it. Make a note of the thoughts and emotions accompanying it. Don't worry if the pain does not go away. Accept that it is there, and see if you can observe it nonjudgmentally.
4. Shift your focus from your left foot to your ankle and repeat the exercise. Repeat on your right foot and ankle. Then slowly and mindfully proceed up the body.

Most Back Pain Is Not Physical

Here is one of the most common questions I receive from patients with stubborn back discomfort: Why won't my pain go away? The latest research suggests that while longstanding back pain may have an initial physical trigger—you picked up a heavy object, say—that pain is perpetuated by your neural circuits, which are the collections of interconnected neurons in the brain and nervous system. As mentioned earlier, this is central sensitization (CS), a condition whereby your nervous system is overly reactive to things that are not typically painful. Even something as innocuous as a handshake can set off CS. In effect, your brain "turns up the volume" in response to stimuli.

Western medicine has been slow to integrate the latest findings about CS. Instead, we often continue to hunt for a structural cause. In most cases, a patient who complains of persistent back pain will get an MRI or CT scan of the spine. If tests reveal a bulging or herniated intervertebral disk at the level that corresponds to their pain, doctors often recommend surgery. But back surgery can lead to months of recovery—and frequently does not alleviate pain. By some counts, as many as 40 percent of the over three hundred thousand lumbar surgeries performed in America every year are unsuccessful in reducing pain long-term.[8] In fact, failure is so common that doctors even invented a new term for it: *failed back surgery syndrome*.

Shockingly, the evidence shows little connection between the physical condition of your spine and whether you feel back pain. In one well-known study[9] published in the *New England Journal of Medicine*, researchers performed MRI examinations on ninety-eight people aged twenty to eighty with no history of back pain. "We found a high prevalence of abnormalities in the lumbar spine on MRI examination of people without back pain," the study concluded. "Only 36 percent of those examined had a normal disk at all levels. About half had a bulge in at least one intervertebral disk, and about a quarter had at least one disk protrusion." In other words, there is often *no radiographic difference* between people with zero back pain and those who cannot get out of bed. This does not negate your pain, but it does mean that how you approach recovery might change.

Note that low-dose naltrexone (LDN), normally used in the U.K. only for helping to treat drug and alcohol addiction, can be used as well to reduce central sensitization. It has been researched as a treatment in multiple kinds of longstanding pain including fibromyalgia, low back pain, and pain from multiple sclerosis.[10] LDN has analgesic and anti-inflammatory effects. The medication Naltrexone is formulated as a 50 mg pill, but LDN is prescribed starting at a dose of 1.5 mg per day, with the most common dose being 4.5 mg per day. This low-dose prescription will usually need to be filled at a compounding pharmacy from a private doctor.

Finally, it is critical for people with CS to own their pain. Too often we feel ashamed of our discomfort and attempt to hide it from others. In my case, sitting often led to a flare-up of pain, but during meetings at work, I would stay planted in my chair alongside my colleagues. My pain levels improved when I became less shy about standing up when I needed to. I now carry a small back pillow and a soft tennis ball (to exert pressure on a tense muscle) around with me so I can adjust chairs to suit my needs.

Don't suffer in silence for the sake of others; if standing up and walking around makes you feel better, do it!

Walking Backwards

The Gokhale Method is a system of healthy posture and movements designed to restore structural integrity. It was developed by Esther Gokhale, who experienced crippling back pain during her first pregnancy and eventually underwent an unsuccessful back surgery. She studied cultures with very low incidences of back pain and relearned how to move and hold her body, developing the Gokhale Method that is now taught throughout the world.

The Gokhale technique that worked wonders for my back was to practice walking backwards. When you walk backwards, your body naturally realigns.[11] You engage the muscles in your pelvis and in your lower abdomen. These muscles are designed to be engaged when walking, but we often let them go slack. When you turn back around and walk forward, you'll be amazed how much better you feel.

Walk This Way

I started having trouble seeing at a distance around the age of eight. My parents got me glasses, but I did not like the way I looked in them. Out of vanity, I avoided wearing them. Instead, I craned my neck forward in class to see the blackboard. It wasn't until I was twenty-one and in medical school—where sharp vision is a requirement—that I finally relented and began wearing glasses regularly. My eyesight was corrected, but my bad posture remained. In medical school, under a critical atmosphere, I instinctively hunched forward and rounded my shoulders to armor myself. Because I cared, I leaned in when speaking with my patients. When I became a mother, I leaned in to soothe my children or hold them in my arms.

Over the years, whenever I would have a massage, the therapist always commented on how tight my neck and shoulder muscles felt. But I never felt pain, so I did not heed their warnings. When our bodies are pain free, we rarely think about how we stand, sit, or walk. It is human nature to ignore the risks inherent in our unhealthy habits until we experience a consequence. When my back pain erupted, I had to unlearn and unwind decades of poor posture.

Modern life makes it difficult to have good posture. Many of us spend an average of seven hours a day typing at our computers and many additional hours with our necks hyperextended as we use our phones or lay sprawled on the couch. Unlearning these habits requires being mindful of how you move. I frequently recommend to my patients the Alexander Technique, which is a movement-education method that teaches you to become more aware of your body habits and to re-educate your movement patterns for improved posture, coordination, and ease of movement. For more information, search online for one of the organizations that offer to teach it.

Migraines and Tension Headaches

For many years, my forty-seven-year-old patient Wendy's migraine headaches were under reasonable control. She was able to prevent flare-ups by avoiding her triggers: red wine and lack of sleep. When she did have a migraine attack, she self-treated with conventional medications, including ibuprofen and sumatriptan. One October, however, she had a spate of back-to-back severe migraines. Nothing she did seemed to prevent them or make them go away. They became unbearable to the point she could hardly get her work done. Wendy's neurologist recommended adding an antipsychotic medication for prevention.

Horrified at the prospect of such a drastic measure, Wendy called me. We zeroed in on the timing of her headaches, which had previously been under control. What had changed in her environment that October? We quickly realized that Wendy's spike in migraines coincided with an increase in wildfires in Northern California, where she lived. She described being housebound due to bad outdoor air quality for days on end. Wendy called in an HVAC technician, who found that her house air filters were completely clogged. Wildfire soot is indeed a trigger for migraines.[12] After replacing the filters, her headache frequency quickly abated.

Migraines are characterized by intense, throbbing pain lasting between four and seventy-two hours, almost always affecting one side of the head and often getting worse with activity. An estimated thirty-nine million Americans live with migraines.[13] As Wendy experienced, they can interfere with daily activities. Beyond the hallmark headache, migraines can present with other neurological symptoms, such as visual disturbances—known as an *aura*—which can precede or accompany the headache; a sensitivity to light and sound; nausea and vomiting; sensory changes, such as tingling or numbness in the face; dizziness or vertigo; and sudden mood changes.

Tension headaches are another common form of headache. They are often described as a tight band or pressure around the forehead or back of the head and neck. Unlike migraines, tension headaches typically occur on both sides of the head. Tension headaches can last from thirty minutes to several days,[14] and are not usually accompanied by visual disturbances, nausea, or vomiting. The episodic form (in which headaches occur fewer than fifteen days per month) is usually triggered by stress, anxiety, fatigue, or muscle strain. Chronic tension headaches can manifest as frequently as fifteen or more headaches per month.

When migraine or tension headaches are severe or occur frequently, they can lead to CS. A significantly reduced threshold for pain in the skin can occur, as well as peripheral sensitization in which migraine headaches are exacerbated by physical activity. The trigeminal nerve (which runs from the brain to the face) can become abnormally excitable as well. All these mechanisms lead to seemingly normal stimuli triggering headaches. If this has happened to you, review the previous section on neural circuit pain and begin instituting steps to retrain your brain to help desensitize it to triggers.

There are many additional steps you can take to activate your recovery reflex and reduce the frequency or intensity of headaches. Here is what I recommend:

Avoid Air Pollution: As we saw with Wendy, air pollution is a trigger for migraines and can exacerbate the frequency and severity of attacks. Before spending time outdoors, check the air quality index, which measures pollution levels and provides information on how safe it is to be outside. On days with poor air quality, opt for indoor exercise to avoid inhaling pollutants that can trigger migraines. Use air purifiers with HEPA filters in your living, working, and sleeping spaces to reduce pollutants. Create a schedule to regularly check your air filters.

Improve Sleep Habits: Insufficient sleep is a common trigger for migraines. A recent study conducted at the University of Arizona confirmed that participants who had poor sleep quality and low energy were much more likely to report having a migraine the following morning. See the "Sleeping Soundly" chapter for more information about improving your sleep habits.

Vagus Nerve Stimulation (VNS): A noninvasive device called gammaCore applies electrical stimulation to the neck overlaying the vagus nerve. The sensor is typically applied for up to twelve minutes per day (alternating sides of the neck), typically in two-minute sessions. It can help prevent and treat migraine attacks,[15] as well as cluster headaches, which are known for causing extreme pain and tend to occur in cyclical patterns, or "clusters."[16]

Exercise: Exercise can be a valuable tool in managing tension headaches, offering both immediate and long-term benefits. Exercises that focus on stretching and strengthening in particular can reduce muscle tension in the neck, shoulders, and back.[17] Exercise also stimulates the production of endorphins, your body's natural painkillers and mood elevators. The relationship between exercise and migraines is murkier. While exercise is a migraine trigger for some people, it has been shown to be prophylactic for others. One study that followed more than forty-six thousand Europeans for over a decade observed that "physically inactive subjects had a higher prevalence of self-reported migraine and/or recurrent headache than physically active subjects."[18]

Explore Acupuncture: Studies have shown that acupuncture may be as good or better than medication for both migraines and tension headaches.[19] For migraines, six to eight sessions are usually required to see a decrease in attacks.[20]

Use Peppermint Oil: Peppermint oil is pleasant and can be an invigorating topical treatment for tension headaches (and potentially migraines).[21] Infuse three to four peppermint tea bags for 10 minutes with a lid on top of the mug to keep the volatile oils from escaping. Then pour the liquid into a bowl of ice cubes. Soak a flannel or washcloth in the ice cold tea and place it on your forehead. Menthol, an active ingredient in peppermint oil, has been shown to reduce pain levels and dilate blood vessels.[22] Apply three or four times daily, or as needed.

Botox Injections: While you may associate Botox with treating crow's feet and smile lines, it is also approved by the NHS for the prevention of migraines. Botox is believed to block neurotransmitters that carry pain signals from your brain, preventing a migraine from being triggered. While Botox is not NHS-approved specifically for tension headaches, studies support its use for chronic tension headaches based on its muscle-relaxing properties.[23] Treatment typically involves multiple injections of Botox around the head, neck, and shoulders every twelve weeks. The exact pattern and number of injections varies, depending on your specific symptoms.

Ketogenic Diet: A ketogenic diet, high in fats and low in carbohydrates, has been used for decades to manage epilepsy. Recent studies have shown it may also be effective in controlling migraines. The keto diet is thought to enhance energy production in your cells, which could help correct underlying metabolic issues associated with migraines. While there are various forms of high-fat, low-carb diets, a meta-analysis involving ten studies found that a very low-calorie keto diet, a classic keto diet with normal calorie intake, and a modified Atkins diet are all effective at reducing the frequency and intensity of migraines.[24] (See page 256 for more information about implementing a keto diet.)

Green Light: Photo-biomodulation with green light–emitting diodes, a therapeutic technique that uses low-intensity light to stimulate cellular processes and promote healing, has been shown to reduce the number of headaches in people with episodic and chronic migraine headaches. In one study, researchers asked participants to expose themselves to photo-biomodulation for one to two hours daily.[25] Their headache frequency dropped from 7.9 headaches per month to 2.4 in the episodic group and from 22.3 to 9.4 per month in the chronic-migraine group.

Manage Stress: Stress is often cited as the primary trigger for migraine attacks, which often come on at the end of a stressful period, known as the "let down." Stress induces the release of hormones that can affect blood-vessel constriction and inflammation. Stress is also a primary trigger for tension headaches, as it can lead to muscle tension. Cognitive behavioral therapy (CBT) can be used to help people revise negative thought patterns, like the ones my twenty-two-year-old patient Darren described. He simply could not shake the thought, *My headache will never get better.* CBT helped him change that to, *I have many ways to manage a headache, should one come on.* CBT has been found effective for both migraines and tension headaches.[26] Other stress-management practices that have been proven to reduce migraines include biofeedback, relaxation training, mindfulness, hypnosis, and yoga.[27]

Supplements: Finally, there are several supplements that can help prevent headaches. Talk to your healthcare team about adding one to your existing care plan. I recommend:

- **Magnesium:** Studies have shown that people who have frequent migraines and tension headaches tend to have lower levels of the mineral magnesium,[28] which is involved in nerve transmission and muscle contraction. Magnesium also affects the regulation of blood flow and can dilate blood vessels, combatting blood constriction, a key factor in the onset of migraines. One trial revealed that people who took magnesium supplements had 42 percent fewer migraines; those given placebo had a 16 percent reduction.[29] I recommend a daily dosage of 400 mg of magnesium citrate.[30] If magnesium citrate is hard on your GI tract (for some people it causes diarrhea), experiment with the same dose of magnesium glycinate. If you have trouble swallowing pills, magnesium also comes in a powder form that is dissolvable in water. I also have many patients who swear by taking a bath with Epsom salts—a relaxing way to absorb magnesium! Buy it in bulk and pour a full cup into the bath water.

- **Riboflavin:** Also known as vitamin B2, riboflavin is a micronutrient essential for the proper functioning of the mitochondria, the cell's energy factory. Because migraines are associated with mitochondrial dysfunction, taking supplemental riboflavin has been explored as a treatment. Several studies confirm that a dose of around 400 mg per day can significantly reduce the frequency and severity of migraine attacks.[31]
- **Coenzyme Q10 (CoQ10):** CoQ10 plays a role in energy production within cells. Like riboflavin, it can help improve mitochondrial function and reduce the frequency of migraine attacks.[32] The typical dose is 100 to 150 mg daily.[33]
- **Butterbur Extract:** Sorry, Harry Potter fans, I don't mean "butter beer." Butterbur (*Petasites hybridus*), with its distinctive broad leaves and lilac-colored flowers, is a perennial plant found in Europe, Asia, and parts of North America. Clinical trials have found that butterbur can reduce the frequency of migraine attacks when taken regularly. A prevention study enrolled people ages eighteen to sixty-five with frequent migraines.[34] Participants who were randomized to take 75 mg of butterbur extract twice daily experienced a 48 percent reduction in migraine attack frequency. Be sure to purchase a brand that removes pyrrolizidine alkaloids (which can cause liver toxicity). As of the time of this writing, there are several brands available online; choose one from a reliable source.

Nerve Pain

My patient Sam asked for a telephone visit a month after she was diagnosed with shingles, a painful rash caused by the same virus that causes chicken pox in childhood. Her doctor prescribed an antiviral medication as soon as he saw the rash, which followed a dermatomal pattern diagonally down one side of her back to her buttock. But now she was having trouble sleeping owing to the persistent burning pain. She was equally bothered during the day, making her feel, as she put it, "grumpy." I recommended acupuncture twice per week and topical treatment with capsaicin cream, which is derived from hot peppers. (More about these treatments later.) Eight acupuncture treatments and four weeks later, her pain had essentially resolved.

Sam's story is typical of post-herpetic neuralgia (PHN), which is a complication of shingles.[35] While aciclovir (or acyclovir) is the most commonly recommended conventional treatment, it has not been shown to reduce PHN.[36] And nerve pain like Sam's, also known as neuropathic pain, can continue long after the initial shingles rash has healed. It's often described as a burning, shooting, or stabbing sensation and may be accompanied by sensations of tingling, numbness, or the feeling of "pins and needles." Nerve pain can also present as a sensation of "lancinating pain," which refers to a sudden and severe stabbing pain that occurs in brief but recurrent episodes; it's sometimes described as feeling like an electric shock. In addition to post-herpetic neuralgia, some of the most common causes of nerve pain include diabetic and trigeminal neuralgia.[37]

To relieve nerve pain, I recommend the following.

Lidocaine Patches: Lidocaine will be familiar to most people as a local anesthetic. Lidocaine patches are available over the counter with a concentration of 4 percent and by prescription at 5 percent concentration. They can easily be cut to fit over the localized area of pain and are a low-risk and frequently effective strategy for nerve pain. (Take care not to leave on longer than twelve hours.) One review looked at 332 patients using lidocaine patches for nerve pain and found that by day seven of treatment, 66 percent reported improvement in pain intensity while 74 percent experienced improved quality of life.[38]

Capsaicin: As we saw with Sam, capsaicin—the component that gives hot peppers their heat—is often effective at treating nerve pain.[39] It's made into creams, gels, and patches, but it may be a bit tricky to use, as it can actually cause pain (which is what it is supposed to treat!) and irritation when first applied. If you struggle to tolerate the sensation, numbing agents (like lidocaine) can be used prior to the application of capsaicin patches.[40] Despite the challenge in applying capsaicin, it may be worth persevering, since the application of one 8 percent patch for up to an hour has been shown to bring relief for up to twelve weeks.[41]

Alpha-Lipoic Acid (ALA): A naturally occurring compound, ALA serves as a powerful antioxidant in the body. It has been studied for its benefits in relieving nerve pain, primarily due to diabetic neuropathy.[42] ALA is thought to reduce inflammation in the body, increase blood circulation to the nerves,[43] and improve insulin sensitivity, which can help alleviate nerve pain among people with diabetes.[44] I have prescribed ALA to many people with peripheral neuropathy from various causes. They tell me it gradually dampens the nerve sensations to the point where they no longer interfere with sleep. I recommend beginning with a dose of 200 mg twice daily, but you may need as much as 600 mg twice daily for relief.

Glutamine: Glutamine is an amino acid found in our bodies, as well as in foods like grains, dairy, fish, poultry, and meat.[45] It plays key roles in various physiological processes, including muscle repair, immune system function, and gut health. In supplement form, glutamine has been shown to reduce nerve pain caused by chemotherapy by helping to repair and maintain nerve tissue and reduce inflammation.[46] Ask your doctor about using glutamine; I recommend you buy it as a powder and take 10 grams in a small amount of water or juice twice daily. A side benefit is that glutamine acts as a nutrient for the intestinal lining and can help support the gut microbiome.[47]

Lion's Mane Mushroom: Lion's mane mushroom (Scientific name *Hericium erinaceus*) is a powerful antioxidant. It can stimulate the production of nerve growth factor (NGF), a protein crucial for the growth, maintenance, and regeneration of nerve cells.[48] Nerves grow slowly, so you will have to stick with lion's mane for at least three months to see benefits. The dose has not yet been standardized, but I usually advise my patients to take one 500 mg capsule twice daily. Lion's mane may also confers side benefits: it reduces stress and can improve cognitive performance in healthy adults.[49]

Cannabis: Although illegal in many countries, cannabis is legal in thirty-eight U.S. states for medicinal use. In the "Unwinding Anxiety" chapter I discuss the use of cannabis for stress;[50] it may also be valuable for treating nerve pain. A 2024, meta-analysis found that plant-based THC alone had the most evidence for alleviating nerve pain.[51] If it is legal where you live, I recommend starting with a low dose and titrating up slowly, if needed. The exact dose will depend on the method of administration (such as smoked, sublingual, or edible). A 25 mg inhaled dose of 9.4 percent THC herbal cannabis used three times daily was found to be effective in reducing chronic neuropathic pain. As a side benefit, it also improved sleep.[52]

Ketamine: Ketamine therapy has been studied for the potential mitigation of severe nerve pain when administered intravenously. The mechanism is twofold, altering transmission along the nerve pathway and reducing inflammation.[53] However, ketamine is illegal in the U.K. except for restricted medicinal use.

Acupuncture: Acupuncture appears to improve conduction in sensory and motor nerves, altering the pain signals sent to the brain. It may also promote the release of endorphins, which reduce the perception of pain. A review of studies that included 680 patients with various forms of neuropathy found that acupuncture was four times more likely to lead to symptom improvement than control subjects.[54]

Electrical Stimulation: There are a number of different tools that deliver small amounts of electrical currents to relieve pain and help heal tissues. The TENS unit is one device frequently recommended by physiotherapists. A lesser-known unit is Alpha-Stim, which has been studied in veterans with chronic or persistent pain lasting three months or longer.[55] Alpha-Stim treatment was associated with reductions in pain severity, improved mood, and less depression and anxiety. It is distributed widely by the Veterans Administration (VA) and is available on the NHS for treating anxiety. Another device, Laser Touch One, was also studied[56] at the VA and found to reduce pain and anxiety. These devices can also be effective for neuralgias. (Note: Talk to your doctor before using one of these devices. Electrical stimulation devices are not recommended if you are pregnant, have a seizure disorder, or have a pacemaker or an implanted defibrillator.)

Hyperbaric Oxygen Therapy (HBOT): HBOT is a medical treatment in which you sit in a pressurized chamber and breathe pure oxygen. This increases the concentration of oxygen in the tissues of the body and can improve the healing of damaged nerves. HBOT has been studied in people with longstanding nerve pain,[57] and has been found to reduce pain and improve quality of life. For full effect, HBOT sessions are typically administered daily for 90 to 120 minutes, for a total of twenty to forty consecutive sessions.

If it persists, nerve pain can also lead to central sensitization. The nervous system becomes overactive in processing the pain signals, and even mild stimuli can cause the hallmark burning, shooting, or stabbing sensations. The recommendations I made earlier for neural circuit pain apply here as well.

Osteoarthritis

About a decade ago, my colleague Andrew Weil, M.D., woke up with excruciating pain in his right knee. There was no triggering event, no accident, no old sports injury from years earlier. One day his knee was fine, and the next he could barely put any weight on it. Andy (what I and most of his friends call him) tried everything from icing to ibuprofen, to bracing, but the pain remained for days. Finally, he booked an appointment with an orthopedist.

Andy feared he had osteoarthritis (OA), which occurs when the smooth, slippery surface at the ends of bones, called *cartilage*, wears down over time. Cartilage normally allows bones to glide smoothly when you move. When it erodes, the bones start rubbing against each other, causing pain, swelling, and difficulty moving the joint. Osteoarthritis tends to occur as people get older, but it can also be instigated by obesity, previous joint injuries, and genetic predisposition.

An X-ray indeed confirmed advanced osteoarthritis of Andy's right knee. The orthopedist told him he had no cartilage left, and that he would likely need a total knee replacement. The pain persisted and made walking difficult, but Andy was not yet ready to undergo surgery. Instead, he sought out a movement specialist trained in yoga, Rolfing, Feldenkrais, and trigger-point therapy. He came to the conclusion that Andy's right side had excessive tension from head to toe that was not evident on his left side. The problem was load distribution, meaning he was using his body in an asymmetric way. After two sessions, during which Andy learned to distribute his weight more evenly across his body, he was completely pain free.

Andy told me he has had a few recurrences over the years that are usually short lived. "Knowing that it goes away quickly makes me not worry about it; it's just an occasional nuisance." He did eventually see a second orthopedic specialist widely sought out by athletes, who told him, "You just have an old knee.... I wouldn't run up mountains, but you should be able to do anything else you want."

Andy's results may not be typical of the nearly thirty-three million Americans who suffer from osteoarthritis,[58] but his experience does challenge our assumptions about the course of arthritis. Often, when a person complains of stiffness and aching in a joint and an X-ray indicates wear and tear, they are told they need a joint replacement. I am struck by research revealing that 373 cases of OA are identified for every ten thousand people screened by X-ray,[59] but of these cases, just fifty are symptomatic. This means only one in seven people with a worn-down knee on an X-ray actually complains of pain. In short, being diagnosed with OA based on an X-ray does not always mean you need aggressive treatment like surgery. As with Andy, arthritis pain can come and go. It may be worse in damp cold weather or after overuse, and it may feel better when the joint has been rested.

Adopting better biomechanics can also make a big difference. People whose legs are knock-kneed or bowed have more arthritis, owing to a malalignment that puts extra stress on one part of the joint. Re-aligning your gait, as Andy did, can reduce this stress. Physiotherapy can also play a major role in reducing arthritis symptoms. Physiotherapists use manual therapy (such as joint mobilization or massage), heat or cold therapy, electrical stimulation (TENS units), and ultrasound. These interventions can decrease pain and inflammation in the affected joints. Studies also routinely suggest that physiotherapy, especially when resistance exercises are included, can slow the progression of osteoarthritis.[60]

Researchers are increasingly casting doubt on the theory that osteoarthritis is solely caused by wear and tear on joints. William Robinson MD, PhD, an associate professor of immunology and rheumatology at Stanford University, has published numerous studies suggesting that low-grade inflammatory processes play a role in osteoarthritis. According to Dr. Robinson, initial damage to a joint can set in motion a chain of molecular events that "escalates into an attack upon the damaged joint by one of the body's key defense systems against bacterial and viral infections, the so-called complement system."[61] In one study, he tore a bit of the cartilage in two sets of mice;[62] this kind of injury typically leads to osteoarthritis. One set of mice was bioengineered to knock out the complement system, and they ultimately developed much less severe arthritis than the normal mice despite having the same injury.

For humans suffering with osteoarthritis, this research suggests that reducing inflammation can help. Adopting an anti-inflammatory diet, taking anti-inflammatory supplements, and even reducing stress—all of which I will discuss more in depth in the following section on rheumatoid arthritis—are all likely to ease your pain.

Conventional treatments for osteoarthritis typically focus on relieving symptoms and improving joint function. If you're overweight, losing weight can significantly reduce stress on weight-bearing joints; it can also reduce pain and prevent further damage. Excess weight puts a disproportionate burden on the knee joints. Simply moving around causes the load on your knee joints to equal four to six times your body weight.[63] So, if you weigh 68 kilograms (10 stone 10 lb/150 lb), your knees support 270–400 kilograms (600–900 lb) of force when you stand or walk! This pressure can be even further magnified when you are walking up steps or squatting to pick up something from the floor.

Pharmaceutical treatments include over-the-counter pain relievers like paracetamol (acetaminophen), nonsteroidal anti-inflammatory drugs (NSAIDs) like ibuprofen, and naproxen sodium. Topical NSAIDs are also effective; apply the ointment directly on the arthritic joint, thereby avoiding some of the side effects of oral NSAIDs, such as GI discomfort. Capsaicin, discussed earlier, is also an effective treatment for OA. When applied to the skin, capsaicin works by gradually depleting substance P, a chemical messenger associated with pain transmission and inflammatory processes;[64] over time, this can reduce the pain signals sent to the brain. Mentholated salves such as Tiger Balm, Bengay, or "Blue" are also commonly used to relieve arthritis pain.

In more severe cases, doctors may recommend injecting a substance directly into the joint to reduce pain and inflammation, including corticosteroids, platelet-rich plasma, prolotherapy, or hyaluronic acid. Steroids must be used sparingly, though; while they are potent anti-inflammatory agents, repeated use can worsen joint damage over time. Not all of these treatments are available on the NHS, but they may be available at a private clinic in your area. Prolotherapy is a treatment in which a dextrose solution (sugar) is injected every two to six weeks over the course of several months. Alternatively, hyaluronic acid injections can help restore fluidity and elasticity to the joint and have been shown to reduce arthritis pain, improve function, and delay the need for surgery. These injectables have been shown to be more effective than NSAIDs or even steroid shots in reducing pain and improving function.[65]

Finally, platelet-rich plasma (PRP) uses the healing properties of your own blood to treat osteoarthritis. The process involves drawing blood, processing it to concentrate the platelets (which are rich in molecules that stimulate tissue regeneration), and then injecting the PRP directly into the affected joint. Early studies suggest that PRP therapy may reduce inflammation and potentially accelerate the repair of damaged cartilage, tendons, and ligaments in the joint affected by osteoarthritis.[66]

My patient Sandra had significant hip pain that limited her ability to walk more than a few hundred meters. She went to a Rolfer, a physiotherapist, and a massage therapist, all with only minimal relief. A physiatrist finally ordered an MRI and diagnosed her with a tear in her labrum, the rim of soft cartilage around her hip joint. When Sandra was treated with PRP, she finally found pain relief. Six months later, she told me with real joy in her voice that she had walked 11 kilometers (7 miles) daily on her visit to Paris.

If you are suffering with OA, choose the type of exercise you do with care. I recommend lower-impact activities like swimming, cycling, and light weight training, which put little stress on the joints, as opposed to running, jumping, and stair climbing. If the strategies described here haven't helped, remarkable advances have been made in orthopedic surgery, and most people with arthritis are delighted with their results. (See the "Recovery from Orthopedic Surgery" chapter for more information.) Most important, if you are in pain, don't wait to take action; there are many ways to address OA and reduce the risk of central sensitization, which can occur if the pain is persistent and severe enough.

Are NSAIDs Dangerous?

Nonsteroidal anti-inflammatory drugs (NSAIDs) are commonly used to treat osteoarthritis. Available over the counter, they are easy to access and can provide rapid relief. Still, I caution against their long-term uses, especially if you have existing kidney disease or a history of stomach ulcers.

NSAIDs can cause irritation of the GI tract, leading to stomach irritation or, more seriously, ulcers and gastrointestinal bleeding. The risk is higher in older adults.[67] When using NSAIDs for arthritis or other pain, use the lowest effective dose for the shortest duration to manage symptoms.

Rheumatoid and Other Inflammatory Arthritis Conditions

When Martha came to see me, her life was in freefall. She was caring for her father, who had advanced Alzheimer's disease, and her husband, who had just been diagnosed with prostate cancer. Her oldest son was going through a divorce, and her youngest had just been charged with a DWI. Her business was failing, and she had been recently forced to declare bankruptcy. She had also gained a significant amount of weight and had terrible knee pain. Her blood work revealed markers for an autoimmune disease, and a rheumatologist diagnosed her with mixed connective tissue disease, which is a form of inflammatory arthritis.

I put Martha on a gluten-free, plant-based diet, and I encouraged her to eat organic foods. We discussed potential environmental chemicals that could be affecting her, and I recommended she do her best to avoid plastics and use a water filter at home. Martha learned daily de-stressing techniques, including 4-7-8 breathing and mindfulness-based stress reduction. Slowly but surely, she got better. Her family life stabilized along with her business. Her knee pain dramatically decreased, and she began walking 5 kilometers (3 miles) per day. When she returned to her rheumatologist to get her blood retested, he was baffled: Her markers for mixed connective tissue disorder had disappeared entirely. "Your numbers are like a twenty-year-old's!" he exclaimed.

Rheumatoid arthritis (RA) is another form of autoimmune arthritis. *Autoimmunity* is when the body's immune system mistakenly sees itself as foreign and launches an attack on its own tissues. In the case of RA, this attack is primarily levied against the joints, causing pain, swelling, and if left unchecked, joint damage. RA usually affects multiple joints in the body in a symmetrical pattern. That means if one finger or thumb is affected, the finger or thumb on the opposite hand is likely to be affected, as well. Central sensitization can also occur in RA, amplifying the pain that was initiated by the inflammation and peripheral joint damage.[68]

An RA diagnosis is made via patient history, a physical examination that shows signs of symmetrical inflammation, and laboratory tests. The first step toward treating RA is to dial back all modifiable risk factors, which include the following:

1. **Smoking:** Smoking cigarettes is the most established modifiable risk factor for RA.[69] It significantly increases the risk of developing the disease and can also exacerbate its severity.
2. **Obesity:** A high body-mass index has been linked to an increased risk of RA.[70] Fat cells produce adipokines (a type of signaling protein),

which promote inflammation. Losing weight can decrease the risk and may improve disease outcomes.

3. **Traditional Western Diet:** Meals rich in saturated fats (including dairy, poultry, and red meat), trans fats, and refined sugars are associated with increased inflammation.[71]
4. **Sugar-Sweetened Beverages:** One study found a 63 percent increased risk of RA in women who consumed one or more sugar sweetened beverage daily compared to those who had less than one per month.[72] This finding was even stronger for women whose RA was diagnosed after the age of fifty-five.
5. **Gum disease:** More commonly called *periodontal disease*, this is an inflammatory condition affecting the gums and the supporting structures of the teeth. The bacteria that cause gum disease can enter the bloodstream, triggering an immune response that can increase inflammation throughout the body, including in the joints.[73]
6. **Air Pollution:** Wildfires and other sources of air pollution can increase the risk of developing RA or exacerbate existing symptoms.[74] For instance, increased inflammatory arthritis was seen in people exposed to debris as a result of the September 11 World Trade Center attacks.[75] Pollution contains particulate matter, volatile organic compounds, carbon monoxide, nitrogen dioxide, and other pollutants that can trigger inflammatory responses in the body.

Before the advent of disease-modifying anti-rheumatic drugs (DMARDs), it was common to see people with misshapen hands owing to the destructive nature of aggressive RA. Older medications, including methotrexate, hydroxychloroquine, and sulfasalazine, often helped put RA into remission and stopped its destruction of the joints. Newer biologic agents,[76] including adalimumab, etanercept, and infliximab, along with medications such as the IL-6 receptor antibody tocilizumab and JAK inhibitor tofacitinib, can have a dramatic impact in driving RA into remission. Still, my colleague Dr. Jill Weintraub, an integrative rheumatologist and graduate of our Integrative Medicine Fellowship, points out that patients achieve clinical remission only about 50 percent of the time when using a conventional medication-based regiment alone, highlighting the need for the integrative approach described here.

Your recovery reflex can help you recover from RA (or other autoimmune diseases). By altering your risk factors and following the integrative-medicine recommendations that follow, it is possible to put your RA into remission or prevent it from worsening. Here is what I recommend.

Fasting: Fasting can reduce the production of cytokines, which are signaling proteins that play a key role in promoting inflammation. Reducing cytokines helps decrease joint inflammation, pain, and swelling. There are many different ways to fast and careful planning enhances success. In one study,[77] thirty-five participants with RA were followed during Ramadan, when observant Muslims fast for thirty days from dawn to dusk. The study found that during the fasting month and for three months following, RA symptoms were significantly reduced. Another study was carried out in which twenty people with RA fasted (drinking tea, broth, and juices only) for seven to ten days and then followed a strict vegan diet. At the end of the study, they reported significantly less pain and an improvement in RA symptoms.

Fasting can change the composition of the gut microbiome, which plays a role in immune system regulation and inflammation. Of course, a fast is not a sustainable long-term strategy. To maintain the benefits of the fast, I encourage you to reintroduce foods slowly, testing them one at a time to see which foods worsen inflammatory symptoms. See "Your Rapid Recovery Toolkit" for further instructions about elimination diets. Note that fasting is not recommended for people who are significantly underweight.

Fasting-Mimicking Diet: Many of my rheumatology colleagues also prescribe a fasting-mimicking diet (FMD) rather than a full fast. This program is designed to provide the benefits of fasting while allowing you to eat about five hundred calories per day for five days. One commercially available product I commonly recommend is the Prolon Five-Day Program (search online for their products in your local area), which has been studied in thirty-two trials; in their preclinical trials, the program was shown to suppress autoimmune cells and activate healthy immune cells.[78] Prolon is pricey, unfortunately, and I wish I could recommend a less-expensive option, but there is not currently another one with sufficient studies supporting it.

Mediterranean Diet: I commonly recommend a Mediterranean diet to my patients with RA. (See "Your Rapid Recovery Toolkit," appendix 1.) Studies show that the Mediterranean diet, which emphasizes vegetables, fruits, fish, and little meat, can reduce RA pain and increase physical function.[79]

ITIS Diet: A variation of the Mediterranean diet known as the ITIS diet, developed by Monica Guma, MD, a rheumatologist and researcher at the University of California, San Diego, is also effective in managing RA symptoms.[80] The ITIS diet includes a homemade shake (green veggies and fruit) each morning; green tea; oily fish (sardines, salmon, or tuna) twice per week; a high daily intake of monounsaturated fatty acids, found in foods such as avocado, nuts, and seeds; unsweetened yogurt and miso; fruits high in enzymes, such as pineapple and papaya; and turmeric. The diet excludes wheat flour and gluten, which some studies show may exacerbate RA symptoms; tomatoes, potatoes, and aubergine (eggplant); added salt; as well as any red meat, sugar, soda, and highly processed foods.[81] In one small study, twenty-two patients with RA followed the ITIS diet for two weeks. Half experienced a 50 percent improvement in symptoms, and some went into complete remission.[82]

Destressing: As we saw with Martha, stress can play an important role in the onset and treatment of RA, as stress hormones can alter the immune system's function. For people with RA, this can mean increased inflammation and pain.[83] I recommend practicing the 4-7-8 breathing twice daily and learning mindfulness-based stress reduction.

Sauna: Here's a feel-good recommendation for arthritis: Studies show that saunas increase blood flow and can limit inflammation and pain.[84] A pilot study of infrared sauna use by people with inflammatory arthritis found that it can reduce pain, stiffness, and fatigue.[85] Adverse effects reported in the Global Sauna Survey were mild, with the top three being dizziness, dehydration, and headache. While a sauna is generally considered safe, people with medical conditions involving unstable blood pressure (such as aortic stenosis or recent cardiac event or stroke), altered temperature-sensing capacity, or abnormalities in their autonomic nervous system (such as a recent spinal injury) should avoid the sauna.[86] Here's another side benefit to saunas: sauna bathing, which alternates hot sauna, cold water, and rest, can lead to intense feelings of happiness (known in Japan as the *totonou* state).[87]

Supplements to Take for OA and RA

The following supplements have been shown to help with some people's symptoms of osteoarthritis and rheumatoid arthritis.

Turmeric: Turmeric's active ingredient, curcumin, is known for its potent anti-inflammatory and antioxidant properties. Turmeric can inhibit the activity of molecules and enzymes that are involved in inflammation, helping to reduce joint pain and swelling.[88] It can take from six to twelve weeks to show effects, so it requires a little patience. The side benefits of turmeric may include improvement in non-alcoholic fatty liver disease, GORD, and depression.[89]

Boswellia: Also known as Indian frankincense, boswellia is an herbal extract taken from the *Boswellia serrata* tree. It has been used traditionally in Ayurvedic medicine to treat chronic inflammatory conditions. Its OA benefits come from its active components, known as boswellic acids, which can contribute to improved joint flexibility and mobility while reducing pain and inflammation, and potentially slowing cartilage damage.[90] The usual dose is a boswellia extract of 100 to 250 mg daily.[91]

Omega-3 Fatty Acids: Omega-3s have been studied in both OA and RA and found to alleviate symptoms by making your immune system work more efficiently, as well as by limiting inflammation.[92] Studies suggest that regular intake of omega-3 supplements may decrease the need for NSAIDs for pain relief and slow the progression of cartilage damage.[93]

I recommend a daily dose of 2 to 3 grams of EPA plus DHA. I have been impressed by patients over the years who have told me how much better their joints feel after a hike or long walk when they are on regular omega-3s (and turmeric).

S-Adenosyl-Methionine (SAMe): A compound naturally produced by the body, SAMe plays a crucial role in many biological processes. It is believed to help OA symptoms by controlling inflammation.[94] Preliminary studies suggest it may even promote cartilage repair and regeneration.[95] Multiple clinical trials have revealed that SAMe at a dose of 400 to 1,200 mg daily works better than placebo and is comparable to NSAIDs in reducing symptoms of OA.[96] SAMe generally has fewer side effects than NSAIDs, but may take longer (thirty days compared to fifteen) to take full effect. Side benefits may include improved liver function and less depressed mood!

Vitamin D: A twenty-six-year-old woman named Sarah came to me complaining of intermittent joint pain in her hands and knees. She had a family history of RA, and her labs indicated elevated levels of anti-citrullinated protein antibody, which is common among people with RA.[97] Notably, her blood work also indicated vitamin D levels well below normal. Sarah was highly motivated and followed my advice to adopt a Mediterranean diet and quit smoking. She also began taking turmeric supplements as well as vitamin D daily. Within six months of making these changes, her joint pain had disappeared. Studies indicate that low vitamin D levels may be associated with a higher risk of RA,[98] so I highly recommend getting your levels checked and supplementing as necessary.

Glucosamine Sulfate and Chondroitin: Two substances found naturally in cartilage—glucosamine sulfate and chondroitin—have been shown in a meta-analysis of almost four thousand people to reduce the symptoms of osteoarthritis when compared to a placebo.[99] They can contribute to maintaining the integrity of cartilage by providing the building blocks needed for repair and regeneration. I recommend a daily dose of 1,500 mg of glucosamine sulfate in combination with 400 mg of chondroitin.[100]

Vagus Nerve Stimulation for Rheumatoid Arthritis

In addition to its success with headaches, vagus nerve stimulation (VNS) has been explored for its potential benefits in treating RA.

VNS has been shown to inhibit the production of cytokines.[101] By reducing cytokines, VNS can potentially decrease inflammation and alleviate the symptoms of RA.[102] A trial of thirty patients of all ages with RA who wore a VNS for up to thirty minutes daily revealed reduced disease activity scores in more than 50 percent of the participants.[103]

Your Rapid Recovery Prescription for Deactivating Pain Signals

The degree of pain that you may experience is not necessarily correlated with the physical injury that initiated the pain. Consider whether central sensitization is contributing to your current discomfort. The following integrative strategies can help you relieve the pain, relax your nervous system, and revise the "story" that heightens your pain experience:

1. For back pain, adopt strategies such as mindfulness, guided imagery, and journaling to help reduce psychological stress. Become aware of your triggers and avoid them. Practice improving your posture and alignment.
2. For migraine and tension headaches, the following integrative strategies can help: avoiding air pollution, improving sleep habits, VNS, exercising, acupuncture, supplements, peppermint oil, Botox, a keto diet, and stress management.
3. Nerve pain may be diminished with lidocaine patches or capsaicin. Useful supplements to discuss with your doctor include ALA, glutamine, and lion's mane mushrooms. Additional strategies to explore are acupuncture, electrical stimulation, and HBOT.

4. For OA, begin by adopting better biomechanics and low-impact exercise. Anti-inflammatory diet and supplements can help. For more significant OA, consider an injection with PRP, hyaluronic acid, or steroids.
5. For RA, fasting (or a fasting-mimicking diet), a Mediterranean diet, an ITIS diet, destressing, and a sauna can all help.
6. Potentially beneficial supplements for both OA and RA include turmeric, boswellia, omega-3s, SAMe, and vitamin D.

11

Reversing Type 2 Diabetes

When I was a medical student on my surgery rotation, I admitted a patient, Roger, who needed a below-the-knee amputation of his leg owing to a diabetic ulcer that would not heal. As I took Roger's history, I observed that his blood sugar levels—which people with diabetes often struggle to keep down—were in the normal range.

"You're doing a good job of keeping your blood sugar under control," I said.

Roger looked at me wearily and then, gesturing to his leg, said, "You call *that* control?" At that moment I suddenly realized I had been indoctrinated with the conventional notion that the goal of medicine is to manage people with chronic disease instead of to restore their health. "Good" numbers provided no solace to Roger, who was about to lose his leg. As it turns out, Roger had a major influence on the doctor I would become, and I think about him often. My goal became first and foremost to partner with my patients and give them options that would help them become healthy.

Five years later, I was in practice in Santa Rosa, California, and I diagnosed another patient, David, with type 2 diabetes. He also had high blood pressure and high cholesterol, and he was dismayed at the thought of taking yet another medication—or, even worse, insulin shots. He asked me if there was anything else he could do. I hesitated for a moment, then I told him about a doctor named John McDougall, who practiced just one town over, in St. Helena. Dr. McDougall was using a novel approach to treat diabetes: a low-fat vegan diet.

Back in 1965, when McDougall was just eighteen, he suffered a massive stroke that left him paralyzed on the left side of his body for two weeks.[1] When his doctors could not explain how this had happened at such a young age, or if he could prevent another stroke, McDougall developed the bold idea that his steady diet of eggs, cheese pizzas, and hot dogs was to blame. He went on to medical school, and later founded the McDougall Program, which advocates a low-fat vegan diet (that is, devoid of animal products). When David heard that Dr. McDougall's diet had helped people reverse their type 2 diabetes, he was excited and committed to make the change. He came back to my office every two months, and over time I watched him lose 18 kilograms (2¾ stone/40 lb) and reverse his elevated cholesterol and high blood pressure diagnosis. Ten months later, David's type 2 diabetes was gone. Plus, he felt amazing. All because he changed the way he ate. His experience stirred something deep inside me. *This* was why I had become a doctor: to help people heal.

For centuries, ancient Greek, Indian, and Egyptian civilizations correctly diagnosed diabetes (although it wasn't yet called by that name) by observing increased urination, as well as excess sweetness,[2] by literally tasting it! Much later, the condition became known as *diabetes mellitus*, originating from the Greek word *diabetes*, meaning "to pass through," and the Latin word *mellitus,* meaning "sweet."[3] Indeed, diabetes is characterized by chronically high levels of glucose, or blood sugar, in the bloodstream. Normally, when your blood sugar rises after eating a meal, your pancreas produces the hormone insulin, which your cells use to convert sugar into energy for immediate use or into fat for long-term storage—a perfect example of your recovery reflex maintaining homeostasis. Diabetes can disrupt this process in two ways. In type 1 diabetes, which afflicts about 1.7 million Americans and many more around the world,[4] the immune system destroys the insulin-producing islet cells in the pancreas, which is why people with type 1 diabetes must take insulin shots to maintain normal blood sugar. In the more common type 2 diabetes, the cells in the body become resistant to insulin's effects, and glucose builds up to unsafe levels.[5] It is this second, potentially reversible, form that we will focus on in this chapter.

My hope is for you, like David, not just to manage type 2 diabetes but also to recover from it fully.

Diabetes Reversal Through Diet

My seventy-five-year-old patient Fred was one of nine siblings. Each of them had developed type 2 diabetes, and Fred believed it was only a matter of time before the same fate befell him. His hemoglobin A1C test (abbreviated to HbA1c), which measures average blood sugar levels over the past three months, was well over 5.7 percent—the threshold for prediabetes, which is the precursor to type 2 diabetes. (An HbA1c of 6.5 percent or more signifies full-blown diabetes.[6])

"Is there anything I can do?" he asked me. We discussed options, and Fred decided to enroll in the Diabetes Prevention Program (DPP), available free of charge through the NHS and other venues across the country.[7] This program, accessible to people with prediabetes and sometimes covered by insurance,[8] is designed to help participants adopt healthy eating habits, start an exercise program, and lose weight. Fred began attending cooking classes, working out three times a week, and keeping track of his diet. After seven months, he lost about 12 kilograms (2 stone/27 lb) and his HbA1c levels returned to normal. Unlike the rest of his family, Fred has not developed diabetes.

Fred's experience is not unique. The DPP's success is evidence you can reverse prediabetes when you make simple lifestyle changes—an intervention far more effective than the standard diabetes medication, metformin. In a landmark study published in the *New England Journal of Medicine*,[9] the DPP enrolled three thousand participants with prediabetes. One-third were assigned intensive lifestyle modifications like Fred's, one-third received metformin, and one-third were given a placebo. By the end of the study, the lifestyle-modification group lost weight and reduced their risk of developing diabetes by 58 percent, compared to just 31 percent for the metformin group. The study concluded simply: "The lifestyle intervention was more effective than metformin."

Your recovery reflex can even reverse established type 2 diabetes with lifestyle changes. For example, in 2017, researchers from Weil Cornell Medicine-Qatar randomized 158 people with type 2 diabetes to receive either standard care with medications or an intensive lifestyle intervention that included exercise and a calorie-restricted diet.[10] At twelve months, the intervention group "had lost an average of twenty-six pounds [almost 12 kilograms/2 stone], 61 percent were no longer considered diabetic, and 33 percent had completely normal blood-sugar levels—all these measures being far better than those seen in the control group."

While a 7 percent weight loss is one of the DPP's goals, weight is just one of many variables involved in developing diabetes. Genetics, age, ethnicity, exercise habits, environmental toxins, and circadian rhythms all play roles, too. In fact, today, the fastest increase in diabetes diagnoses is among people who are not overweight; since 2015, cases of so-called lean diabetes have grown by 17.8 percent.[11] Some people who are significantly overweight never develop diabetes, and others who are at a normal weight do. While losing weight can help reverse type 2 diabetes, the focus in this chapter is on ways to restore blood sugar levels with dietary changes. You may lose weight as a side benefit, but this is not the primary goal.

As the McDougall program that David adopted showed, a low-fat vegan diet can be effective at reversing diabetes. In a recent study published in the *American Journal of Lifestyle Medicine*,[12] researchers analyzed the health records of fifty-nine patients with type 2 diabetes who were treated with a low-fat, whole food, "plant-predominant" diet at a health clinic. The diet consisted primarily of vegetables, pulses (legumes), whole grains, fruits, nuts, and seeds. More than a third of the participants achieved total remission from diabetes, while the number of people who required blood-sugar-lowering medication fell from forty to twenty-nine.

While many people benefit from a low-fat vegan diet, a seemingly opposite approach—namely, a low-carbohydrate diet—has also been proven to be effective. About a decade ago, a British doctor named David Unwin was concerned when one of his patients stopped refilling her type 2 diabetes medication. When she arrived at his surgery a full year later, he was shocked to find that she had gone into remission by dramatically cutting down on carbohydrates. She was also furious. "You've given me metformin for about ten years and you never once asked me about the side effects or gave me an alternative," she exclaimed. "I've now learned about cutting the carbs. I've lost weight and I feel fabulous."[13]

He had not, in fact, known just how dramatically carbohydrates impact diabetes. Subsequently, Dr. Unwin and his wife, Dr. Jen Unwin, a clinical psychologist, started a program to teach their patients how to use low-carb diets to reverse type 2 diabetes. Drs. Unwin followed 186 of their patients with diabetes for thirty-three months, finding that a low-carb diet led to a complete remission in 51 percent of cases, including more than three-fourths of patients who had been diagnosed in the previous year.[14] Another study followed 262 people with diabetes aged twenty-one to sixty-five over a two-year period.[15] They measured their blood sugar up to three times a day while receiving health coaching to help them adhere to the low-carb diet. At the end of a year, 60 percent had reversed their diabetes, with side benefits including lower incidences of fatty liver, obesity, and depression.

So which diet works best? This complex question was tackled by researchers at Stanford Medicine by studying the effect of either a ketogenic diet or a Mediterranean diet.[16] The keto group consumed high-quality animal- and plant-based protein and nonstarchy vegetables while avoiding nearly all other carbs, including pulses (legumes), most fruits, all grains, and all added sugars. Conversely, the Mediterranean diet group ate copious amounts of vegetables (including starchy ones), fruits, pulses (legumes), whole grains, nuts, seeds, and olive oil while avoiding animal-based protein except fish. (Studies reveal that eating omega-3-rich fish like salmon and sardines may help improve insulin sensitivity.[17]) Both groups avoided unhealthy processed carbs, including added sugars, anything made with white flour, and breakfast cereals. Despite taking very different approaches, at the end of the study, the keto and Mediterranean diets were equally helpful in reducing blood sugar levels.

However, while the keto diet was effective at lowering blood glucose levels, researchers found that many participants had trouble maintaining it after three months. "Even the participants who had followed the keto diet nearly perfectly during the trial largely gave it up afterward," the study concluded.[18] Another concern is the lack of long-term studies confirming whether keto diets prevent—or more important, if they might cause—heart disease. On the other hand, evidence shows that people who lose weight eating a Mediterranean diet tend to keep the extra weight off for the long term compared to other diets.[19] (For more information about the Mediterranean diet, see "Your Rapid Recovery Toolkit," appendix 1.)

Choosing organic food—especially organic produce—also reduces the risk of developing type 2 diabetes. The French NutriNet-Santé study found that for each 5 percent incremental increase in organic food intake, the risk of diabetes decreased by 3 percent.[20] Overall, people with the highest percentage of organic food consumption had a 35 percent lower risk of type 2 diabetes.

When it comes to diabetes reversal, no matter which diet you ultimately choose, avoiding ultra-processed foods is paramount. As we've seen repeatedly in this book, processed foods increase inflammation and interfere with your recovery reflex. These products have been highly transformed from their original state and contain ingredients like artificial colors, flavors, preservatives, sweeteners, and other additives. One meta-analysis from 2022 comprising almost 1.1 million people found that, compared with people who don't eat any ultra-processed foods, people who had a moderate intake of ultra-processed foods increased their risk of diabetes by 12 percent; those with a high intake increased their risk by 31 percent.[21]

To demonstrate how dramatically ultra-processed foods affect our health, Kevin Hall, PhD, and his research team at the U.S. National Institutes of Health (NIH) assigned twenty adults to eat an ultra-processed diet for two weeks, followed by an unprocessed whole-food diet for another two weeks.[22] Participants lived on the NIH campus and were allowed to eat as much or as little as they wanted at each meal. When on the ultra-processed food diet, the participants ate roughly five hundred more calories per day and gained 900 grams (2 lb), on average. (A few people gained as many as 6 kilograms/13 lb when eating the ultra-processed food!) When on the unprocessed diet, they lost the equivalent amount of weight.

The GI Index

When reversing prediabetes or diabetes with diet, it is critical to avoid foods that rank high on the glycemic index (GI), which measures how quickly a specific carbohydrate food is digested. Half the daily calories in a typical Western-style diet comes from carbohydrates, 80 percent of which come from high-GI foods like soda, bagels, crackers, biscuits and cookies, white bread, and breakfast cereals.[23] Also high on the GI scale are refined carbohydrates, which have been processed to remove parts of the grain, such as the bran and germ, resulting in a loss of fiber, vitamins, and minerals.

High-GI foods are digested and absorbed quickly, leading to a more immediate and significant rise in blood sugar. For people with diabetes, insulin does not work as well, so spikes in blood sugar are especially concerning. Low-GI foods, conversely, are digested and absorbed very slowly, leading to a gradual and more manageable rise in blood sugar. Think of the glycemic index as a fireplace: High-GI foods are like kindling, which burns up in minutes, while low-GI foods resemble heavy logs that burn slowly for hours. Here's a good rule of thumb: When you eat carbs, choose whole foods without a laundry list of ingredients. Healthy, low-GI options include soy products, pulses (legumes), and most vegetables. (Potatoes and parsnips are notable unhealthy exceptions.)

What about whole fruits? Even though they contain natural sugars, high fruit consumption is associated with a reduced risk of type 2 diabetes and overall mortality—with exceptions.[24] Fruits like mangos and pineapples are higher on the GI index. Apples, in contrast, are high in fiber, which slows digestion.[25] Different fruits affect people in different ways, and I recommend using a continuous glucose monitor to understand your blood sugar response. (I'll discuss these monitors later in the chapter.)

While the food you choose is important for diabetes reversal, we'll see next that timing your meals may be just as critical.

Reducing Blood Sugar Spikes with Vinegar

When you are craving a high-GI treat, here's a trick: Add 2 teaspoons of vinegar to your meal before eating the high-GI food. (You can add it to your salad before eating your main dish.) This can lower the postprandial (post-meal) bump in blood sugar by 20 percent, simply by delaying the emptying of the stomach and thereby slowing the carbohydrate absorption.[26]

Time-Restricted Eating

My patient Trey had struggled with weight for most of his life. At age thirty-six, routine blood tests indicated that his HbA1c level was in the prediabetes range. When I asked him to describe a typical day, he explained that he woke up at 4 a.m., ate a bagel and cream cheese and had coffee, then commuted an hour to work. Lunch was fast food, and his last meal was typically a ready meal around 7 p.m. When Trey balked at changing his diet, I suggested an experiment: Instead of eating first thing in the morning, he would stick to black coffee and have breakfast on the job around 9 a.m.

I had good reason to believe this change could work well for Trey, as resting the gut for twelve hours or more supports the circadian rhythm and restores equilibrium to the metabolic system. A review paper of multiple human trials suggests[27] that eating within a consistent window of eight to ten hours can help reverse diabetes. In one randomized controlled trial,[28] researchers enrolled thirty-six people with type 2 diabetes and asked them to follow an intermittent fasting plan. Remarkably, after three months, 90 percent of participants were able to reduce their blood-sugar-lowering medication, and 55 percent went into full diabetes remission and discontinued their medications entirely! Moreover, the majority were not people with new diagnoses: 65 percent of the participants who achieved remission had diabetes for more than six years.

Indeed, Trey had a similar experience. Even though he kept his diet the same, incorporating a fourteen-hour overnight fast brought his blood sugar back into the normal range. Over the following eighteen months, he lost 9 kilograms (20 lb) and felt better than he had in years. He was even inspired to sign up for a meal-prep service that made it possible for him to cook healthy meals for the first time in his life. What he loved was the ease: "All those other diets that doctors pushed on me were hard, and I couldn't eat any of my favorite foods. Time-restricted eating is easy for me to follow, and I can eat what I want."

Time-restricted eating (TRE) means consuming all your calories—including meals, snacks, and caloric beverages—within a certain window of time and fasting for the remaining hours. (Water, black coffee, and tea are all allowed during fasting hours.) TRE is a form of intermittent fasting, which includes a variety of strategies to limit the periods of eating. While three large meals per day with minimal fasting is a staple of modern society, it is not how human bodies evolved over millions of years. For most of our history, we may have eaten once or twice a day and fasted for sixteen hours or more.[29] While not everyone accepts this evolutionary theory, most scientists agree that it's healthy to have a respite at night, when the digestive system can reboot. Eating in alignment with your circadian rhythm can optimize metabolism, improve gut health, more effectively regulate glucose, and support your recovery reflex overall.[30]

TRE can be especially beneficial for the estimated 30 percent of Americans who are considered shift workers and many others around the globe. Staying awake during the night and early-morning hours disrupts your natural circadian rhythm, increasing the risk of obesity, type 2 diabetes, heart disease, and other long-standing conditions.[31] If you are a new parent, your frequently interrupted sleep schedule may put you in the "shift work" category, too. A clinical trial by the Salk Institute and UC San Diego Health examined 150 firefighters who worked night shifts, many of whom had elevated blood sugar levels.[32] Without changing their working hours, half the firefighters were instructed to eat within a ten-hour window, and the others ate within a fourteen-hour window. Both groups were encouraged to follow a Mediterranean-style diet. Here's the conclusion: The firefighters who limited their eating window to ten hours saw "significantly improved blood sugar and blood pressure . . . [TRE] may provide even greater benefit for those at risk for cardiometabolic disease and other chronic diseases."

If your goal is to lose weight, time-restricted eating is generally much easier than calorie counting—but it can be just as effective. In a 2023 study published in the *Annals of Internal Medicine*,[33] seventy-seven adults with obesity completed a calorie-restricted diet, a time-restricted diet, or no diet at all. After twelve months (six months of active weight loss and six months of weight maintenance), both the calorie-restricted and the time-restricted groups lost roughly the same amount of weight—4.5 kilograms (10 lb)—compared to the control. As the lead researcher concluded: "You can basically achieve the same amount of energy restriction by counting time instead of counting calories."[34]

How long do you have to fast each day to see health benefits? I recommend a minimum of twelve hours for everyone, and ideally fourteen if you are controlling your blood sugar. Talk to your doctor about whether this approach is right for you, and if so, how to monitor any medications you are taking. As for *when* to fast, I suggest experimenting with various eating windows to find your sweet spot.

Exercising After Eating

Blood sugar levels usually peak within ninety minutes of eating, a phenomenon known as your postprandial glucose level. However, research shows that if you exercise shortly after eating, you can greatly attenuate this spike.[35] This is because physical activity increases muscle contractions, which trigger glucose absorption. Additionally, exercise is thought to improve insulin sensitivity, meaning your body is better able to use available insulin to absorb glucose after meals.

The effect of exercise on blood sugar levels will vary depending on its timing, intensity, and type. Aerobic exercises such as walking, running, and cycling tend to lower blood sugar faster, compared to anaerobic exercises like weight lifting. Even a five-minute walk is enough to lower blood sugar after a meal, according to one 2022 meta-analysis.[36] Exactly how long after eating should you exercise? Research shows that beginning exercise within a thirty-minute window after eating will most effectively blunt the postprandial glucose spike.[37] Circadian rhythms are also relevant: A 2018 study revealed that afternoon exercise was more effective in reducing blood glucose levels than morning exercise.[38]

Most important, exercise can help prevent diabetes. This is true even in people whose genetics make them nearly two and a half times more likely to develop the disease. The UK Biobank trial[39] found a 74 percent reduced rate of type 2 diabetes in people who exercise for sixty-eight minutes a day, compared to those who clocked less than five minutes.

The speed at which you walk can also impact your health. In a 2023 meta-analysis, people who were measured walking at a speed of 3–5 kilometers per hour (2–3 mph) had a 15 percent lower risk of diabetes compared with those who strolled along at 3 kilometers per hour (2 mph).[40] And those who walked more briskly—5–6.4 kilometers per hour (3–4 mph)—had a 24 percent lower risk!

Supplements

While diet and exercise are two of the most valuable tools in your arsenal when it comes to reversing diabetes, a number of supplements have also been shown to be beneficial for stabilizing blood sugar levels. Here are some of the most effective.

Vitamin D: Numerous studies have shown that insufficient levels of vitamin D can lead to insulin resistance. A 2023 meta-analysis comprising more than four thousand people concluded that vitamin D was effective in decreasing risk for diabetes in adults with prediabetes.[41] A clinical trial from 2021 recruited 130 people with type 2 diabetes.[42] Half were instructed to supplement with vitamin D in addition to taking their prescribed medication (metformin); the other half continued solely with the metformin. At both three- and six-month follow-ups, HbA1c levels were significantly improved in people who supplemented with vitamin D. For more information about vitamin D supplements, including dosage, see "Your Rapid Recovery Toolkit" (appendix 1).

Chromium: A trace mineral, chromium has been shown to help manage type 2 diabetes by improving glucose metabolism and insulin sensitivity.[43] A meta-analysis of twenty-eight studies found significant reductions in HbA1c levels following chromium supplementation in patients with type 2 diabetes.[44] I recommend chromium picolinate (or chromium-rich yeast), starting with a dose of 200 mcg and gradually increasing as needed to a maximum of 1,000 mcg per day.

Alpha Lipoic Acid: Alpha lipoic acid (ALA) is a naturally occurring compound vital for cellular energy production. It's both fat and water soluble, allowing it to enter every cell in the body. ALA has been shown in studies to enhance the body's response to insulin and increase uptake of glucose into the cells.[45] I recommend starting with a dose of 200 mg per day. ALA can also be used to treat diabetic neuropathy (nerve damage induced by diabetes, causing symptoms such as numbness, tingling, and burning);[46] in this case, you will likely need a higher dose of 600 mg or more each day.[47]

Berberine: Berberine is a compound extracted from various plants, including shrubs of the *Berberis* genus. It has a long history of use in traditional Chinese and Ayurvedic medicine. In recent years, it has gained attention for its potential benefits in managing type 2 diabetes. In studies, berberine has been shown to manage blood sugar levels as effectively as metformin.[48] Berberine has multiple positive effects, including lowering glucose production in the liver, enhancing insulin sensitivity in cells, improving blood sugar by promoting the growth of good bacteria in the gut,[49] and acting as an anti-inflammatory.[50] The usual dose is 500 mg twice per day. Be aware that berberine can speed up the metabolism of commonly prescribed statins, making them less effective.[51]

Magnesium: Magnesium plays an important role in glucose metabolism and insulin sensitivity. Studies show that many people with type 2 diabetes have a magnesium deficiency,[52] so consider taking 200 to 400 mg of magnesium citrate or glycinate to improve insulin sensitivity and regulate blood sugar levels. Magnesium can loosen up your bowel movements—a welcome side benefit for many—but if it's too much, lower your dose or choose the glycinate form, which is less likely to cause diarrhea.[53]

Can Aspirin Lower Your Blood Sugar?

Aspirin, commonly used for its pain-relieving, anti-inflammatory, and blood-thinning properties, has not typically been used as a treatment to lower blood sugar levels. However, there is evidence that taking low-dose aspirin may reduce the risk of type 2 diabetes among older adults.

The Aspirin in Reducing Events in the Elderly (ASPREE) trial was a double-blind, randomized controlled trial of healthy adults aged sixty-five or older.[54] Participants took 100 mg of aspirin daily, and after a median follow-up of nearly five years, the aspirin group saw a 15 percent reduction in diabetes. However, note that aspirin can also cause gastrointestinal bleeding.

Medications

Two classes of medication have been shown most beneficial for controlling diabetes as you work toward reversing it, and these are the drugs I typically recommend.

Metformin: This is an NHS-approved medication for both prevention and treatment of type 2 diabetes. It is generally the first medication prescribed for diabetes because, while it effectively lowers both basal (fasting) and postprandial glucose levels, it does not usually cause hypoglycemia, a condition in which your blood sugar drops to unsafe levels. Metformin may have additional benefits:[55] In people with diabetes, it reduces the risk of all-cause mortality, cancer, and cardiovascular disease, while increasing longevity and health span (your total number of healthy years).

Common side effects of metformin include GI upset, which can often be managed by switching to an extended-release form. Metformin can also increase the production of lactic acid, which can be a problem for people with kidney disease. Metformin may also cause a deficiency in two important nutrients—B12 and magnesium—so be sure to have regular blood tests to check levels or take a supplement.

Glucagon-Like Peptide-1 (or GLP-1) Receptor Agonists: These drugs have received significant press in recent years for their ability to induce weight loss. They work by triggering an insulin release from the pancreas, thereby lowering blood glucose; blocking glucagon (another hormone that raises blood sugar levels); delaying stomach emptying, which slows digestion and the consequent rise in blood glucose; and increasing the sense of satiety after eating. There is evidence as well that GLP-1 medications can prevent heart attacks and strokes and improve kidney function.[56]

This class of medication includes semaglutides (Ozempic and Wegovy), which are now widely used as a weight-loss medication, as well as exenatides, liraglutides, lixisenatides, and dulaglutides. A similar medication, tirzepatide,[57] is a combination GLP-1 and GIP (glucose-dependent insulinotropic polypeptide) that has one additional mechanism: It helps regulate food intake. In addition to better blood-sugar control and weight loss, its side benefits include reducing atherosclerosis and heart failure. While these can sometimes seem like miracle medications—reducing people's craving for food—if they are stopped, weight gain almost always reoccurs. Additionally, not everyone tolerates these medications well, with abdominal bloating, nausea, vomiting, and diarrhea.

Multiple other classes of medications may be prescribed alone or in combination depending on your HbA1c level, response to other medications, heart-protective mechanisms, or side-effect profile. Sulfonylureas, which includes the medicines gliclazide, glipizide and glimepiride, are also commonly prescribed. While these medications help normalize blood sugar, they often have the unwanted side effect of weight gain and can cause hypoglycemic episodes, especially in older people. And thiazolidinediones, meglitinides, alpha-glucosidase inhibitors, SGLT2 inhibitors, and insulin are all used to treat, rather than reverse, diabetes.

Continuous Glucose Monitoring

In this chapter, I have discussed a variety of dietary patterns and their impact on blood sugar. I have also suggested that people can react differently to the same foods. While regular HbA1c tests—the blood test that measures your average glucose level over the course of three months—are useful for the diagnosis and long-term management of type 2 diabetes, they will not tell you which specific foods are spiking your blood sugar.

For this reason, I advise using a continuous glucose monitor (CGM), which I strongly believe will soon be a cornerstone of medicine. These are small wearable devices that provide personalized feedback about how your body reacts to the foods in your diet in real time. One of our fellowship graduates, Dr. David Cannon, an internal medicine specialist in Virginia, told me, "One thing that I think is really a game changer is continuous monitoring. I've seen several people who have just about totally reversed their diabetes using them. When they had that kind of feedback, they know exactly what does what and they're motivated."

For example, my thirty-four-year-old patient Kate was able to detect several foods that spiked her blood sugar into an unhealthy range when she used a CGM. She was surprised to learn that freshly pressed orange juice, which she had always considered super healthy; potatoes (she was from Idaho, known for its potatoes!); and rice all led to warning messages about spikes in her blood sugar. By eliminating these specific foods, Kate was able to keep her HbA1c stable and prevent a progression to diabetes. Curiously, when I wore a CGM, I saw that my blood sugar surged whenever I ate porridge made with coarse Scottish oats, but not cake or dark chocolate. Consequently, I gave up porridge as a breakfast food. But, before you rush to your local confectionery shop, remember that every body is different; what spikes my blood sugar may not spike yours, which is why I encourage you to experiment with a glucose monitor.

Your Rapid Recovery Prescription for Reversing Type 2 Diabetes

Prediabetes and type 2 diabetes can be reversed in most people using a host of strategies, including diet, exercise, medication, and supplements.

1. The most effective way to reverse type 2 diabetes is with dietary changes. Vegan, Mediterranean, and low-carbohydrate diets can all reverse diabetes in some people. The one that will work best for you over the long term is the one you are willing to adhere to.
2. No matter which diet you choose, limit your consumption of high-GI foods.
3. To get personalized feedback about your food choices, use a continuous glucose monitor. This will tell you the foods that increase your blood sugar the most.
4. Time-restricted eating can reverse or prevent type 2 diabetes. I recommend fasting for a minimum of fourteen hours daily if your goal is to better control your blood sugar.

5. Exercising within thirty minutes after a meal reduces blood sugar spikes.
6. Vitamin D, chromium, alpha lipoic acid, berberine, and magnesium supplements can help stabilize blood sugar levels.
7. Metformin has been proven to prevent progression from prediabetes to diabetes and may have other health benefits.

12

Easing Asthma

Can a healthy microbiome prevent asthma?

In 2016, researchers revealed the curious results of a study contrasting the rates of asthma in two traditional farming communities in the United States: the Amish of Indiana and the Hutterites of South Dakota.[1] The two populations share a similar genetic ancestry, lifestyles, customs, and diet; they do not allow household pets or get childhood vaccinations. The key difference: The Amish typically have small farms near their homes and rely on horses for fieldwork, whereas Hutterite farms are farther from home and use modern, industrialized farm machinery.

The study uncovered a "whopping disparity in asthma,"[2] with just 5 percent of Amish children having the condition, compared to 21.3 percent among the Hutterites. (Of note, 6.5 percent of American children have asthma.[3]) The reason? Amish children tend to run barefoot through barns near their houses and frequently interact with farm animals, leading to greater exposure to microbial products that confer protection against asthma. To confirm the link, the researchers exposed mice to the dust from both Amish and Hutterite homes. Sure enough, the airways of the mice that inhaled Amish dust were better protected against asthma-like responses to allergens.

Don't worry, I'm not going to recommend you adopt a horse or a cow to treat your asthma symptoms (although having a dog may help), nor will I suggest sprinkling house dust from Amish farms on your floors (although spending time in a home garden will help you develop a more diverse microbiome). Rather, what I'd like you to understand from this study is that asthma is influenced by many different factors, including your early microbe exposure, genetics, environmental agents, lifestyle factors, immune system makeup, and underlying health conditions. As we'll see, you can make the most of new scientific discoveries about the microbiome, inflammation, and even breathing practices to attune your recovery reflex and greatly reduce asthma symptoms.

Globally, more than 260 million people suffer from asthma, a longstanding condition characterized by the inflammation and narrowing of the airways that allow air to enter and exit the lungs.[4] For many years, we believed asthma had two distinct forms: *intrinsic asthma*, in which nonallergic factors, including infections, exercise, stress, cold air, or irritants like smoke, cause airways to constrict; and *extrinsic asthma*, in which airways close after being exposed to allergens like pollen, dust mites, pet dander, mold, or certain foods.[5]

Today, we recognize asthma as a highly complex condition with overlapping triggers, some allergic (extrinsic) and others nonallergic (intrinsic). There are many types of asthma, with different causes and different responses to treatment. Modern asthma care looks beyond intrinsic and extrinsic classifications and attempts to manage the condition in a more nuanced way. Still, for most people, the treatment approach is largely similar: bronchodilators and corticosteroids, delivered either via inhaler or orally. While corticosteroids—I'll just call them steroids from here on—can be a lifesaving treatment, they are rife with negative side effects, especially when given long term.

For patients, the severity of asthma and the type of treatment are determined by several criteria: how often patients require quick-relief medication, if they are awakened at night by asthma symptoms, whether their lung function is normal, if they have needed urgent or emergency care, or if they required a course of oral steroids. Asthma is typically categorized as *intermittent* or *persistent*, and under those two categories, cases are classified as *moderate* or *severe*.[6]

This chapter explores how integrative therapies can prevent the symptoms of asthma or reduce their severity. While you may not be able to cure asthma altogether, you may be surprised to see how your symptoms wane.

As Randy Horwitz, MD, PhD, the medical director at the Andrew Weil Center for Integrative Medicine, specializing in integrative therapies for asthma, explains, "What we find in adults is people who have asthma as a child will usually go through a period of time when it subsides." And, even if you have more severe symptoms, it is certainly possible to live a full life. Consider that an asthma diagnosis did not prevent David Beckham becoming a world-renowned football star, nor did it prevent Jackie Joyner-Kersee winning six Olympic athletics (track-and-field) medals.

Identify and Avoid Asthma Triggers

If you have asthma, I urge you to learn and avoid your specific triggers to best practice prevention. The most common asthma triggers include the following:

- **Tobacco Smoke:** When you inhale tobacco smoke—whether by smoking yourself or being exposed to secondhand smoke—irritating chemicals aggravate the delicate lining of your airways.[7] Vaping can also cause asthma symptoms.[8]
- **Dust Mites:** These are microscopic bugs, too small to see with the human eye, but easy for a person with a sensitized immune system to react to. Purchase and encase your pillows and mattresses in allergen-proof covers. Avoid down-filled pillows and blankets. Use a vacuum with a HEPA filter to clean your carpets, rug, and floor.
- **Air Pollution:** I have become a regular user of my smartphone's air-quality updates, and I recommend you use this feature, too. If there is an alert that the outdoor air quality is unhealthy or that people with health conditions should stay indoors, minimize your time outdoors. Indoor air can also contain pollutants that irritate the lungs; using a HEPA air filter removes these chemicals.
- **Pollen Counts:** If you are sensitive to particular plants, avoid exposure when they are in bloom.
- **Pets:** Some people know they have a cat or dog allergy and will not adopt one. Others adopt a pet that is nonshedding to greatly reduce

their exposure to animal dander. If you know you are sensitive but can't resist having a pet, keep it out of the bedroom.
- **Mold:** Indoor mold can be found in damp areas, including your kitchen, bathroom, cellar or basement, or any area with water damage. It is best to wear an FFP2 face mask, gloves, protective glasses, and long sleeves and trousers when you scrub mold off surfaces; use detergent and water, then dry completely.[9] Repair leaks as quickly as possible. Remediate any mold in a wall, cellar, or loft (attic). Mold can not only trigger asthma but also cause chronic sinus infections, fatigue, and many other symptoms.[10]
- **Cleaning Products:** Disinfectants and harsh cleaning products can trigger asthma. When you use them, open windows to create ventilation. Rather than spraying (which aerosolizes the product), pour a small amount onto a cloth or absorbent paper.
- **Infections:** Colds, respiratory syncytial virus (RSV), influenza, and other infections can trigger asthma.
- **Acid Reflux:** Asthma and acid reflux often occur together. If you have asthma, avoid any known acid-reflux triggers, including spicy foods or big meals before bed, drinking alcohol, or using tobacco products.
- **Fragrance:** Scents and certain chemicals in perfumes, deodorants, and air fresheners can worsen asthma.[11] As many as fifty-five million Americans are sensitive to scented products, for example.[12] Fragrance-free offices are becoming more common, and if you are reacting at your workplace, consider initiating such a policy.
- **Physical Exercise:** Exercise can trigger asthma symptoms in some individuals—a condition known as exercise-induced bronchoconstriction or exercise-induced asthma. If exercise is one of your triggers, you can take omega-3 supplements (as described later) or use your inhaler 10 to 15 minutes before activities.
- **Breathing Cold, Dry Air:** Cold air entering the lungs can cause airways to constrict. This is especially true during intense exercise, when you tend to breathe more through your mouth, bypassing the natural humidifying effect of the nose (more on this in the following section).
- **Emotional Stress:** When you are feeling anxious, your body releases the stress hormones adrenaline and cortisol.[13] This can cause a tightening

of the airway muscles, making it harder to breathe. Additionally, stress can lead to increased inflammation in the airways.

The Importance of Nasal Breathing

Breathing through your nose can help reduce symptoms of asthma. Unfortunately, a survey of 1,001 Americans suggests that as many as 60 percent of people regularly breathe through their mouth,[14] even though the human nose is brilliantly designed to accomplish all these functions:

- Filtering out foreign particles by tiny hairs called *cilia*. Unwanted particles include dust, allergens, and pollen, which could otherwise enter the lungs and trigger asthma.
- Humidifying and warming the inhaled air.
- Producing nitric oxide, which dilates blood vessels and increases blood circulation in the body.
- Lowering blood pressure and reducing anxiety.[15]

There are other benefits to nose breathing; for instance, while it might seem counterintuitive, you inhale more air when nose breathing than when mouth breathing.[16] Mouth breathing can exacerbate asthma, while breathing through your nose during exercise has been shown in studies to reduce exercise-induced asthma.[17] Last but not least, mouth breathing can cause sore throat, dry mouth, and even bad breath.[18]

One strategy that can encourage nose breathing is to place a small piece of paper tape (6 × 12 millimeters (¼ × ½ in)) vertically across your upper and lower lips before bed, essentially taping them shut. This will be a gentle reminder to keep your mouth closed while you sleep. It may take some getting used to; the first few nights I tried it, I ripped the tape off within twenty minutes. Over time, however, you will adjust, as I did, to sleeping with the tape on and learning to nose-breathe.[19] In addition to all the benefits of nose breathing noted here, studies support the effectiveness of mouth taping in reducing snoring and even mild sleep apnea.[20] For more information about the science of breathing, I highly recommend reading James Nestor's excellent book *Breath: The New Science of a Lost Art*.

Breathing for Asthma Relief

An asthma attack produces the sensation that you cannot get enough air, which, depending on its severity, can be an incredibly stressful experience. When you encounter a trigger, whether it's an allergen, emotional stress, physical exercise, infection, or poor air quality, the bronchial tubes in the lungs become inflamed, which causes your cell linings to produce excess mucus. Triggers can also cause a constriction of the muscles that line the airways, known as bronchospasms. The combination of inflammation, mucus, and bronchospasms narrows the airways during an attack, reducing the available space for air to flow.

As discussed, learning to breathe through your nose may reduce the risk of an asthma attack. But there are other types of breathwork that can help, too. A metanalysis published in 2020 that reviewed twenty-two studies of breathwork found that people who did breathing exercises—in which they were taught how to breathe through their noses, relax their chest and abdominal muscles, and pay attention to the amount of air inhaled with each breath—were found to reduce hyperventilation and improve quality of life and lung function when compared to people who had usual asthma care.[21] Among the modalities studied were yoga breathwork (pranayama), breathing retraining, Buteyko, Papworth, and deep diaphragmatic breathing. Trained yoga teachers can help you learn these principles, as can smartphone apps; there are a number of apps available, and Breath Ball is an effective one that is also free.

Often in this book I encourage you to practice deep-breathing exercises. However, asthma may be one of the few exceptions, where shallower breathing may be preferable. During an attack, the airways are inflamed and narrowed, and taking deep breaths can lead to increased wheezing or coughing. Instead, I recommend looking into Buteyko breathing, which teaches you to consciously reduce either the volume or the frequency of your breathing.

Developed by Ukrainian doctor Konstantin Buteyko in the 1950s, the Buteyko Breathing Technique (BBT) is based on the theory that hyperventilation depletes carbon dioxide (CO_2) in the blood,[22] which may exacerbate symptoms of asthma, as CO_2 is known to play a role in controlling blood vessel diameter. While deep breathing can promote hyperventilation, which lowers CO_2 levels and makes asthma symptoms worse, BBT trains you to maintain and tolerate higher levels of CO_2 in the body with slow, calm, and shallower breaths; inhaling and exhaling through the nose; and incorporating breath holding.

There is evidence that Buteyko breathing can be effective for adults and children with asthma, decreasing symptoms of asthma while reducing bronchodilator inhaler use[23] and improving overall quality of life.[24] To learn Buteyko breathing, I recommend working with a skillful practitioner; you can search online for more information in your area.

Reducing Asthma Symptoms with Diet

Many vegetables and fruits contain compounds with anti-inflammatory properties, such as flavonoids and carotenoids. One large meta-analysis concluded that eating fruits and vegetables appeared to be protective against asthma.[25] This might be because many fruits and vegetables are prebiotics, meaning they contain nondigestible compounds called *oligosaccharides*, which support the growth of beneficent bacteria in the microbiome.[26] Garlic, onion, asparagus, pistachios, wheat, oats, and soybeans are all prebiotic foods. Notably, human breast milk also contains oligosaccharides, which serves as a prebiotic supporting the development of the infant's microbiome.[27]

A six-month study of children by Johns Hopkins University researchers found that having more omega-3 fatty acids in the diet—which are found primarily in cold-water fish, walnuts, linseeds (flax seeds), and purslane—resulted in fewer asthma symptoms from indoor air pollution, such as that caused by cooking, cleaning activities like sweeping, and cigarette smoke. The study also found that eating more inflammatory omega-6 foods, which are found in vegetable oils—including corn, soybean, safflower, and sunflower oil—increased the risk of more severe asthma.[28] See "Your Rapid Recovery Toolkit" (appendix 1) for more information about omega-3s.

Evidence also suggests that the typical Western diet, which is high in refined grains and processed meats, may have pro-inflammatory effects that exacerbate symptoms of asthma.[29] If you have mild to moderate asthma, an anti-inflammatory Mediterranean-style diet could help. See "Your Rapid Recovery Toolkit" (appendix 1) for more information on how to get started.

Supplements

A number of supplements have been shown to help reduce asthma symptoms. Here are my recommendations to explore.

Omega-3 Fatty Acids: As discussed, omega-3s in food are beneficial in reducing inflammation and asthma. If you have exercise-induced asthma, also known as *exercise-induced bronchoconstriction* (EIB), studies support the value of taking omega-3 supplements. As many as 90 percent of asthma sufferers also experience EIB,[30] which is caused by the loss of heat and water from the airways when breathing in dry air during exercise. (Remember, nose breathing humidifies breath while exercising!) This in turn triggers an inflammatory response, causing shortness of breath, wheezing, chest tightness, coughing, and other symptoms. In a landmark study out of Indiana University, the post-exercise lung function of participants with mild to moderate persistent asthma improved by about 64 percent, and their use of emergency inhalers decreased by 31 percent when they consumed a diet supplemented with fish oil for three weeks.[31]

Dr. Randy Horwitz, mentioned earlier, explains that omega-3s in conjunction with vitamin C can eliminate the constriction that occurs in some people with exercise-induced bronchospasm. Omega-3 fatty acids may also be beneficial for other forms of asthma. Dr. Horwitz puts the majority of his patients with asthma on 2 grams of supplemental omega-3s daily, no matter what kind of asthma they have, and most get better.

Vitamin D: A key vitamin that helps regulate the immune system, vitamin D plays a role in controlling inflammation. A recent study found that supplementation reduced symptoms in asthma patients with low vitamin D levels.[32] See "Your Rapid Recovery Toolkit" (appendix 1) for more information about vitamin D supplementation and optimal dosage.

Butterbur: Butterbur contains the compound petasin, which is believed to have anti-inflammatory effects, and reduces allergy-induced asthma owing to its impact on histamine release. In one study of a butterbur root extract supplement, the duration and severity of asthma attacks decreased and lung function improved to such a degree that 40 percent of the patients were able to reduce their asthma medications.[33] Be sure to check with your doctor and consider a product that is pyrrolizidine alkaloid–free.[34] (This will be on the label.) I recommend a dosage of 25 to 75 mg two to three times daily, with a maximum total dose of 150 mg per day.[35]

Quercetin: My patient Miriam, who had mild asthma, asked me during her annual visit about natural alternatives. I suggested quercetin at the recommended dose of 400 mg twice a day.[36] At her next visit, Miriam reported she was able to completely discontinue the use of her asthma inhaler. Her exact words were: "I want to maintain my status as a prescription-free old fart as long as possible!" (I did recommend she keep an inhaler on hand for emergencies.)

Miriam's experience is supported by research. Quercetin has been studied in people with mild to moderate asthma as an addition to their standard medication; it was shown to reduce the need for supplemental asthma medication and to decrease daytime and nighttime symptoms.[37] It is used for prevention only—it will not work during an attack—and needs to be taken regularly. A side benefit is that it can also reduces allergic rhinitis (runny nose caused by an allergen).

Make an Asthma Action Plan

I urge you have a plan worked out with your healthcare provider to amp up your medications if your asthma worsens. Action plans are usually divided into green, yellow, and red zones.[38] *Green* signals that you feel fine and that your peak flow measurement (how much air you can forcibly exhale) is at 80 percent or more of your highest peak flow reading. The recommendation for the green zone is to continue to take your regular medicine.

Yellow means that your asthma is getting worse. You may be experiencing coughing, wheezing, chest tightness, or trouble breathing, and these symptoms may be waking you up during the night. Your peak flow measurement is at 50 to 75 percent. I recommend that you talk to your doctor about adding quick-relief medicine to your long-term control medicine and keep an eye on your symptoms. If they are better after an hour or so, keep checking them and continue your regular asthma control medicine.

Red is a problem! Your peak flow meter is less than half your best peak flow. You may be having a lot of trouble breathing or your quick-relief medicines are not helping. Alternatively, it could be you have been in the yellow zone for twenty-four hours and are not getting better. I recommend you call your doctor, in addition to taking any other medicines they have prescribed. If your symptoms don't get better and you can't reach your doctor, go to the hospital for evaluation and treatment.

How the Mind–Body Connection May Improve Asthma

In 1999, researchers from the State University of New York at Stony Brook School of Medicine revealed a fascinating finding: Writing about stressful life experiences could improve symptoms of medical conditions, including asthma and rheumatoid arthritis.[39] In their study, a group of people with asthma or rheumatoid arthritis were asked to journal about the most stressful moments of their lives, while another group simply journaled what they did each day. As the study concluded, patients with mild to moderately severe asthma who wrote about stressful life experiences saw improved symptoms after four months compared with those in the control group.

How does this work? It is possible that expressing our emotions about a traumatic event in a safe environment leads to a sense of control over the trauma.[40] Written expression may also desensitize us from that trauma. Research suggests that writing about both the facts and the emotions related to a traumatic event often leads to higher resolution of the stress compared to focusing on facts or emotions alone.[41] For example, you can write a letter (that you will not send) in which you express feelings of anger, sadness, or grief towards another person.[42] You can also write to yourself and express compassion for the situation you experienced.

You can choose to discuss this writing with your doctor or therapist. This can be an intense exercise, and it has been proven to improve symptoms for months after the disclosure. As we've seen in this book, emotional stress can affect the body in specific ways. Some people carry stress in their back, others carry it in their gut, and some carry it in their airways. As written-disclosure research indicates, there is a profound mind–body connection that can greatly affect how we react to triggers.

Many years ago, in a study that would not be considered ethical today, a team of researchers asked forty people with asthma what their triggers were.[43] The researchers secretly put saline in a bottle and asked each person to inhale the contents. "These are your asthma triggers," participants were told after inhaling, and nearly half the people immediately began wheezing, while twelve developed full-blown asthma attacks. They were treated with what they believed to be bronchodilating nebulizers—once again just saline—and their symptoms improved. The mind triggered the asthma attack, and the mind also made it go away.

We know that stress and anxiety can lead to a tightening of the muscles around the airways, increased inflammation, and heightened sensitivity to triggers, all of which can exacerbate asthma. In other words, you may be surprised by the role the mind plays in improving or exacerbating asthma symptoms. To activate your recovery reflex, I recommend stress-reduction techniques, including breathing exercises, meditation, yoga, progressive muscle relaxation, hypnosis, and guided imagery. I discuss these techniques and many more in the "Unwinding Anxiety" chapter. Choose a strategy that resonates with you and that you know you will do regularly.

Medications for Asthma

Sodium cromoglicate is a medication that, like the supplement quercetin, works by stabilizing mast cells in your airways. Available by prescription only, it is taken daily via nebulizer or inhaler as a preventive medication. Studies have shown that sodium cromoglicate is effective and safe. For instance, one meta-analysis concluded that sodium cromoglicate is effective in controlling the symptoms of mild to moderate chronic asthma in as many as 70 percent of people.[44] Additionally, it has few known side effects and is well tolerated by most people. Be aware that sodium cromoglicate is not a rescue medication and will not be effective during an acute asthma attack. Like quercetin, it generally takes several weeks before you begin seeing results.

The most commonly prescribed medications for asthma are bronchodilators and steroids. Inhaled bronchodilators relax the bronchial muscles and expand the air passages. They work quickly, relieving the symptoms of breathlessness within a few minutes and lasting for three to five hours or longer. In contrast, inhaled steroids reduce inflammation in airways. They work more gradually and are prescribed to be used regularly to prevent attacks from occurring. The most common forms of steroids—inhaled corticosteroids—are typically used daily to prevent the release of substances that trigger asthma symptoms. Oral corticosteroids, meanwhile, are usually used for short-term relief during an asthma exacerbation or for long-term management of severe symptoms.

Given how commonly bronchodilators and steroid inhalers are prescribed, it may surprise you to learn that up to 94 percent of people do not use their inhalers correctly.[45] Ask your healthcare provider to review your technique so that the medication goes into your air passages and does not end up on your tongue or the back of your throat.

When asthma symptoms are persistent and severe, people may be put on either high-dose inhaled corticosteroids or extended courses of oral steroids, both of which may have negative long-term effects. Research has shown that when used for extended periods, high-dose steroids may reduce the body's ability to absorb calcium, increasing the risk of osteoporosis and bone fractures;[46] can elevate the risk of cataracts and glaucoma;[47] can cause skin thinning;[48] and may cause diabetes or adrenal suppression.[49] In light of these potential negative effects of steroids, many asthma patients want to discontinue their use.

Dr. Horwitz recently cared for a patient named Sandra with severe asthma symptoms. She had become dependent on an extremely high dose of the steroid prednisolone, which caused multiple side effects, including cataracts, weight gain, swelling, and high blood pressure. Only fifty-two years old, Sandra was horrified. She traveled from Helena, Montana, to our integrative-medicine clinic in Tucson, desperate to reduce her use of steroids—or, even better, to get off them entirely.

The good news is that getting off steroids in close coordination with your doctor is possible and beneficial. With Sandra, Dr. Horwitz used a broad treatment approach to get her off steroids safely. Using a combination of mind–body exercises, omega-3s, and sodium cromoglicate, he was slowly able to reduce her prednisolone dosage from 60 mg a day to just 7 mg, over the course of eighteen months. (One potential side effect of high-dose steroids is adrenal suppression, so a lengthy slow tapering is needed to jump-start the adrenal glands, which are responsible for the body's natural production of steroids.) Eventually, Sandra was able to get off steroid medications entirely and rid herself of the side effects that had plagued her.

Bear in mind that studies routinely show that lower-dose inhaled corticosteroids are safer than oral steroids. This is because inhaled steroids are delivered directly to the lungs, where they work with little systemic effect. By contrast, oral steroids circulate throughout the body and can impact many organ systems. If you are on a low-dose inhaled corticosteroid for mild asthma symptoms, the risk of dangerous side effects—whether you are an adult or a child—is low. This was confirmed by the Childhood Asthma Management Program Study, which followed more than one thousand children aged five to twelve, and revealed that long-term use of the inhaled steroid budesonide for persistent asthma was safe. (Higher doses sometimes lead to a marginal decrease in height in adulthood.[50]) This finding has been replicated in large-scale meta-analyses, which consistently show that the benefits of low-dose inhaled steroids outweigh the risks, especially when used at the lowest effective dose.[51]

Biologics: The Future of Asthma Treatment?

Biologics, or biological therapies, for asthma are a new category of immunological drugs that provide highly targeted treatment. Biologics are at the forefront of the shift toward personalized medicine, targeting the exact cells in your body that cause inflammation. They are administered via injection or intravenous infusion. The results are promising for people with moderately severe asthma, with studies showing that biologics are consistently able to reduce symptoms while reducing the need for other medications.[52]

Still unanswered are questions about which is the best biologic or how long to treat. Long-term side effects are also not certain,[53] and some research has suggested that biologics can increase the risk of certain cancers.[54] Biologics are one of the hottest areas of active medical research and are likely to emerge as a potent strategy for managing moderate and severe asthma in addition to other medical conditions.[55]

Your Rapid Recovery Prescription for Easing Asthma

Remember that an asthma diagnosis need not prevent you from having a normal, active life:

1. Understand your triggers. Many asthma attacks can be prevented by avoiding common triggers like tobacco smoke, dust, pollen, and pets.
2. Learn to breathe through your nose, which humidifies and warms inhaled air, making it easier for your lungs to use.
3. Practice breathing exercises.
4. Adopt an anti-inflammatory Mediterranean-style diet, which supports the growth of helpful bacteria in the microbiome.
5. Omega-3, vitamin D, butterbur, and quercetin supplements can help reduce asthma symptoms.

6. Build a clear asthma action plan together with your doctor so that you know how to advance your medications, if needed.
7. Harness the mind–body connection by journaling, as well as practicing mindfulness.
8. Reduce high-dose steroids by working closely with your doctor on a plan to taper medications.

13

Building Stronger Bones

Several years ago, a fifty-nine-year-old woman named Amy came to see me. She brought along the results of a routine scan revealing low bone density in her right hip, putting her at a high risk of osteoporosis—a serious disease that makes someone susceptible to bone fractures.

Amy's doctor had prescribed bisphosphonates—medications designed to help slow bone loss—but Amy was concerned about the possible side effects, which include GI (gastrointestinal) reflux and, in rare cases, damage to the jaw bone and unusual fractures. She was extremely active—walking daily and cycling over 160 kilometers (100 miles) per week—and told me she would prefer to try to strengthen her bones naturally before resigning herself to a life of prescription drugs. I recommended a regimen of yoga, Pilates, and weight-lifting exercises, including lat pulldowns and squats. Amy performed them faithfully, and on her follow-up bone scans, done one and three years later, her bone density had stabilized. Without taking a single medication, she was able to maintain her bone density and avoid the progression to osteoporosis.

Most of us know that bones make up our skeletal system. But what we often forget, and what Amy's story makes clear, is that bones are living tissue. Throughout our lives, bones are in a constant state of turnover, called *bone remodeling*. Old bone tissue is constantly being broken down by cells, a process known as *resorption*, while new bone tissue is constantly being formed. Our bodies continuously form more bone than they resorb until we reach peak bone mineral density (BMD), then it usually shifts and our bones tend to lose density. If too much bone is lost, we develop osteoporosis, a disease that affects about ten million people over the age of fifty.[1] A further forty million people have osteopenia—the precursor to osteoporosis—a condition characterized by lower-than-average bone density.[2]

Your recovery reflex can slow, stop, or even reverse the natural decline in BMD. For some people with very low bone density or a history of fractures, medication may be the best course of action. For others, the focus will be on diet, supplements, and exercise. Bones, like muscles, are dynamic and they grow strong in response to their workload, whether it's carrying heavy things or working out with weights. No matter which group you're in, as you read through this chapter, remember that your bones are amazingly adaptive. With attention to them, reaching a new homeostasis with stronger, healthier bones is possible.

Who Is at Risk for Osteoporosis?

Doctors look at many variables in addition to a bone scan to determine your risk of a fracture, starting with the following:

- **Gender:** Women's bones are typically less dense than men's, and women begin losing BMD at an earlier age and at a faster rate. Menopause increases the risk. On average, women aged fifty or older have four times the rate of osteoporosis and two times the rate of osteopenia compared to men of the same age.[3]
- **Age:** Men and women begin losing BMD in their thirties, so the risk of a fracture for everyone goes up with aging.
- **Body Size:** The heavier you are, the stronger your bones have to be to support your body. Women with a body mass index (BMI) under 19 are at the highest risk for osteoporosis,[4] but underweight men also have an elevated risk.[5]
- **Ethnicity:** Caucasian and Asian women have a higher risk of developing osteopenia and osteoporosis than African American women.[6]
- **Family History:** Anyone with a parent who suffered a hip fracture has an elevated risk of osteoporosis.[7]

- **Men with Low Testosterone:** Testosterone helps keep bones strong, and men with low levels are at a higher risk for fracture.[8]
- **Smokers and Heavy Drinkers:** Adults who smoke or have more than two alcoholic beverages per day may be accelerating bone loss.[9]
- **Inflammatory Conditions:** Anyone diagnosed with inflammatory conditions such as inflammatory bowel disease, rheumatoid arthritis, or periodontal disease may have a higher risk of osteoporosis.[10]
- **Medication Use:** People who take corticosteroids on a daily basis (such as for asthma or arthritis), thyroid hormones (if on too high a dose[11]), immunosuppressant drugs, or blood-thinners may have a higher odds of fracture.

How Do You Determine Your Risk of Fracture?

Doctors can measure bone density with a dual-energy X-ray absorptiometry (DEXA) scan of your hip and spine. Your DEXA will report both a T-score and Z-score. Your T-score compares your BMD to the average peak bone density of a young adult of the same sex; this is the primary score used to diagnose osteopenia and osteoporosis in older adults. The Z-score compares your bone density to an average person of the same age, sex, and ethnicity; this is sometimes used to determine secondary causes of bone loss in premenopausal women, in men, and in children (such as hyperparathyroidism, medication side effects, or bed rest). A T-score above -1.0 indicates normal bone density; a score between -1.0 and -2.5 indicates osteopenia; and a score below -2.5 indicates osteoporosis. For Z-scores, a normal reading is above -2.0.[12]

Another resource your doctor will use to assess your bone health is an online risk calculator such as QFracture or the Fracture Risk Assessment Tool (FRAX). These online resources calculate the ten-year probability a person will suffer a bone fracture because of osteoporosis. For example, FRAX is determined on the basis of risk factors such as age, weight, family history, previous fracture history, steroid use, and rheumatoid arthritis. The American National Osteoporosis Foundation Guide recommends medication for people whose FRAX score indicates a ten-year hip fracture risk of 3 percent or higher, or a risk of at least 20 percent for another major fracture.[13]

While a DEXA scan measures bone density, and FRAX assesses your risk of fracture, there is no definitive way to predict whether *you* will have a fracture. This adds to the complex decision-making about treatments to pursue if your bone density is on the low side.

Osteoporosis Medications

If osteoporosis medications had no potential risks, I would recommend them to everyone with low bone density. Unfortunately, these drugs do have some challenging side effects, like the ones my patient Amy was concerned about. As discussed earlier in this book, I typically introduce two concepts with my patients when weighing the pros and cons of taking a given medication: NNT and NNH. The first, Number Needed to Treat (NNT), measures a drug's effectiveness. It is determined by calculating the number of people who need to be treated with a particular medication to prevent one additional bad outcome—in this case, a fracture. The lower a drug's NNT, the more effective it is. The NNH, or Number Needed to Harm, measures how many people receive a particular treatment before one person experiences a harmful side effect. A higher NNH is better, as it means fewer people are harmed by the treatment. (You can find NNT and NNH for the most common medications at www.thennt.com.)

I usually have long conversations with patients about the risks and benefits of taking medication for osteopenia or osteoporosis, which are different for each person. (We will review medication effects and side effects later in the chapter.) For instance, I do not typically recommend medications for postmenopausal women who don't have a history of fracture or severe osteoporosis. For those postmenopausal women who do have a history of a fracture, I often recommend bisphosphonates, the most common class of bone density medications. But it's important for women to understand that these medications have an NNT of 100 to prevent a hip fracture, even for women with a history of fracture.[14] This indeed means that 99 percent of women see no benefit at all but still are exposed to the risks.

Consider that osteoporosis medications have about a 50 percent relative risk reduction, which sounds impressive—after all, who wouldn't want their risk of fracture cut in half? But your *absolute* risk—meaning the actual probability of a fracture occurring while taking the medication—is the more important figure. For instance, if your absolute risk of a fracture was calculated at 4 percent, the medication cuts that figure in half to 2 percent. For some, this is a compelling reason to take the medication. For others, it is not.

Amy was prescribed bisphosphonates when a DEXA scan of her hip indicated osteopenia with a T-score of -2.3. Per the FRAX calculator, Amy's ten-year probability of a hip fracture was about 2.8 percent. Bisphosphonates could reduce her relative risk by half, bringing her absolute risk down to 1.4 percent over ten years. But several things suggested to me that her true risk was actually lower than 2.8 percent—namely, her healthy anti-inflammatory diet and her vigorous physical activity level. Even though her doctor recommended bisphosphonates, in my view her T-score did not warrant a strong need to prescribe medication. In our visit, we determined that her preference to manage her osteopenia without medications was reasonable, and the benefits of bisphosphonates did not outweigh the risks. She ultimately thrived—and her T-score improved—by adding a robust weight-training regimen.

Regardless of their DEXA or FRAX results, women with a fracture history have demonstrated that their bones are susceptible to fracture. If this describes you, I encourage you to consider the following medications:

- **Bisphosphonates:** These are the typical first-line medications prescribed for both the prevention and the treatment of osteoporosis. Bisphosphonates reduce the risk of a fracture and increase BMD by inhibiting osteoclasts, which are the cells that degrade bone during the remodeling process. Common side effects include heartburn, nausea, esophagitis, and abdominal pain. Rare, but serious, adverse effects include atypical femur fractures, esophageal cancer, and osteonecrosis of the jaw, in which bone cells in your jaw die off. NHS-approved bisphosphonates include alendronic acid, risedronate, etidronate (but newer, better options are preferred), ibandronate (ibandronic acid) zoledronate (zoledronic acid). They can be dosed daily, weekly, monthly, or yearly, and taken either orally or intravenously. They are usually prescribed for five years or longer. One fascinating study found that women on bisphosphonates may be able to take a "drug holiday" after five years with a maintenance of bone density benefits for an additional five years.[15]

- **Denosumab:** The generic name for several brands, denosumab is usually a second-line treatment for women who don't tolerate bisphosphates. Denosumab is an immune-system protein, known as a monoclonal antibody, that also works by inhibiting osteoclast activity, decreasing bone resorption, and increasing bone density.[16] NICE has approved for both the treatment and prevention of osteoporosis. Side effects of denosumab may include urinary and respiratory infections, cataracts, constipation, rashes, and joint pain. Rare but serious side effects include osteonecrosis of the jaw and atypical fractures.[17] One downside of denosumab treatment is that when it is discontinued, bone loss reoccurs and the higher risk of fracture resumes, so it will most likely be replaced by another prescribed drug.[18]
- **Parathyroid Hormone:** Teriparatide and abaloparatide are medications that stimulate bone formation and bone remodeling; they have been shown in large trials to reduce vertebral and nonvertebral fractures in postmenopausal women.[19] Teriparatide is injected daily for up to two years. Side effects include nausea and headaches. Because of the high cost and frequent injections, these medications are usually reserved for people with severe osteoporosis, although they are the most effective medications for stimulating new bone growth.

As you can see, while these medications are effective, they do carry some risk. This might explain why one study found that among 126,000 women with osteoporosis who had health insurance coverage in the United States, just 28 percent began drug therapy within a year of diagnosis.[20]

No matter which medication you take, how do you know if it's working? Doctors have two painless ways to determine if the medication is effective. One is to repeat a DEXA scan after about one year to assess whether your bone density has improved. A faster approach is to check a bone turnover marker (via a blood CTX test) to see whether the breakdown of bone has diminished.[21] This will require one baseline blood test and another three months later.

Putting Risk in Context

When discussing whether to begin medication for low bone density with your doctor, it is important to put the risks of severe side effects into context.

A task force of fourteen professional organizations of dentists, doctors, and bone scientists found that each year, just 0.001 to 0.01 percent of people on oral bisphosphonates like alendronic acid, ibandronate, or risedronate develop jaw necrosis—a number that Harvard Medical School has pointed out is "only slightly higher than among people not taking those medications."[22] The risk is higher, however, for cancer patients on certain medications or people who have poor dental hygiene or suffer from diabetes or rheumatoid arthritis.

Note that some dentists will not perform invasive procedures, such as extractions, on patients taking bisphosphonates owing to a higher risk of necrosis. For this reason I recommend having a complete dental checkup before beginning these medications.[23]

Nutrition

The most important mineral for bone health is calcium, which plays a central role in the structure and maintenance of our bones.

Another critical nutrient for bone health is vitamin D. Without sufficient vitamin D, the body struggles to effectively absorb and use calcium from food. Other important nutrients for bone health include phosphorous, which works in conjunction with calcium to maintain bone density; vitamin K, which is central to bone mineralization; protein, which provides structure for bone collagen; magnesium, which contributes to bone mineralization and effective absorption of vitamin D; and vitamin C, which supports calcium absorption and aids in the regeneration of bone after a fracture.

The connection between these nutrients and bone health is not necessarily a straightforward case of cause and effect. Surprisingly, studies show that countries with the highest consumption of calcium from dairy products also tend to have the highest rate of bone fractures.[24] So, there seems to be another factor at play: inflammation.[25] Research has increasingly linked osteoporosis with chronic low-grade inflammation. When inflammation is present, the body produces molecules called *cytokines*, some of which promote the activity of bone-resorbing osteoclasts. Chronic inflammation can also increase the levels of the hormone cortisol, which can interfere with the formation of *osteoblasts*, the cells that form new bones. This may explain why people with inflammatory conditions like rheumatoid arthritis and inflammatory bowel disease tend to have a much higher risk of bone loss and osteoporosis.

When it comes to avoiding inflammation, the answer is, again, nutrients. The following foods fight inflammation and are excellent sources of bone-healthy vitamins and minerals:

- **Leafy Greens:** Dark leafy greens such as spinach, kale, spring (collard) greens, and Swiss chard are rich in calcium and other bone-supporting nutrients, like vitamin K and magnesium. Studies show that eating two to three servings of green leafy vegetables every day can improve BMD among middle-aged men and women.[26] A serving is about 100 grams (3½ oz) of greens.
- **Other Vegetables and Fruits:** Many vegetables and fruits are good for your bones and are considered BRIFI, or bone resorption inhibitory food items.[27] BRIFI foods include garlic, parsley, dill, onion, rocket (arugula), fennel, orange, leek, wild garlic, red cabbage, and celeriac. In addition to reducing the body's acid load, these plant foods have active compounds that have been shown in animal studies to prevent

bone loss.[28] While this effect has not yet been definitively proven in humans, these are healthy foods with many side benefits!

- **Soy Foods:** Studies reveal an association between soy food intake and higher BMD.[29] This relationship is especially strong at menopause, when bone loss accelerates. I recommend 75 mg per day of soy isoflavones. For context, 240 milliters (8½ fl oz) of soy milk contains about 24 mg; a quarter-block of tofu contains around 25 mg; 80 grams (3 oz) of tempeh contains about 36 mg; and 75 grams (2½ oz) of steamed edamame contains around 18 mg. Depending on what you eat, reaching 75 mg means having two to three servings of a soy-based food daily.

- **Omega-3 Fatty Acids:** Research shows that populations who eat the most fish, which are rich in omega-3 fatty acids, tend to have lower rates of osteoporosis.[30] By reducing inflammation in the body, omega-3s can tame osteoclast activity and help prevent bones from breaking down. Omega-3s have also been shown to promote collagen formation and improve calcium absorption in the intestines. For more information about the best sources of omega-3s in your diet, see "Your Rapid Recovery Toolkit" (appendix 1).

- **Nuts and Seeds:** Almonds, chia seeds, and sesame seeds are excellent sources of calcium and magnesium, which promote bone health. I recommend a handful of seeds and 30 grams (1 oz) of nuts (or a handful) per day. This roughly equals 14 walnut halves, 24 almonds, 16 cashews, 28 peanuts, or 45 pistachios.[31]

- **Prunes:** Prunes (dried plums) are rich in vitamin K and antioxidants, which may positively affect bone quality. In one study, Penn State researchers evaluated the bone density of 235 postmenopausal women and assigned them to eat varying amounts of prunes each day.[32] After a year, women who did not eat any prunes saw a 1.1 percent decrease in bone density, while those who ate five to six daily did not have any measurable bone loss. "Prunes may help prevent bone loss, especially at the hip and tibia," the study concluded.

- **High-Quality Dairy:** In particular, fermented dairy such as yogurt, kefir, and cheeses can be excellent sources of calcium. (Fermented products feed your microbiome and are better tolerated among people with lactose intolerance.) Having 225 grams (8 oz) of natural full-fat yogurt contains about 450 mg of calcium; Greek yogurt contains 260 mg; and kefir contains 317 mg.[33] Cheddar, Monterey jack, provolone, and romano cheeses all contain 200 to 300 mg of calcium 30 grams (1 oz). Parmesan has a bit more, at around 335 mg per per 30 grams (1 oz). Avoid low-quality dairy products containing added sugars, artificial flavors, preservatives, or other additives. Examples of these include American cheese, flavored milks, instant powdered milk, and aerosol creams.

- **Fortified Plant Milks:** While we commonly associate dairy milk with high levels of calcium, the "milks" made from oats, almonds, and soy are typically fortified with calcium, too. Having 240 milliliters (8½ fl oz) of almond milk, for instance, contains as much as 470 mg of calcium, compared to around 300 mg in low-fat dairy milk.

Are Plant-Based Diets Healthy for Bones?

Studies routinely show that high consumption of vegetables and fruits is associated with greater bone density and a lower risk of osteopenia and osteoporosis.[34] The Women's Health Initiative, which tracked tens of thousands of women for approximately fifteen years, found that a Mediterranean diet—which is rich in healthy fats, whole grains, beans, vegetables, and fruits—"is associated with a lower risk for hip fractures."[35]

But some studies also indicate that plant-based diets might put people at a higher risk of bone fracture. For example, in one 2009 meta-analysis, vegetarians were found to have 4 percent lower bone density, and vegans to have 6 percent lower bone density, compared to omnivores.[36] Additionally, the EPIC-Oxford study, which followed approximately fifteen thousand vegetarians, two thousand vegans, thirty thousand meat eaters, and eight thousand fish eaters, found that vegans had more than double the risk of fractures.[37]

Does this mean that plant-based diets lead to a higher risk of fractures? Not necessarily. The EPIC-Oxford study also found that the fracture risk disappeared among vegans and vegetarians who ate foods with sufficient amounts of calcium and took supplemental vitamin D.

My conclusion: If you do follow a plant-based diet, be sure to eat foods rich in calcium. I recommend tracking the amount of calcium you eat daily. The International Osteoporosis Foundation offers a handy calculator on their website. If you are consuming less than 700 mg of calcium daily, add additional calcium-rich foods to your diet or talk to your doctor about taking a 500 mg calcium supplement.

Just as some foods can strengthen bones, others can accelerate bone loss. Here is what I recommend avoiding:

- **Too Much Caffeine:** Studies suggest that caffeine increases the excretion of calcium in the urine. A University of South Australia study found that people who consumed 800 mg of caffeine—about eight cups of coffee—over the course of a day had a 77 percent increase in calcium in their urine.[38] I recommend drinking no more than four cups of coffee or caffeinated tea each day to minimize your risk while also avoiding other caffeine sources, such as soda and energy drinks.
- **Alcohol:** Studies show that consuming three alcoholic drinks a day increases the risk of hip fractures.[39] Alcohol can interfere with the absorption of essential nutrients, including calcium, vitamin D, and magnesium.
- **Meat-Heavy Diet:** Meat, particularly red meat, produces acid when digested.[40] Because maintaining a blood pH level between 7.35 and 7.45 is critical for good health, the body deploys a variety of mechanisms to neutralize excess acid, including releasing calcium, a strong base, from your bones.[41] Over time, this can lead to a decrease in bone density, increasing the risk of osteoporosis and fractures.
- **High-Sodium Foods:** Too much sodium in your diet can lead to increased excretion of calcium in the urine,[42] as well as contribute to an unhealthy acid-forming pH level in the body. I recommend consuming no more than 2,300 mg per day.

What About Calcium Supplements?

I advise my patients to maximize the amount of calcium they consume by choosing healthy foods. Still, some women may need a supplement. (I do not recommend that men take any form of calcium supplement. A study of nearly thirty thousand men in Finland found that consuming 2,000 mg or more of calcium daily markedly increased the risk of prostate cancer.[43])

For women under fifty, I generally recommend an inexpensive calcium carbonate supplement. As we get older, however, our stomachs produce less acid and may not break down the calcium carbonate effectively. For older patients, I recommend calcium citrate supplements, though they usually cost more than calcium carbonate. I also advise people to avoid oyster shell, dolomite, bone meal, and coral calcium because they contain trace amounts of lead.

If you do take supplemental calcium, how much should you take? The maximum daily dose of calcium absorbable at any one time is about 500 mg.[44] I rarely find that anyone needs a larger dose, considering the daily recommended intake is 1,200 mg of calcium and the fact that most people get at least 700 mg from their diet. Moreover, some experts believe that 700 mg daily is enough.[45] Dr. Walter Willett, professor of epidemiology and nutrition at Harvard University, and one of the world's leading nutritional experts, says: "Essentially, I think that adults do not need 1,200 mg of calcium a day. The World Health Organization's recommendation of 500 mg is probably about right. The United Kingdom sets the goal at 700 mg, which is fine, too. It allows for a little leeway."[46]

There is concerning evidence that calcium supplements (but not calcium in our foods) increase the risk of heart disease. A meta-analysis of thirteen randomized controlled trials comprising almost twenty-nine thousand participants found that calcium supplements increased the risk of cardiovascular disease by about 15 percent in healthy postmenopausal women.[47] Whether the benefits of a supplement outweigh the risks depends on your specific risks of heart disease versus osteoporosis.

For adults with osteopenia or osteoporosis, I often recommend a bone health supplement, which typically contains a range of nutrients important for bone health. This ensures that they consume the essential minerals and vitamins for bone formation, including boron, magnesium, and vitamin K2. There are many different brands and combinations of minerals and vitamins available; for some women, a multivitamin with minerals may be enough, but others who need additional calcium should choose ones that target bone health.

Exercises to Increase Bone Density

As we saw with my patient Amy at the beginning of this chapter, it's possible to use exercise to slow the body's natural decrease in bone density. This is because bone is dynamic—it responds to what we ask it to do. This is a wonderful example of our recovery reflex leading our body to adapt to new demands.

A meta-analysis from 2023 examining postmenopausal women concluded that "high-intensity and high-impact exercises are effective in improving, or at the very least maintaining, bone density in the lumbar spine and femur in postmenopausal women."[48] In one clinical trial from Germany, 246 women aged sixty-five or older were put on an eighteen-month program with both high-intensity and low-intensity exercises.[49] At the conclusion of the trial, when compared with a control group, the exercise group "significantly improved BMD" especially at the lumbar spine and femoral neck; they were also much less likely to experience a fall.

Improving bone density and lowering your fracture risk without medications is possible, even if you have experienced significant bone loss. Weight-bearing and resistance exercises are the most effective at promoting bone growth and maintaining bone strength, but even walking can go a long way. Data from the Nurses' Health Study, which followed tens of thousands of registered nurses beginning in 1976, found that simply walking for four hours per week was associated with a 41 percent lower risk of hip fracture compared to those women who walked less than an hour per week.[50]

Here are some exercises that can improve bone density.[51]

Weight-Bearing Aerobic Exercises (30 Minutes, Most Days of the Week): These include both high- and low-impact activities that make you work against gravity while staying on your feet:

- Jogging and running
- Jumping rope
- Playing tennis, pickleball, and other racquet sports
- Stair climbing
- Walking on pavement or hiking along uneven terrain, which also improves balance

While walking on a treadmill is good for your heart, it is not commonly recommended as a bone-stimulating exercise because the rubber surface of the treadmill reduces the force of impact on its surface.

Strength Training (Twice Per Week): Resistance exercises—whether with weights or your own body—are an excellent way to prime your recovery reflex and demand more from your bones and muscles.[52] Strength training increases the demand on the bones, which respond by becoming denser. If possible, I recommend meeting with a physiotherapist or a trainer who can instruct you on proper form. Here are examples of exercises to ask them about:

- Weighted lunges, hip abduction/adduction, knee extensions, back extensions, and dumbbell reverse fly. I also recommend compound exercises like deadlifts and squats, which target the major muscle groups attached to the hip and spine.
- Resistance bands, which are lightweight elastic bands used for strength training, stretching, and physical rehabilitation, can be used to achieve similar results as weight training while putting less pressure on the joints. While they are especially helpful for people with limited mobility, a 2020 meta-analysis of a large number of trials showed that they are not as effective as free weights for building bone strength.[53]
- Bodyweight exercises including press-ups or push-ups, squats, and planks.

Balance Exercises: These are particularly important to help prevent falls. Some of my favorite examples include:

- Tai chi (one to two times per week).
- Yoga (daily). In one study of both men and women in Massachusetts, a twelve-minute daily yoga regimen was found to reverse osteoporotic bone loss.[54]
- Pilates (weekly).

The "BEST" Exercises for Improving Bone Strength

Nearly thirty years ago, the University of Arizona College of Medicine recruited 320 women aged forty-five to sixty for the Bone, Estrogen, Strength Training (BEST) study.[55] The multi-year program concluded that the most effective prevention program for osteoporosis included weight-bearing and weight-lifting exercises, hormone therapy, and a calcium supplement. The study found that women who took 800 mg per day of calcium citrate and followed the structured exercise program increased their muscle mass while also boosting their BMD by roughly 2 percent.[56]

To this day, I continue to recommend the six bone-strengthening exercises from the BEST trial: wall squats, one-arm dumbbell military press, leg press, lat pulldown, seated row, and back extensions. When my patient Diana was found to have low BMD, she signed up for a program at our local community center that taught the BEST exercises and then integrated them into her weekly workout routine. On her DEXA scan two years later, her bone density was markedly improved—and as a side benefit, her mood and overall sense of well-being had improved, too. Ideally, I recommend taking a class, as Diana did, or working with a trainer or physiotherapist who can teach you to do the exercises correctly and with good posture while safely increasing the amount of weight.

Your Rapid Recovery Prescription for Building Stronger Bones

Keep in mind that bones are dynamic and there are many steps that you can take to make them stronger:

1. Determine your personal risk of a future fracture with a QFracture or FRAX score and a DEXA scan.
2. Find an exercise regimen you enjoy and commit to a regular practice. Include a mix of weight-bearing, resistance, and balance training.
3. Enjoy foods that fight inflammation and support your bones, including SMASH fish, soy foods, minimally processed yogurt and cheeses, nuts, seeds, fruits, and vegetables.
4. Avoid food and drinks that may accelerate bone loss, including excessive caffeine, alcohol, red meats, and foods high in sodium.
5. Supplement with vitamin D if your blood levels are low and with calcium (women only) if you do not get 700 mg per day from your diet. Consider adding a bone health supplement to ensure you get adequate vitamin K2 and trace minerals.
6. Take bone-strengthening medication if you have already had an osteoporotic fracture or are at a very high risk of one based on your QFracture FRAX and DEXA scores.

14

Defeating Depression

A few years ago, a thirty-four-year-old woman named Sandra came to see me. She felt sad and anxious, had difficulty sleeping, and experienced daily crying spells seemingly for no reason. She felt too exhausted to cook or exercise; as a result, she frequently resorted to fast food and had gained nearly 7 kilograms (15 lb), which only added to her anxiety.

Sandra was alarmed—she had no *reason* to be this sad. After all, she had friends and family who loved her. She and her husband were hoping to have kids soon, her sister lived close by, and she loved her job as a paralegal. Sandra told me she had been diagnosed with depression during college and she had been successfully treated with an antidepressant. When she reduced her dosage or tried to stop taking her pills altogether, though, the depression symptoms returned. "I want to feel well again," she explained to me, "just without medication."

Depression is a complex and multifaceted condition that can manifest differently from person to person. The best description I've come across of the internal felt state is by Andrew Solomon, author of *The Noonday Demon: An Atlas of Depression*:

> It's an experience of finding the most ordinary parts of human life incredibly difficult. Finding it difficult to eat. Finding it difficult to get out of bed. Finding it difficult and painful to go outside. Being afraid all the time and being overwhelmed all the time. And it's frequently quite a sad

experience to be afraid all the time and overwhelmed all the time ... [but depression] isn't primarily an experience of sadness.[1]

Like Sandra, you can have a robust support network, a loving family, and a great job, and still develop depression for no apparent reason. It isn't necessarily linked to a specific event, and there is no blood test or brain scan that can definitively diagnose it. Instead, it is typically diagnosed based on self-reporting of at least five of the following symptoms:[2]

- Changes in appetite
- Weight loss or gain
- Poor or too much sleep
- Constant fatigue and low energy
- Feelings of worthlessness, guilt, or hopelessness
- An inability to focus or concentrate that interferes with daily tasks at home, work, or school
- Movements that are noticeably and unusually slow or agitated
- Frequent thoughts about death
- Suicidal ideation or suicide attempts

Unlike recovering from, say, the flu, there is no simple treatment for depression. You cannot will yourself to "cheer up," "look on the bright side," or easily perform any of the helpful actions discussed later in this chapter. Today, the most common treatment is antidepressant medication. For people with severe depression, or those with suicidal thoughts or hallucinations, these medications can be lifesaving. But as we'll see later in the chapter, if you have mild to moderate depression, and if your symptoms come and go, there may be other options that can help relieve symptoms.

Sandra and I spoke about the importance of self-care, and we reframed the time spent on these activities not as a burden, but as an investment in her health. She and her husband began taking long evening walks together, watched less television, and paid closer attention to the subtle changes in the beautiful fall desert. I recommended she take two supplements, St. John's wort and omega-3 fatty acids, which improved her symptoms. She listened to a guided imagery track when she felt anxious. With time, her energy levels increased, and so did the length of her walks. Gradually she found herself able to cook again. She stopped eating processed foods and began a Mediterranean diet. She lost weight and slept better. No single one of these treatments was a silver bullet, but within four months, Sandra reported she felt her depression was lifting and her anxiety was mostly resolved. Within six months, she felt a sense of ease and vitality.

In this chapter, I will present many integrative approaches that can treat depression effectively and with fewer side effects than antidepressants. It is essential to work with a care team who can help support you. No matter your symptoms or how long you've suffered from depression, I remind you that if one treatment is not working, do not lose hope; it may just be time for a new strategy.

Finally, while this chapter will focus on many varied integrative strategies to deal with depression, remember that psychotherapy is often of great value. A therapist can help you learn skills to more effectively cope with life's stressors, gain insight into the causes of your depressed mood, or resolve past trauma.

What Is Depression and What Causes It?

It is estimated that more than one in five Americans will experience a major depressive episode in their lifetime,[3] so it is worth considering in greater depth what depression is and why it's so common.

The prevailing theory for many years was that depression was caused by a neurotransmitter imbalance. Neurotransmitters are chemicals that regulate everything from mood to emotions, to muscle movement and cognition. There are well over one hundred neurotransmitters, and three are thought to be especially associated with depression: serotonin, dopamine, and norepinephrine.

The chemical imbalance theory is what initially led Sandra—and millions of other people with depression—to antidepressants, which work by altering the levels of neurotransmitters in the brain. They are not only widely prescribed, but also the rate of prescriptions are increasing dramatically, especially in young people; between 2016 and 2022, for instance, the number of young people aged twelve to twenty-five taking an antidepressant increased by 66 percent.[4] Today, approximately 12.7 percent of Americans over the age of twelve take them.[5] The main classes include selective serotonin reuptake inhibitors (SSRIs), serotonin-norepinephrine reuptake inhibitors (SNRIs), and monoamine oxidase inhibitors (MAOIs).[6]

However, research has largely debunked the theory that depression is caused by a chemical imbalance in the brain. One study suggested that as much as 80 percent of the perceived benefits of antidepressants may be related to the placebo effect.[7] But if depression isn't caused by chemical imbalances in the brain, then what causes it?

It turns out that inflammation may play a role. The immune system typically responds to infection or injury by releasing tiny proteins called *cytokines*,[8] which are tasked with initiating the body's inflammatory response. When cytokines remain elevated, they can affect brain function by breaking down the blood-brain barrier, triggering an inflammatory response in the brain known as *neuroinflammation*.[9] This may explain why as many as 30 percent of people diagnosed with depression also have elevated levels of inflammation.[10] Indeed, many studies have shown that patients with no history of depression can develop symptoms with the onset of an inflammatory condition like rheumatoid arthritis or when given interferon,[11] a "pro-inflammatory" medication used in the past to treat viral infections like hepatitis C. Research suggests that a blood test for inflammation—called *C-reactive protein*—can be useful in identifying if you are likely to respond to an anti-inflammatory treatment for depression.[12]

Finally, a rarely considered theory concerns our loss of spiritual life. I ask my patients if they have a religious or spiritual practice that gives them strength during difficult times. I often quote a favorite Zen saying: "Meditate for fifteen minutes every day unless you are too busy. In that case, meditate for an hour."

Religious practices may help insulate people against depression and enhance grit, optimism, and resilience; this is a finding described in the book *The Awakened Brain*, by Columbia University psychology professor Lisa Miller, PhD. In her research,[13] she found a 90 percent reduced risk of major depression in adults with a family history of the disorder and who said that religion or spirituality was highly important to them. She also found that adolescents with strong spirituality were less prone to depression and had an 80 percent lower risk of addiction.[14]

Dr. Miller hypothesizes we have a kind of spiritual biological clock that may lead to depression but can also prime us for spiritual growth. The awareness that a mental-health challenge may be a trigger for deeper spiritual development has the potential to help prevent us from spiraling into despair. In one study, participants were asked about a time when they felt a deep connection to a higher power.[15] Later, when a recording of their responses was replayed to them while in an MRI machine, their brains responded in much the same way that a baby's brain reacts to a mother's embrace. Dr. Miller describes depression and spirituality as two sides of the same door: when we experience depressed mood, "We can open the door to a reshuffling of meaning to the foundational, felt awareness that we are loved and held and part of it all."[16]

For some people, religion is central to their sense of what makes existence meaningful. Others find a sense of connection to a higher power in the beauty of nature, music, mindfulness exercises, or creative expression. I encourage you to think deeply about the practices or people who make you feel the most connected with the world and your community. How can you integrate them into your everyday routine?

What Hormone Testing Can Show You

The thyroid gland produces thyroid hormone, which plays an important role in regulating metabolism, energy levels, and mood. When the thyroid is not functioning properly—usually when it produces too little hormone, known as *hypothyroidism*—it can lead to symptoms that resemble depression. For this reason, I recommend thyroid blood tests before beginning treatment for depression.

Additionally, for depression symptoms that begins in the perimenopausal period,[17] I generally recommend a trial of hormone replacement therapy as a first approach. The brain is sensitive to the changes in estrogen and progesterone, and replacing those hormones can be the most effective treatment.

How Effective Are Antidepressants?

Despite the research concluding that chemical imbalances in the brain are unlikely to cause depression, the typical treatment in the United States for depression is antidepressant medication. The most commonly prescribed drugs are SSRIs, which work by blocking the reabsorption of serotonin in the brain. By allowing more serotonin to circulate in the brain, SSRIs—including fluoxetine, sertraline, citalopram, and escitalopram—are thought to improve mood, relieve anxiety, and overall reduce the symptoms of depression.

How well they work is a complicated question that can really vary from person to person. Some patients complain that SSRIs cause weight gain and flatten their full range of emotions, making it harder for them to feel joy. Others cite the sexual side effects, which include a loss of desire, erectile problems, and difficulty having an orgasm (anorgasmia).[18] Additional side effects include fatigue, headaches, and agitation. Antidepressants may also stop working after a period of time.[19] While the exact mechanism is not clearly understood, one theory proposes the brain's neurons may adjust to increased levels of serotonin by reducing the number of serotonin receptors. The placebo effect may also play a role; as the novelty wears off, the psychological boost from taking a medication may wane.

If you are on antidepressants and are considering getting off them, work closely with your treating healthcare provider. Together, you can discern whether to taper and the best timing. Factors to consider include: Has your depression resolved? For how long have you felt well? Is life overly stressful? (For example, if you are going through a difficult divorce or beginning a new job, this may not be the best time.) Are you having unwelcome side effects from the medication? Have you improved your nutrition and exercise habits? Do you have adequate social support?

It's important to remember these medications affect our biochemistry and alter our neurotransmitters. Indeed, a large meta-analysis found that the twelve-month relapse rate was 45 percent in patients who discontinued their antidepressants compared with 19.5 percent in those who continued them.[20] In my experience, you can significantly lower the relapse rate when you add nonpharmacologic therapies (described later in this chapter) before discontinuing your medication.

Going off antidepressants can also lead to a range of withdrawal symptoms known as antidepressant discontinuation syndrome. This is distinct from a recurrence of depression. Some of the most common effects include flu-like symptoms, frequent dizziness, sensations of electric shocks (often described as "brain zaps"), anxiety, intense mood swings, and sleep disturbances.[21] In some cases, especially among young adults and adolescents, suicidal thoughts can occur.[22] For these reasons, avoid stopping antidepressants cold turkey; work closely with your doctor if you are having an adverse reaction or are switching to a new medication.

Understanding Medication Tapering

It can take much longer than you might expect—months or even years—to discontinue antidepressants. In one 2017 survey following 250 long-term users of psychiatric drugs, primarily antidepressants, researchers found that about half who attempted to reduce up to two prescribed medications rated the withdrawal as "severe."[23] This is because the receptors in the brain may have adapted to the presence of the pharmaceutical.[24]

Two researchers who had their own struggles tapering off antidepressants, Dr. Mark Horowitz and Dr. David Taylor, published a major study in *Lancet Psychiatry* arguing that the taper process should last several months at a minimum—even years sometimes—to avoid withdrawal syndrome.[25] Unfortunately, the commonly advised guidelines for stopping antidepressants calls for just a four-to-eight week taper period.[26] This may be woefully inadequate.

Based on the science, reports from patients, and his own experience, Dr. Horowitz suggests that prescribing healthcare providers looking to advise patients on reducing or stopping psychiatric medication consider making a small reduction, monitoring for withdrawal effects or destabilization, and once the patient is stable, making a further reduction. He strongly recommends that dose reductions be made in smaller and smaller increments, with the final dose being very small.[27] The tapering process will likely require much smaller doses than are commonly available in pharmacies, and may require prescribing either incremental or liquid doses, or small tablet formulations called tapering strips.

Improving Symptoms with Diet

In late 1944, physiologist Dr. Ancel Keys began a series of trials known as the Minnesota Starvation Experiment to understand the effects of severe dietary restrictions.[28] Conducted on volunteer conscientious objectors, the goal of the experiment was to recreate conditions in wartorn Europe and learn the most effective methods for refeeding populations who had been starved. Thirty-six healthy men were placed on a severe calorie-restricted diet—around 1,500 calories per day—for twenty-four weeks, losing around 25 percent of their body weight before being gradually refed. The findings provided valuable insights into the treatment of starvation victims and had lasting impacts on understanding eating disorders and the psychological effects of dietary restrictions, including how diet affects mental health. As the months of underfeeding progressed, the men became irritable, lethargic, and socially withdrawn, and they had difficulty concentrating.

The human brain may account for only 2 percent of our body weight, but it burns 20 percent of the total energy available to us, in the form of glucose.[29] This is because complex cognitive functions like decision-making, planning, reasoning, and memory formation require a constant supply of energy. You may be familiar with the term "hangry"—a portmanteau of "hungry" and "angry"—and the feelings of irritability it describes. Skipping a meal can lead your blood glucose level to drop, which the brain perceives as a dangerous situation, triggering the release of stress hormones that lead to aggressive feelings and irritability.

But the total number of calories you consume is only one part of the puzzle. Research suggests that the quality of the food you ingest may impact the chance you will experience depression. As one major review comprising twenty-one studies from ten countries concluded: "A dietary pattern characterized by a high intake of fruit, vegetables, whole grain, fish, olive oil, low-fat dairy and antioxidants and low intakes of animal foods was apparently associated with a decreased risk of depression. A dietary pattern characterized by a high consumption of red and/or processed meat, refined grains, sweets, high-fat dairy products, butter, potatoes and high-fat gravy, and low intakes of fruits and vegetables is associated with an increased risk of depression."[30]

This probably sounds familiar by now. Once again, the Mediterranean diet supports your recovery reflex, as research shows it can both reduce the risk of depression and restore mental health equilibrium. The SMILES trial (Supporting the Modification of Lifestyle in Lowered Emotional States) was a groundbreaking study conducted to investigate the impact of dietary improvements on depression.[31] All participants ate a diet rich in sweets, processed meats, and salty snacks and deficient in fiber, lean protein, and vegetables and fruits—in short, they ate unhealthfully. The trial randomly placed people with depression into one of two groups: a dietary intervention group that consumed a modified Mediterranean diet, and a control group that received social support alone. By the end of the trial, 32 percent of those in the diet group experienced remission of major depression, compared to just 8 percent in the social-support group.

The AMMEND (A Mediterranean Diet in Men with Depression) trial focused on eighteen- to twenty-five-year-old men: It found that adopting a Mediterranean diet may improve symptoms of depression within twelve weeks.[32] This is significant because in the United States, depression is most prevalent in adults aged eighteen to twenty-four,[33] and just 13 percent of young men experiencing a mental health problem are likely to seek help.[34] Nearly 10 percent of men have daily feelings of depression or anxiety, and the suicide rate among men is four times higher than among women.[35]

Why might the Mediterranean diet be effective at treating depression? For one, research indicates that polyphenols—compounds found in many plants—have antioxidant and anti-inflammatory properties, which help reduce oxidative stress and inflammation; these are factors thought to contribute to depression. Polyphenols also affect brain function by influencing neurotransmitters and improving blood flow. Additionally, they can have a positive impact on gut health, which is closely linked to mental health through the gut–brain axis. I recommend eating organic produce, which has been shown to have more iron, magnesium, and vitamin C, as well as less pesticide than conventionally grown varieties.[36]

Fatty cold-water fish are also a key component of the Mediterranean diet's ability to treat depressive symptoms. The first clue is that depression occurs less commonly in the countries in which people eat the most fish.[37] This is thought to be because SMASH fish (salmon, mackerel, anchovies, sardines, herring) contain high levels of omega-3 fatty acids, particularly EPA and DHA, which are known for their anti-inflammatory properties and ability to enhance brain function. Omega-3s can easily navigate the blood-brain barrier and interact with mood-related molecules in the brain.[38] Fish are also an excellent source of iodine, low levels of which have been associated with a higher risk of depression, and vitamin D, which is covered further later.

The Mediterranean diet is also notable for what it excludes: ultra-processed foods. A recent study coauthored by researchers at Harvard T.H. Chan School of Public Health examined the eating patterns of more than thirty-one thousand middle-aged women, finding that those who ate nine or more servings of ultra-processed foods per day had a 50 percent higher risk of developing depression compared to those who ate the least (four to five servings per day).[39] And women who consumed the most artificial sweeteners also had a 26 percent higher risk of depression compared to those who consumed the least. Additionally, the Global Mind Project, an initiative that has sampled three hundred thousand participants worldwide, found that those who consume ultra-processed foods several times a day are "three times more likely to have serious mental health struggles compared to those who rarely or never do."[40]

Dr. Bonnie Kaplan, professor emerita at the University of Calgary and the co-author of *The Better Brain*,[41] points out that ultra-processed foods lack the micronutrients the brain needs to function optimally. Zinc, copper, iron, selenium, and vitamins D, C, B1, B2, B6, and B12 are all recognized as protective nutrients for the brain yet are deficient in ultra-processed food.[42] Dr. Kaplan's pioneering work builds on that of Dr. Bruce Ames, who described fifty different genetic mutations that can change brain metabolism making it sluggish.[43] You may have one or more of these mutations, but the good news is that Dr. Ames also showed that they can be counteracted by taking high doses of the appropriate vitamins or minerals.[44] The bottom line is that some of us need higher amounts of vitamins and minerals for optimal brain function.

Ultraprocessed foods also lack dietary fiber, which feeds the good bacteria in your gut. As your gut bacteria ferment dietary fibers in the colon, they produce short-chain fatty acids, which play a crucial role in reducing inflammation and regulating brain function.[45]

A growing number of studies have also been conducted on the ketogenic diet, which emphasizes high-fat, low-carb foods. Eating a keto diet pushes the body into a state of ketosis, where the body burns fat instead of carbs for energy, a shift that can stabilize the brain's electrical activity.[46] The classic keto diet, which has been proven to treat hard-to-manage epilepsy in children, contains 90 percent fat, 6 percent protein, and 4 percent carbohydrates. Scientists theorize that because anti-seizure medications have been shown to help hard-to-treat depression, the keto diet, which stops hard-to-treat seizures, might also work for depression.

Recent studies have affirmed this theory. One analysis found that switching thirty-one adults with treatment-resistant depression to a ketogenic diet that emphasized more protein (15 to 20 percent of calories) was "associated with significant and substantial improvements in depression and psychosis symptoms and multiple markers of metabolic health."[47] (Multiple new studies of the keto diet are in progress.[48]) Note that it is challenging to follow a strict ketogenic diet, as food quantities must be exact, at least initially. Happily, metabolic psychiatrist Dr. Georgia Ede, author of *Change Your Diet, Change Your Mind* and a leading proponent of ketogenic diets for mental health, finds that many patients see their depression lift on a modified ketogenic diet (sometimes called a modified Atkins diet) containing 75 to 80 percent fat, 15 to 20 percent protein, and just 5 percent carbs.[49]

It's not known exactly why the keto diet works so well. One theory is that it increases levels of GABA, a neurotransmitter that blocks impulses between nerve cells in the brain.[50] (Research suggests that low levels of GABA are associated with mood disorders.[51]) Another theory is that the keto diet significantly increases energy production (by enhancing mitochondria) in the brain.[52] Additionally, a high-fat, low-carb diet stimulates the production of ketones, a chemical created by the liver as it breaks down fats. Ketones are thought to reduce inflammation, which both protects the brain and improves mood. Finally, the keto diet largely forgoes sugars and starches, which are metabolized to sugar and increase inflammation in the body.

It is important to note that not everyone feels well on a keto diet. Initially, some people experience flu-like symptoms while their body adjusts to using ketones rather than glucose for energy.[53] But this should pass in two to three days. Some people struggle also with nausea, vomiting, constipation, or simply find the diet too restrictive. Others experience fatty liver, kidney stones, or vitamin deficiency. Work with your doctor to avoid these side effects or address them should they occur.

Supplements

If you are interested in adding supplements to your treatment plan, talk with your doctor about the options. As described earlier in this chapter, both individual genetic variation and insufficient dietary nutrition leads researchers like Dr. Bonnie Kaplan, mentioned earlier, and doctors like me to recommend a combined multi-mineral multivitamin (MMMV) supplement. In research primarily focused on children, they have been shown to improve depression.[54] Here's one more reason to supplement with a MMMV: Some medications can deplete minerals and vitamins. For example, mood-stabilizing meds can lower levels of folate, copper, selenium, zinc and vitamins D, B6, and B12.[55] Metformin, widely prescribed to prevent and treat diabetes, can also reduce vitamin B12.[56] Birth control pills can deplete the mineral magnesium and vitamins C, E, B6, and folate.[57]

Several other dietary supplements have been shown to help manage symptoms of depression. Here are some of the most effective options to discuss with your doctor.

St. John's Wort: As we saw with my patient Sandra, mentioned at the beginning of this chapter, St. John's wort, a botanical supplement, can be used to treat mild to moderate depression. It is believed to work by altering levels of neurotransmitters in the brain, including serotonin, norepinephrine, and dopamine. A meta-analysis of thirty-five studies with close to seven thousand patients with major depression found that St. John's wort is more effective than a placebo and in some people may be similarly effective to antidepressant medication with fewer side effects.[58] One caution: St. John's wort can rev up the metabolism of medications,[59] thereby reducing their blood levels and thus their effectiveness. The affected medications include birth control pills and immunosuppressants. It can also increase the effect of other medications. If you are on any prescribed medications, be sure to ask your doctor or pharmacist about interactions. With this important caveat, I typically recommend from 900 to 1,500 mg per day taken in two or three divided doses. Read the label to be sure it contains a standardized extract of 0.3 percent hypericin and/or 3 to 5 percent hyperforin. Some people have side effects, such as an upset stomach, sensitivity to light, feelings of restlessness, or mild sedation.[60]

Probiotics: Many microbiome studies are still in their infancy, but strains of *Lactobacillus* and *Bifidobacterium* at doses of 1 to 10 billion units per day have been studied and found to be effective in treating depression and boosting the effects of antidepressants. Other strains of bacteria have been noted to be more or less prevalent in people with depression and anxiety,[61] but have not been as well studied for treatment.[62]

Omega-3s: I recommend these supplements to anyone with depression who has high levels of inflammation or is not getting enough omega-3s in their diet via fatty fish, walnuts, and linseeds (flax seeds). Studies suggest that the best outcomes result from omega-3 products with an EPA content of at least 60 percent. I recommend a daily dosage of 1 to 2 grams of EPA,[63] and 400 to 800 mg of DHA. Read the label carefully: all high-quality omega-3 supplements will state the amount of EPA and DHA they contain.

Vitamin D: Low levels of vitamin D are associated with an increased risk of depression, especially among people with a prior history.[64] Vitamin D plays a role in neurotransmitter synthesis, as well as in protecting the brain from inflammation and oxidative stress, all of which are believed to impact mood. The main source of vitamin D in our diet is fish, which may be another reason eating them is good for the brain. Doses of 1,500 to 4,000 IU per day have been used in trials;[65] please speak with your doctor to help identify the proper dosage that will be suitable for you.

Methylfolate: This is the active form of folate, a B vitamin critical for protein metabolism. Methylfolate has been proven in meta-analyses to be an effective "booster" of antidepressants.[66] Talk to your doctor about whether this is a supplement you should consider, and at what dosage.

Zinc: This is a common mineral I discuss extensively in "Conquering Colds and Vanquishing Viral Infections," as it can enhance immune function. In doses of approximately 25 mg per day, zinc has been shown to boost antidepressant effectiveness.[67] It is usually well tolerated, but can sometimes cause nausea when taken on an empty stomach.

S-adenosylmethionine (SAMe): SAMe is a naturally occurring molecule in the body that produces and breaks down neurotransmitters.[68] SAMe supplements are used to treat osteoarthritis, fibromyalgia, and liver disease. It is not usually used alone to treat depression,[69] but it can significantly boost the effect of antidepressants. If you have been diagnosed with bipolar disorder, *do not* take SAMe, as it can trigger manic episodes.[70] Please discuss with your doctor if you want to take SAMe. I recommend beginning with just 200 mg twice daily and increasing every five to seven days as needed up to 800 mg twice a day.

Exercise

Recent studies confirm that exercise can be just as effective in treating depression as taking an antidepressant. Researchers in Amsterdam recruited approximately 141 people with depression or an anxiety disorder and gave them the option to either take an SSRI or participate in a running group. At the end of the study, 43.3 percent of the runners saw their depression go into remission compared to 44.8 percent of those who took antidepressants.[71] And the runners experienced side benefits! They lost weight, improved their lung function, and reduced their blood pressure.

The only problem was adherence: While 82 percent of the antidepressant group continued their medications during the course of the study, just 52 percent of the runners adhered to the exercise routine.

This makes intuitive sense; most of us find it easier to swallow a pill than to maintain a running practice, and this is even truer if you have a condition that impairs your energy and motivation—like depression. The good news is that even low-intensity exercise can create a surge of endorphins and release feel-good neurotransmitters.[72] Taking walks can reduce symptoms of depression.[73] A German study found that bouldering—a form of rock climbing without ropes that you can do in a gym—was effective in alleviating depressive symptoms.[74] And a 2024 meta-analysis reviewed 218 studies with more than fourteen thousand participants and revealed dancing to be an effective exercise for major depression.[75]

I recommend finding an activity you enjoy and will look forward to—perhaps one you did regularly in the past. It could be jogging, walking the dog, gardening, cycling, hiking, yoga, dancing, resistance training, or Pilates.

The Importance of Sleep

Getting enough sleep is crucial for mental health. Poor sleep can disrupt mood regulation, exacerbate stress and anxiety, and negatively impact cognitive function. Studies suggest that people with insomnia may be as much as ten times more likely to develop depression compared to those who regularly get a good night's sleep.[76] Moreover, among those who do have depression, three-fourths struggle to fall or stay asleep. I highly recommend you read the "Sleeping Soundly" chapter, where you will find strategies to improve your sleep.

The Surprising Role of Light

One fascinating finding about circadian rhythms and depression has to do with our reaction to light. While some people experience *seasonal affective disorder* (with the appropriate acronym SAD), a kind of depression that occurs when the days get shorter and there is less daylight, all of us are impacted by our exposure to light.[77] For many years I have recommended my patients expose themselves to sunlight upon awakening by going outdoors for five to ten minutes. It helps set their circadian clock. I have also recommended avoiding bright light and blue light (from your cellphone, computer screen, or television) at night so as not to suppress the sleep hormone melatonin.

Research from the UK Biobank supports my recommendations.[78] Not only has it confirmed that increased outdoor light exposure during the day improves mood and significantly reduces the risk of major depression, but it also found that nighttime light exposure was a risk for major depression. Nevertheless, many of us will spend 90 percent of their time indoors, in no small part because many of our jobs require us to.[79] Making a point of getting outside a few times each day will put you ahead of the game.

My thirty-year-old patient Eric studied for his master's degree in British Columbia. Arriving from sunny Tucson, Arizona, he was accustomed to an abundance of sunlight—not something there's a lot of during the Canadian winter. He called me one day, explaining he was having trouble getting out of bed in the morning. He said he simply had no energy and was in a fog all day. Suspecting he was suffering from seasonal affective disorder, I recommended a light box, which is designed to mimic sunlight. Eric reported that results were immediate: Turning the box on felt like stepping out into the sun. It was as stimulating as a strong cup of coffee (which he had tried and found unhelpful), and his symptoms disappeared.

While light-box therapy is a proven treatment for SAD, studies show that it can help nonseasonal depression as well.[80] I recommended a "dose" range of 7,000 to 10,000 lux (a measure of light intensity) for 30 to 60 minutes every morning for up to five weeks.[81] It is important to note that simply turning on a bright light bulb is unlikely to help. A typical lit room has roughly 500 lux,[82] depending on how close you are to the light source. (If you are curious, there are free apps that measure the lux in various parts of your home or office.) In contrast, full sunlight can be as high as 100,000 lux.[83] A light box with 10,000 lux is bright enough to mimic the sun's rays.

Some people experience headaches or mild nausea from their light box, so do consult with your doctor first. I recommend starting with 10 minutes per day and gradually increasing the intensity. Don't look directly at the light; project the box upward or downward to avoid glare, and be sure to follow the instructions carefully to avoid injury.

Whole-Body Hyperthermia

When Dr. Charles Raison, a psychiatrist and mental health expert for CNN, arrived in the Himalayas to study Tibetan Buddhist monks, he became intrigued by their *tummo* meditation practice, which includes a specific way of breathing that increases body temperatures.[84] Dr. Raison, a former University of Arizona colleague of mine, has researched the causes of depression extensively. He theorized that the pathways the body uses to regulate heat are also involved in depression, and that by dramatically raising your core temperature you may be able to "reset" your body's thermostat and improve your mood. He and other researchers have shown that a technique called *whole-body hyperthermia* (that is, overheating—the opposite of hypothermia) can quickly and effectively reduce symptoms of depression. In one double-blind study conducted by Dr. Raison,[85] a group of participants lay in a device that safely heated the body to 38.5°C (101.3°F). Not only did their symptoms improve when evaluated five days after the treatment, but the group also showed "significantly reduced" depression symptoms even six weeks after the single hypothermia treatment.

You can now access hyperthermia equipment outside of a clinical study. In one trial, a commercially available infrared sauna was studied to see if it could raise body temperatures to the same degree that reduced depression in whole-body hyperthermia studies.[86] Twenty-five healthy adult participants increased their core body temperature to 38.5°C (101.3°F) and stayed there for two minutes (the target in the research trial). It took participants an average of eighty-two minutes to raise their temperature. Side effects are generally mild and transient and include feeling hot, headache, and nausea.[87]

Other traditional methods to raise your core temperature have long been used in societies with cold, dark winters. The Viking Bath, for instance, is a centuries-old therapy that involves transitioning from extremely cold environments to a hot bath or sauna—an experience that is often described as "euphoric."[88] One study involving forty-five people with moderate to severe depression had groups either exercise or take a 40°C (104°F) bath for thirty minutes twice per week.[89] The bathers' depression was reduced more significantly and faster when compared to the exercise group. And far fewer participants dropped out of the bath group than out of the exercise group. No surprises there! For many people, it is a treat to soak in a tub and a lot of work to exercise.

Treatment-Resistant Depression

Treatment-resistant depression (TRD) is the diagnosis generally used for people with depression who do not respond adequately to typical treatments, including multiple courses of antidepressants and psychotherapy. People with TRD sometimes go through multiple treatments without significant improvement in their symptoms. The usual approach to TRD is called *augmentation*, in which a treatment that uses a different mechanism of action is added to the currently prescribed pharmaceutical. For example, mirtazapine, buspirone, and lithium, which work by changing various neurotransmitters in the brain, may be used to augment SSRIs. Less commonly, MAOIs or electroconvulsive therapy (ECT) are used. As discussed earlier, the ketogenic diet is increasingly being used to address TRD.[90]

If you have TRD, I recommend genetic testing, which can identify variations in genes that impact your response to antidepressants (and other drugs). Genetic variants can be assessed in *pharmacokinetics*, which focuses on absorption and metabolism of medications, and *pharmacodynamics*, which measures drug sensitivity and response. These newly emerging tests in psychiatric practice can help your doctor tailor medication choices for you. In an unblinded trial of 685 patients, genetic testing was used to select an appropriate medicate.[91] Of the more than two-thirds of participants who had taken two or more meds for their mood without success, there was a 91 percent clinical improvement observed by their doctors. The patients also noted significant improvement in depression, anxiety, medication side effects, and an enhancement of their quality of life.

Additionally, one of the best examples of rapid recovery is emerging from a series of studies on using psychedelics—a class of psychoactive substances that produce changes in perception, mood, and cognitive processes—to treat TRD.[92] During trials, psychedelic medicines are administered by a professional after several preparation sessions with a psychotherapist. The medication is given in a clinical setting with one or two guides sitting with the patient. Follow-up integration sessions are also a key part of the protocol.

One of the first promising studies for treating depression using psychedelics was carried out at Johns Hopkins University among people with cancer.[93] The trial found that one dose of psilocybin relieved depression in 80 percent of the participants for six months. Furthermore, 67 percent described the experience "as one of the top five meaningful experiences in their lives, and about 70 percent reported the experience as one of the top five spiritually significant lifetime events."

Another recent trial explored the use of psilocybin for TRD.[94] Approximately 230 patients with TRD were randomized to receive either a 1 mg, 10 mg, or 25 mg dose. The study revealed that the highest dose led to fewer sad feelings, better energy levels, better self-esteem, and improved concentration. Ketamine, an anesthetic that has some hallucinogenic effects, may be used off-license to treat TRD.[95]

While TRD is an extremely challenging condition, these integrative approaches do provide hope for its resolution.

Your Rapid Recovery Prescription for Defeating Depression

Depression is a complex condition with numerous causes, and there are many treatment options that are effective and may have fewer side effects.

1. For people with severe depression, or those with suicidal thoughts or hallucinations, antidepressants can be lifesaving.
2. Diet can make a difference. Both the Mediterranean diet and the keto diet have been shown to be effective. In contrast, ultra-processed foods increase the risk of depression.
3. St. John's wort, probiotics, omega-3 fatty acids, vitamin D, methylfolate, zinc, and SAMe supplements can be used to treat depression or to boost the effectiveness of antidepressant medication.
4. Regular exercise can be as effective as antidepressants—without the negative side effects. Choose an activity you enjoy and, ideally, gets you outside or onto the dance floor!
5. Light-box therapy can help alleviate both seasonal and nonseasonal depression.
6. Whole-body hyperthermia treatments that raise your core temperature to 38.5°C (101.3°F) can quickly and effectively improve mood.
7. Treatment-resistant depression may respond to augmentation with another medication, hyperthermia, a ketogenic diet, or psychedelic medication.
8. If you are currently on antidepressants and are no longer depressed, ask your doctor about developing a tapering plan.

15

Taming Post-Traumatic Stress Disorder

A few years ago, a long-term patient, Kate, confided in me that she had been raped. It had happened nearly three decades prior, when she was twenty-five years old. A fiercely resilient person, Kate was determined to move on with her life. And she did. She attended a support group and saw a psychiatrist, and the trauma slowly faded from the surface.

Kate's healing, however, was incomplete. Her sense of self had been violently ripped away. Starting in her early thirties, she began to feel distress while making love. Sometimes the distress came on when she moved close to her husband; at other times a certain smell would trigger her, and occasionally so would touch. One moment she felt normal, and the next she felt she was on the precipice of a cliff. Kate returned to counseling, and learned eye movement desensitization and reprocessing (EMDR), a therapy designed to alleviate distress associated with traumatic memories.

Still, her triggers remained, and the nightmares came and went. Despite her husband's warmth, she sometimes felt terribly isolated. One day, after a breakdown that came seemingly out of nowhere, her counselor said: "I think you are experiencing post-traumatic stress disorder."

Post-traumatic stress disorder (PTSD) has long been recognized, if not understood. During the American Civil War,[1] many soldiers returned home from battle with symptoms that couldn't be explained by their wounds, including palpitations, chest pain, shortness of breath, fatigue, tremors, and anxiety. Believing the condition was related to cardiac problems, doctors dubbed it "soldier's heart." In World War I, "shell shock" was used to describe the symptoms of psychological trauma displayed by soldiers returning from trench warfare.[2] The condition was renamed "battle fatigue" following World War II. It wasn't until the aftermath of the Vietnam War,[3] along with growing understanding of other traumatic events, that there was a push to recognize and diagnose the condition.

PTSD is now understood as a condition that develops after a person experiences or witnesses a traumatic event.[4] It is believed to occur in one-third of people who are exposed to extreme stressors and the symptoms can emerge within days, weeks, months, or even years.[5] PTSD symptoms can include intrusive thoughts like flashbacks and nightmares; avoidant behavior; persistently negative thoughts; and sudden mood swings. Symptoms occur for at least a month (and typically much longer), and they interfere with multiple areas of your life, including work, school, or relationships. Around half of people with PTSD will get better on their own within a year, while others will suffer for many years.[6]

For example, in a study of how PTSD has affected 9/11 first responders,[7] one participant noted, "I don't even ride a train because of anxiety. I get . . . I get fear . . . I start sweating. I can't board the train." Another explained how, even years after 9/11, their symptoms have gotten worse: "My problem didn't start for a few years after, and then . . . when it started, the . . . the sounds and . . . and it was so horrible and so loud, and I hear the . . . from that and it gets louder and louder and I have to get up. I can't sleep."

If you have read this far, you'll know I am an optimist who believes in human resilience and the body's incredible ability to recover. So, I want to explicitly acknowledge how challenging PTSD can be. Trauma can leave a lasting imprint on the brain. Memories of the traumatic event can be vivid, intense, and emotionally charged. People who suffer with PTSD may be at a higher risk of suicide and addiction.[8] Even as a person recovers, they may feel at times as if they are taking two steps forward and one step backward. All seems well, and then a flashback pulls them back down. In some ways, the most challenging task is to get up, start again, and value the progress that has been made. Still, the brain is neuroplastic, which means it contains the potential to heal from trauma.

What Is Trauma?

I like the definition developed by the psychiatrist Dr. Paul Conti. He describes it as "anything that causes us emotional or physical pain. [Anything] that surpasses our coping mechanisms, that makes us feel then overwhelmed, often overwhelms our nervous system, both body and mind, and then really leaves a mark on us as we move forward."[9] To understand the feeling state of a person with PTSD, consider the experience of a journalist named Mark, who spent nearly five months in a Turkish jail, where he "saw brutality beyond what anybody could imagine":[10]

> I wasn't aware that I had post-traumatic stress disorder. When I returned to Australia my mental state manifested in anxiety and nightmares and night terrors and fear. I started to avoid people, I lost my job, I lost my home, I lost the beautiful young woman that I'd married and the two young children that we had. . . . It cost me a lot.

Trauma is often described as consisting of *big T* events, *little t* events, or both. Big T events are more commonly associated with PTSD and can include serious injury, sexual violence, or life-threatening experiences. Trauma can also be an accumulation of less significant events. Such little t traumas may include divorce, death of a family member or friend, non-life-threatening injuries, bullying or harassment, emotional abuse, and other losses.

My mother died suddenly and unexpectedly. I found out about her death when my sister called me and blurted out the news, just as I was leaving a movie theater. For years afterwards, I couldn't go back there because it stirred up painful memories of that horrible moment. This is certainly a little t trauma, but it shows how PTSD can be triggered by many things. Lucky for me there were many other movie theaters in Tucson. But not everyone can completely avoid their triggers.

People vary in their capacity to handle trauma of either variety, and what is highly distressing for one person may not cause the same reaction in someone else. Gabor Maté, MD, author of *The Myth of Normal*,[11] points out that trauma is not the event itself; rather, it is your internal reaction to the event. Trauma leads people to disconnect from their emotions and from their bodies. It makes it hard to be present in the moment. The essence of trauma is a lost sense of self, and recovery constitutes finding the self again.

> ### PTSD vs. Moral Injury
>
> I want to make a distinction between PTSD and another situation that may create similar responses. *Moral injury* refers to the psychological toll of participating in, witnessing, or failing to prevent actions that transgress someone's moral or ethical code. It occurs in situations where people have had to make impossible choices under extreme conditions.
>
> Examples include soldiers who must decide whether to kill or be killed, or medical professionals whose triage decisions may lead to life or death. Moral injury can result in persistent negative emotions, including guilt, shame, and remorse, and it may make it hard to derive pleasure from activities you previously enjoyed. Treatment for moral injury is usually centered on psychotherapy, support groups, and mindfulness exercises that emphasize self-compassion.

Common Treatments for PTSD

PTSD is often treated with psychotherapy that addresses thoughts, feelings, or memories of the trauma, or by using a more indirect route. There are many approved therapies, in part because no one therapy proves useful for everyone.[12] If you are suffering from PTSD and not benefiting from a specific therapy or treatment, I suggest you discuss other options with your care provider. For many people, noncognitive approaches that do not directly stir up the trauma are gentler and more effective. Here are the treatments I recommend starting with.

Cognitive Behavioral Therapy (CBT): This is one of the best-researched forms of psychotherapy. It helps people understand their own thinking about something that challenges them and then teaches them how to restructure their thinking into more useful patterns and to develop new behaviors. I love therapist and comedian Loretta La Roche's explanation of CBT, who once said at a conference that I attended: "Think of your mind as a bus and ask yourself, 'Who's driving the bus?'" My answer is usually my father. When I ask my patients, they often tell me it's their ex-husband or ex-wife—or someone else who has been critical of them. Indeed, a less humorous way of looking at CBT is to consider your inner critic. How loud, mean, or nasty is your inner critic? How often do you beat yourself up?

CBT teaches you to identify and then challenge that inner critic. You can ask: "Is this thought true?" or "What evidence supports or contradicts it?" CBT then helps you reframe negative thoughts with more balanced, realistic, and compassionate ones. For example, you may learn to shift your inner narrative from "I always fail" to "I sometimes make mistakes, but I also learn and grow from them."

When it comes to PTSD, CBT challenges distorted thoughts like "It was all my fault," or "I will never feel safe again," and encourages a more a balanced and compassionate perspective, such as "I did the best I could in a terrifying situation." CBT also teaches grounding exercises and relaxation to manage overwhelming emotions.

Studies show that CBT can help reduce symptoms of PTSD among many people,[13] but it is not for everyone. If CBT causes you to dissociate, if you go completely numb, or if you simply cannot bear to tell the story of what happened, CBT—or any talk therapy—may not be of benefit.

Cognitive Processing Therapy (CPT): CPT is quite similar to CBT, however it is delivered over twelve sessions following a manual that includes education and writing exercises about the trauma.[14] It helps people identify their "stuck points,"[15] which are fixed ideas that prevent recovery. These thoughts may be about issues of safety, trust, power, control, esteem, or intimacy. The goal of CPT is to replace distorted and unconstructive thoughts with more helpful ones.

Prolonged Exposure (PE): During prolonged-exposure therapy, patients are gradually exposed to thoughts, feelings, and situations related to their trauma in a controlled way. This can be extremely difficult, as it involves reliving distressing moments. PE is a specific type of CBT that asks a person to imagine their trauma and recount the narrative out loud to a therapist, as well as confront trauma-evocative situations in real life. Prolonged exposure typically lasts for about three months; the goal is to diminish the power of trauma-related memories and reduce avoidance behaviors.

CBT, CPT, and prolonged exposure are considered confrontational therapies because they address the root of the trauma head on. Indirect forms of therapy, on the other hand, do not directly target the feelings and thoughts related to the trauma. Less confrontational approaches are often necessary, as many people do not follow through with CBT, CPT, or PE because they are too painful. One Veterans Administration study revealed that out of 796 patients attending a PTSD and anxiety clinic, barely 11 percent of referred patients initiated either CPT or PE, and an even smaller percentage (7.9 percent) completed either treatment.[16] Some of the most useful indirect therapies include eye movement desensitization and reprocessing (EMDR), somatic experiencing (SE), and acupuncture, as described next.

Eye Movement Desensitization and Reprocessing (EMDR): EMDR is an indirect form of psychotherapy that does not require talking in detail about your trauma. Instead, a therapist guides you to focus on emotions, thoughts, or behaviors while directing you to move your eyes back and forth. This may sound strange—or even a little woo-woo—yet evidence shows it is strongly effective. It has been listed as a first-line treatment and a best practice for trauma by the U.S. Veterans Association, the U.K. Ministry of Defence and the World Health Organization.[17] EMDR is based on the theory that the brain stores traumatic memories quite differently from normal ones,[18] creating a kind of mental wound that cannot heal, always keeping you on high alert. EMDR uses bilateral sensory input, such as side-to-side eye movements, hand tapping, or auditory tones, leading your brain to reprocess memories and integrate them in a more adaptive way. Your therapist will have you select a positive belief to replace negative thought patterns. As one participant in an EMDR trial reported, "Negative memories I tend to remember with less hatred and anger and they feel less directly emotive as though they weren't happening to me."[19]

Often, PTSD has psychological and physical symptoms, a feature of the condition that any treatment plan needs to take into consideration. Dr. Bessel van der Kolk, a psychiatrist and researcher who studies how children and adults adapt to traumatic experiences, emphasizes that PTSD is not just a psychological disorder, but also a physiological one where the body continues to hold onto and respond to traumatic memories. As he writes in *The Body Keeps the Score*, "We have learned that trauma is not just an event that took place sometime in the past; it is also the imprint left by that experience on mind, brain, and body."[20] While talk therapy is important and beneficial, Dr. van der Kolk explains that it might not be enough for trauma treatment because it does not always reach the emotional and physical effects of trauma.

So, how can you activate your recovery reflex to address body, mind, and spirit? My patients have had success with the following treatments.

Somatic Experiencing (SE): Developed by Dr. Peter Levine, somatic experiencing helps people release and resolve the physical tension and energy trapped in their body due to trauma.[21] SE is based on the theory that trauma can lead to dysfunction in the nervous system, which prevents you from fully processing the experience. Many people with PTSD are thought to be stuck in the "freeze response"—the third element of the sympathetic nervous system. (The others are fight, flight, and a final element called fawn.) This is reminiscent of prey animals that "play dead" when threatened.[22] The therapy involves gradually guiding patients to develop awareness of their bodily sensations and renegotiating their physiological response to stress. While there is not as much evidence for SE's effectiveness compared to other psychotherapies,[23] in my experience, people often prefer it because it does not require direct confrontation with trauma.

Acupuncture: Another nonconfrontational approach to PTSD treatment that has been well studied is acupuncture. A 2023 meta-analysis of eight randomized controlled trials included 656 patients, 330 of which received acupuncture while the remaining 326 received either medications or psychotherapy.[24] The study revealed that acupuncture outperformed both medications and psychotherapy for PTSD.

Medications for PTSD

The NHS has approved only two medications for the treatment of PTSD: sertraline and paroxetine. Both are selective serotonin reuptake inhibitors (SSRIs), a class of drugs commonly used to treat depression and anxiety. These medications may alleviate symptoms including intrusive thoughts, avoidance behaviors, and hyperarousal. Overall, however, between 40 and 60 percent of people with PTSD do not respond to either drug.[25] I believe these medications do have a place and that they can reduce several of the worst symptoms for some people, but I prefer other approaches that get to the root of and help resolve PTSD.

Trauma-Releasing Exercises

In 1979, while working with a Catholic missionary group, Dr. David Berceli sat in a Lebanese bomb shelter with dozens of refugees as missiles exploded overhead. He was struck by the difference between the petrified children who trembled violently and their parents, who, determined to be strong, held still.[26] Years later, Dr. Berceli again noticed the phenomenon while working with refugees in Sudan. During intense moments, the children trembled and held their parents, while the adults willed themselves to stay calm.

Some time later, Dr. Berceli tracked down the Sudanese families to see how they had coped in the aftermath of the violence. He observed that while the children had completely bounced back, the adults displayed symptoms of PTSD. This led him to theorize that due to cultural and social norms, humans suppress their intrinsic tremor response during trauma, leading to the accumulation of stress and tension in the body.

Consider that animals naturally tremor to release stress and return to a state of equilibrium after a traumatic event. When an antelope is cornered by a lion, for instance, it freezes in place, awaiting its fate. If the lion is distracted or frightened off, the antelope begins tremoring violently as it processes its near-death experience. But after thirty seconds or so, its trauma discharged, the antelope bounds away as if nothing had happened. Humans, too, have this ability to discharge trauma, Dr. Berceli theorized, but we may be conditioned not to use it.

Dr. Berceli later developed Tension & Trauma-Releasing Exercises (TRE) to assist individuals in releasing tension and trauma from the body.[27] TRE is based on the idea the human body—just like the antelope—has an innate ability to release tension through involuntary shaking or tremoring. Dr. Berceli recommends performing TRE together with a trained professional if you have PTSD. For more information about TRE, including detailed how-to videos, I encourage you to visit Dr. Berceli's website.

Yoga

In addition to TRE, yoga can help release tension and provide relief to people whose unresolved trauma has caused them to get stuck in a perpetual "freeze" response. Studies by Dr. van der Kolk, mentioned earlier, and others have shown that yoga is as beneficial as medication for alleviating symptoms of PTSD by helping the autonomic nervous system adapt more effectively to triggers and stimuli.[28] And a meta-analysis found that practicing yoga helped to reduce physiological arousal in PTSD patients.[29]

Several styles of yoga have been shown to be beneficial for PTSD. These styles typically emphasize gentle movements, mindfulness, and breath work:

- **Hatha Yoga:** Focusing on physical postures and breath control, Hatha yoga is often recommended for beginners and can be particularly suitable for individuals with PTSD, owing to its slower pace and emphasis on relaxation and mindfulness.[30]
- **Trauma-Sensitive Yoga:** Developed specifically for trauma survivors, trauma-sensitive yoga is adapted to emphasize making choices about movements, focusing on bodily sensations, and developing a more grounded and empowered relationship with the body. This style of yoga was designed to enhance feelings of safety and body awareness. As one major review concluded, trauma-sensitive yoga's "emphasis on mindful movement and interoceptive awareness helps to regulate affective arousal, increases ability to experience emotions safely in the present moment, and promotes a sense of safety and comfort within one's body," and "may assist in both symptom reduction as well as personal growth."[31]
- **Kundalini Yoga:** Kundalini Yoga combines postures, breath work, and the chanting of mantras to awaken and channel energy that is said to be located at the base of your spine, known as Kundalini energy. Compared to Hatha and other forms of yoga, Kundalini yoga is a more spiritual practice that deemphasizes physical movements in favor of chanting, singing, movements, and breathing in specific patterns. Studies have shown that this style can be effective in reducing PTSD symptoms, likely due to its focus on the connection between physical movement, breathing, and mental focus.[32]

I love yoga and have practiced it for many years. I frequently recommend it to my patients, though it is not for everyone. Some people tell me, "I am not flexible." (This is actually a *good* reason to go.) Others are uncomfortable being in a room with lots of people in skintight yoga clothes. You can always wear loose, comfy clothes, or even attend virtual classes with your video off! If you have an intuition that yoga might be helpful for you, choose your class with care. Find one that offers trauma-sensitive yoga.

Another possibility is a "nervous system reset class," sometimes called *restorative yoga*, which is intended to create a soothing and balanced practice that allows the nervous system to down-regulate from the fight-or-flight state. It creates a renewed sense of energy, clarity of mind, and a feeling of peace. These classes are normally gentle and beginner-friendly, good for those who are recovering from injury or illness, or for those who struggle with anxiety and feeling overwhelmed.

> ### Deep-Breathing Exercises
>
> Deep-breathing exercises can help people with PTSD manage their symptoms. These exercises work on several levels—physiological, psychological, and emotional—to provide relief and promote relaxation. Deep, slow exhalations can quiet the nervous system and counteract the hyperarousal symptoms common in PTSD. Breathing exercises also activate the body's relaxation response and lower stress hormone levels.
>
> Studies show that deep-breathing exercises, meditation, and other mindfulness exercises can be integrated into daily routines.[33] I cover three of them in "Your Rapid Recovery Toolkit" (appendix 1).

Written Disclosure

Written disclosure is a therapeutic technique in which a person writes about a traumatic event. Writing provides a way to express and process the trauma by organizing and making sense of the events and their impact. Putting feelings onto paper can provide emotional catharsis.

Even a few short sessions can produce lasting results. In one study conducted by Dr. James Pennebaker, who pioneered the field of research on written disclosure, forty-six students were asked to write about either personally traumatic life events or trivial topics for fifteen minutes on four consecutive days.[34] The material was private; neither a teacher nor a researcher read it. Afterwards, "for six months following the experiment, students who wrote about traumatic events visited the campus health center less often, and used a pain reliever less frequently, than those who wrote about inconsequential matters." Another study revealed that written disclosure led to a more positive outlook among female sexual-assault survivors.[35] At three months follow-up, the women described significant reductions in interpersonal distress as well reductions in avoidance behaviors associated with PTSD.

There are several studied formats; you can write for fifteen to twenty minutes once a day for four consecutive days, or once a week for four weeks. The prompts ask you to write about your traumatic experiences, including details about the event, your thoughts, feelings, and the impact on your life. Writing can lead to greater insight and integrates the traumatic experience into your life story; it becomes part of a larger narrative, which can foster a sense of wholeness and continuity. Of course, writing about trauma can be an intense experience in and of itself. I recommend waiting at least two months after a traumatic event to begin journaling in this way. And, you may choose to do it together with a therapist.

Post-Traumatic Growth

While PTSD can exact a huge toll on a person, it also contains the potential for growth. The concept of post-traumatic growth (PTG) was developed by the psychologists Richard Tedeschi and Lawrence Calhoun.[36] They theorized that trauma could ultimately lead to increased personal strength, improved relationships, and greater appreciation for life. And, indeed, PTG has been observed in people who have suffered serious illness or injury, job loss, bereavement, war, and natural disasters.[37]

PTG can occur on its own, and there are five action steps you can take to stimulate your recovery reflex and increase the likelihood of it occurring:[38]

1. **Education:** Understanding trauma and its effects is the first step toward PTG. Paying attention to your body and learning how stress and adversity impact your brain can help normalize the experience and offer a roadmap for healing.
2. **Emotional Regulation:** Trauma can leave you feeling overwhelmed, even when making small, low-stakes decisions. Developing skills like mindfulness,

deep breathing, and cognitive reframing helps you manage your emotional responses and build resilience.
3. **Disclosure:** Sharing your story—whether with a trusted friend, therapist, or support group—can reduce shame and isolation. Talking about trauma in a safe space can help you process emotions and integrate the experience into your identity in a healthy way.
4. **Reframing Your Narrative:** Instead of seeing yourself as a victim, PTG involves reshaping your story into one of strength and transformation. You may come to find meaning in your struggles and recognize the ways that trauma has served as a catalyst for personal growth—and potentially a renewed sense of purpose.
5. **Service:** Giving back to others solidifies your growth. There are many ways to serve, including mentorship, advocacy, or community involvement. Helping others who have experienced similar struggles reinforces resilience, deepens purpose, and can provide a sense of empowerment.

Finally, some people find it helps to learn about famous individuals who overcame great adversity to become leaders—think Oprah Winfrey enduring an abusive childhood or Nelson Mandela spending twenty-seven years in prison. Within your new narrative, you may discover a different set of priorities or a novel way to serve.

Psychedelics

Even though it had been many years since my patient Kate's sexual assault, she had not fully healed. Talk therapy, EMDR, and written disclosure had worked to an extent, but "something is still not right," she explained when she saw me.

"I think you may be a candidate for psychedelics," I said.

Psychedelics are a class of psychoactive medicines that can produce profound changes in perception, mood, and cognitive processes. They can alter a person's thinking, sense of time, and emotions while causing visual and auditory hallucinations. People often describe entering a unitive state during their trip, in which their ego melts away and they feel connected to everyone and everything.

Psychedelics include psilocybin (mushrooms); ibogaine, peyote, mescaline, and Ayahuasca (plants); 5-MeO-DMT (an animal venom[39]); and LSD (a synthetic compound).[40] They have been tightly controlled and highly debated for decades. Two other synthetic compounds—ketamine, which is an anesthetic, and MDMA, which is an empathogen—are not true psychedelics, although they act similarly.

I put Kate in touch with a colleague, Michael, a medical doctor with extensive training in psychedelic therapeutic practices. They began with ketamine, which has shown promise in treating PTSD, particularly in reducing symptoms such as anxiety, depression, and intrusive thoughts.[41] This is possibly due to its ability to increase the levels of the neurotransmitter glutamate, leading to enhanced neuroplasticity—the brain's ability to adapt and change. Ketamine is a controlled substance; its use is illegal except when administered by a qualified healthcare provider. You can receive treatment in privately or through the NHS.

In Kate's case, the ketamine sessions did help with her symptoms, but her trauma still felt unresolved and her triggers remained. She believed there was still some below-the-surface issue she needed to express. When she explained this to Michael, he suggested they do a session with MDMA.

MDMA, short for 3,4-methylenedioxymethamphetamine, is a synthetic drug that alters mood and perception. It has chemical similarities to both stimulants and hallucinogens, and can produce feelings of increased energy, pleasure, emotional warmth, and distorted sensory and time perception. You may know it colloquially as "ecstasy" or "Molly." Despite its reputation as a party drug, MDMA has gained attention for its potential therapeutic benefits when used in a controlled setting, particularly for treating PTSD.

Michael followed the protocol established in the U.S.A. by the Multidisciplinary Association for Psychedelic Studies (MAPS). When Kate was ready, her husband and sister joined her, and under Michael's guidance, she took a dose of MDMA in her living room. About forty minutes later, as the MDMA increased the activity of the neurotransmitters in her brain, vivid traumatic childhood memories surfaced. Over the course of her sessions, Kate began to process her experiences and memories as Michael guided her with the protocols. In her third and final session, Kate saw herself lying alone as an infant in the hospital; she had been born premature and spent six weeks in the NICU. "I saw myself as this little premature bird and experienced my older self teaching my younger self how to fly." Gazing at herself as a tiny, vulnerable baby, she suddenly felt stronger. She was a survivor. Despite multiple traumas, she had pushed through and endured. "Not even survived—I flourished, even in the wake of all of this stuff that was not even accessible to me."

Three months later Kate wrote in her journal: "It's been three-plus months since my last MDMA experience. My heart continues to open and is more expanded and able to receive the messages of the great mystery that we're all connected to. I recognize the fragility of life, and I don't have time to waste. I want to keep peering into the darkness, to transmute it, so that I may live with more light and more space . . . and continue to be touched by the sacred. It's all around me . . . the signs are everywhere."

In trials, other people have responded to MDMA as profoundly as Kate did. In 2017, U.S. authorities awarded MDMA breakthrough status based on research supporting its significant value in treating PTSD when used in conjunction with psychotherapy.[42] Unfortunately, in August 2024, when reviewing the randomized controlled trials, they declined to approve MDMA-assisted psychotherapy, instead requesting further research studies.

Ketamine is not technically a psychedelic but, rather, an anesthetic that has dissociative effects. It has been U.S. FDA-approved since 1970 as an anesthetic, and was approved in the U.S. in 2019 in a nasal form (esketamine) for treatment resistant depression. Dr. Tamara Stoner is an anesthesiologist and a graduate of the Andrew Weil Center's Integrative Medicine Fellowship who uses intravenous ketamine in conjunction with psychotherapy as a treatment for people with PTSD, complex pain, depression, and other conditions. She notes that for seventy-two hours after IV treatment, people tend to feel safer, less anxious, and are more neuroplastic, meaning they can more easily form new neural connections in their brains. A meta-analysis from late 2023 examined six randomized controlled trials comprising 259 patients with moderate to severe PTSD, finding that one injection of ketamine was able to reduce symptoms by about 25 percent at one day and at one week.[43] In the U.K., ketamine is most often administered for treating this form of depression by giving it intravenously during a forty-minute session. Typically, people are treated several times over multiple weeks.

Can Vitamins and Minerals Prevent PTSD?

In 2011, Dr. Julia Rucklidge made a remarkable finding: People who experience trauma may be able to avoid PTSD entirely by taking B vitamins plus minerals. That year, the citizens of Christchurch, New Zealand, experienced a series of intense earthquakes over a five-month period. Dr. Rucklidge, who lives and works there, measured the effect of a broad-spectrum multivitamin-multimineral in sixty-four adults.[44] When PTSD symptoms were assessed one month later, only 19 percent of the people who took the B vitamins plus minerals qualified for the diagnosis compared to 48 percent of the control group.

Another researcher, Dr. Bonnie Kaplan, had a similar opportunity two years later, when heavy flooding devastated southern and central Alberta, Canada. Her randomized study found that compared to people who received vitamin D alone, those who took a B complex or a broad-spectrum mineral-vitamin formula showed significantly greater improvement in stress and anxiety within four to six weeks.[45] This is a low-risk intervention with the potential to short-circuit the initiation of PTSD, so I strongly recommend discussing it with your healthcare provider if you or anyone you love experiences a traumatic event.

The Role of Set and Setting

Two widely accepted influences on the outcome of psychedelic-assisted psychotherapy are the set and setting. The former refers to our internal mindset, while the latter refers to the external environment. In studies, a great deal of attention is usually paid to these factors. Participants are asked to clearly define what they hope to get out of the session,[46] and two therapists commonly sit with them to provide comfort and support if needed. The participant usually wears a blindfold and listens to carefully curated music while lying on a comfortable bed or couch. In some studies of veterans the experience is processed in a group setting, as the support of peers is recognized as deeply meaningful.[47]

Many Indigenous populations, from whom Westerners learned about psychedelics, consider the plant medicines (Ayahuasca, peyote, mescaline) and mushrooms to be sacred.[48] They are consumed communally and administered by a shaman or curandero with extensive experience in a spiritual ceremony that may include singing personalized healing songs called *Icaros*. In the weeks leading up to the ceremony, participants are asked to restrain from sexual activity and eat only certain foods. It's important to point out that many Indigenous people are concerned about the extraction of these plant medicines from their larger cultural context, because of both cultural appropriation and a loss of effectiveness. In response, thought leaders are coming together to create a set of ethical principles that acknowledge and respect Indigenous people and their knowledge, intellectual property, and practices as the root of Western psychedelic medicine.[49]

The legality of psychedelics in the United States is evolving. Ibogaine is a schedule I-controlled substance and is not approved for any therapeutic use in the United States. However, it is unregulated in Mexico, where it has grown in popularity as a treatment for opioid addiction. MDMA and psilocybin are not yet legal in the United States, although they have been decriminalized in the states of Oregon and Colorado and in several cities.[50] (In Oregon, psilocybin is legal for mental health treatment under supervision.[51]) Additionally, in 2006, the U.S. Supreme Court ruled that religious use of traditional psychedelics by Native American people and other churches is legal.

In 2024, Kate was invited to participate in a church ceremony, and here she was legally administered Ayahuasca. While she was given a low dose, she had a profound experience in which she felt a sense of absolute clarity. As she described it, "Nothing that ever happened to me broke me. What happened externally never touched the essence of who I am." Since that ceremony she has felt a sense of lightness of being and a profound deepening of her healing.

The decision to use psychedelics for trauma is not to be undertaken lightly and unless given by the appropriate health care provider, many are illegal in the U.K. as well as in many other countries. Before psychedelics, take time to establish a trusting relationship with your healthcare provider. Avoid using psychedelics if you have a medical history of heart, liver, or kidney disease, as well as a history of psychosis, mania, active substance abuse, and severe personality disorders.

Vagus Nerve Stimulation

Because people with PTSD have chronically overactive sympathetic nervous systems, it has been theorized that vagus nerve stimulation (VNS) could reduce heart rate, respiration rate, and blood pressure by activating the parasympathetic nervous system. This was confirmed in a 2020 study that found the gammaCore device "attenuates sympathetic arousal associated with stress related to traumatic memories as well as mental stress in patients with PTSD."[52] Another gammaCore study found that people with PTSD using the device for three months experienced 31 percent fewer symptoms compared to placebo.[53]

In 2022, the U.S. authorities granted breakthrough designation for gammaCore to be used in the treatment of PTSD.[54] Other vagus-nerve-stimulating or toning methods are also being explored, including an auricular (on the ear lobe) device with 9/11 first responders at the World Trade Center.[55] I have recommended the use of different VNS devices to many of my patients. My patients frequently report back their anxiety has diminished and their sleep is improved. I believe VNS will soon be recognized as one more useful tool for people struggling with PTSD.

Settling our nervous system is a key component of addressing trauma and is an underlying dimension of many of the strategies described in this chapter. VNS devices can play a meaningful role in quieting or resetting a nervous system that is chronically on high alert.

Can a Dog Help?

Dogs truly make everything better, including PTSD! Service dogs have been studied as a treatment for veterans who experience PTSD. For instance, these dogs have been taught to interrupt flashbacks and nightmares by gently licking their owner's face. Dogs can help monitor an environment, thereby reducing hypervigilance in their owner. And they have even been shown to reduce negative thoughts and mood by providing friendship and love.

A clinical survey found that vets with service dogs report lower PTSD severity and better mental health, with less depression, anger, anxiety, and absenteeism from work.[56] Dogs have been shown to restore the normal physiological rise in morning cortisol levels in people with PTSD.[57] (During chronic stress, this rise is blunted.) Interactions with dogs can also raise levels of oxytocin,[58] which is known as the "love hormone." If you are a veteran or worked for the emergency services, you can obtain a dog from Service Dogs UK, Veterans with Dogs and Bravehound.

Please note that not all dogs can fulfill these roles. Service dogs are carefully selected and trained,[59] and anxious animals are never good candidates.

Your Rapid Recovery Prescription for Taming Post-Traumatic Stress Disorder

PTSD symptoms can be caused by a single event or multiple events; they can emerge quickly or take months or years to appear after a traumatic event. While dealing with PTSD can be extremely difficult, it also contains the potential for growth.

1. If your trauma occurred recently, taking B complex vitamins with minerals can reduce the risk of developing PTSD symptoms.
2. A variety of forms of psychotherapy, including CBT, CPT, or prolonged exposure, have proven to help people with PTSD.
3. Less-confrontative methods that address PTSD are preferred by many people. They include trauma-releasing exercises, EMDR, yoga, and somatic experiencing.
4. Practice deep-breathing exercises to quiet the nervous system and counteract the hyperarousal symptoms associated with PTSD.
5. Written disclosure may help organize and make sense of your trauma and its impact.
6. A growing body of research supports the value of psychedelic-assisted psychotherapy for PTSD.
7. VNS devices can help activate the parasympathetic nervous system, quieting symptoms of PTSD.
8. While no one ever welcomes trauma, it is possible to retrain the brain and even ultimately experience post-traumatic growth.

16

Overcoming Long Covid

My sixty-five-year-old patient George came to my office three months after contracting the Covid-19 virus. His symptoms had been relatively mild thanks to immediate treatment with an antiviral medication. However, he felt overwhelmingly fatigued despite sleeping eight to ten hours each night, and he had developed joint pain and brain fog. It was clear to me that George was one of the estimated 7 percent of American adults who experience long-Covid symptoms after acute infection.[1]

First, we worked on George's sleep. Even though he believed he was sleeping well, I asked him to use a sleep tracker, which discovered a thirty-minute latency (the time it took for him to fall asleep), frequent awakenings, and insufficient REM and deep sleep. (For more information about improving sleep, see the "Sleeping Soundly" chapter.) George was spending a lot of time in bed, but he clearly was not getting high-quality sleep. I suggested he avoid drinking alcohol until his symptoms resolved, as it can interfere with normal sleep architecture. I also asked him to stop taking afternoon naps, get exposure to early morning sunlight, dim his lights in the evening, and take a 1 mg nightly melatonin supplement. He also began taking an adaptogen and a mitochondrial support supplement (to improve his energy levels) and turmeric for his joint pain and brain fog.

Gradually, George's symptoms improved, and within seven or eight weeks he returned to good health. Happily, George's positive outcome is common, according to the ComPaRe long-Covid e-cohort,[2] which followed more than two thousand people with long Covid lasting at least two months after an acute infection. (Every sixty days participants were asked about their symptoms; 91 percent improved slowly over a two-year period.)

Covid-19 (coronavirus disease 2019) is an infectious disease caused by the SARS-CoV-2 virus, which of course needs little introduction. Most people recover within two to four weeks,[3] unless they've had a severe illness. Some, like George, have lingering symptoms that persist for weeks, months, or even years after the acute phase of a Covid infection has resolved. Long Covid is diagnosed when signs and symptoms that develop during the initial infection continue for more than twelve weeks and are not explained by an alternative diagnosis.[4] Long Covid can affect men and women of all ages, and it can happen after a severe bout with the virus, a mild one, or even if you were asymptomatic.[5]

There are as many as two hundred different symptoms associated with long Covid; common ones include a profound sense of tiredness that doesn't improve with rest, exertion-induced symptom worsening, brain fog, shortness of breath, autonomic dysfunction, allergic reactions, joint pain, sleep disturbances, neurological problems, and digestive issues.[6] Research also shows that as many as two out of three people with long Covid suffer from mental health challenges, like anxiety and depression. Because we still do not know the exact cause—or causes—of long Covid, determining the best treatment is a challenge. Happily, for the vast majority of people, the body's recovery reflex kicks into gear, and its healing response rids the body of symptoms. If, however, you are struggling with long Covid, this chapter is filled with strategies to boost your recovery reflex.

What Causes Long Covid?

If only the answer to this question were simple! The initial Covid-19 infection is much easier to explain. When an infected person talks, coughs, sneezes, sings, or even breathes, tiny droplets containing the virus are expelled into the air. If you inhale these droplets, the virus can begin to infect the cells of the respiratory tract. You're probably familiar with the classic symptoms—fever, cough, shortness of breath, fatigue, loss of taste or smell, sore throat, muscle or body aches—which usually subside within a few weeks.

While the Covid-19 virus is well studied, long Covid remains enigmatic. There are several theories about what causes it,[7] starting with viral persistence: In some cases, the immune system may not fully clear out the virus. This lingering viral material can continue to provoke the immune system or cause damage to organs, leading to prolonged symptoms. A second theory holds that the body's immune system overreacts to the initial infection, leading to autoimmunity. Inflammation, including in the brain (neuroinflammation), is a common response to the acute Covid infection, but in some people it persists even after the virus is gone. Finally, it is possible that certain nutritional deficiencies play a role in long Covid.[8]

The cause of your long Covid may be one of these factors, all of these factors, or perhaps none of them. Furthermore, there may be many different subtypes of long Covid that require different treatment approaches. As studies progress, we will likely learn the underlying causes of, and most effective treatment approaches for, long Covid. There are more than seven thousand such studies in progress worldwide,[9] including the U.S. NIH's RECOVER (Researching COVID to Enhance Recovery) Initiative, which has invested more than $1.6 billion in research dollars since 2021.[10] Until we have definitive answers, we can use the principles of integrative medicine, which has an important approach to helping people recover even when the underlying mechanisms of an illness are not fully understood.[11]

Prevention of Long Covid

It is always better to prevent illness than to have to treat it. We have strong data to support two measures that can greatly reduce your risk of developing long Covid, and one measure that may.

The first is vaccination. For instance, by early 2022, when the Omicron family of variants predominated, the rate of long Covid declined to just 3.5 percent among vaccinated adults,[12] compared to 7.7 percent for unvaccinated adults. The takeaway is this: You can halve your risk of long Covid by getting a vaccine!

The second method to prevent long Covid is to take metformin as soon as the symptoms begin. As we saw in the "Reversing Type 2 Diabetes" chapter, metformin is a first-line medication for preventing and treating type 2 diabetes. It also has antiviral and anti-inflammatory properties that may improve mitochondrial function[13]—potentially addressing the underlying mechanisms that cause long Covid. A study among overweight people infected with Covid aged thirty to eighty-five found that metformin reduced the risk of developing long Covid by 41 percent.[14] Researchers are looking into the potential benefit of taking metformin if you have recently been diagnosed with Covid-19.

Another treatment that might prevent long Covid is Paxlovid, which is the only oral medication approved for treating a Covid infection. It combines two antivirals, nirmatrelvir and ritonavir, and is currently recommended for treating mild to moderate Covid in people who have a high risk of progressing to severe disease. (In general, this means people aged fifty years or older, especially those with other longstanding diseases.) I took Paxlovid when I caught Covid for the first time in September 2022, partly because data at the time suggested it might help prevent long Covid. The Paxlovid rapidly eliminated my sore throat, headache, and fever, and I did not develop any lingering side effects.

Today, research is less clear about how effective Paxlovid actually is at preventing long Covid. A 2024 study compared roughly 165,000 people treated with Paxlovid within five days of infection and nearly 308,000 who were not treated with any antiviral medication.[15] Compared with the nontreated group, higher-risk patients on Paxlovid had a 12 percent lower risk of developing long Covid, as well as a 30 percent reduction in hospitalization and a 47 percent reduced risk of death. Another trial of more than four hundred thousand people treated with Paxlovid found it somewhat helpful in preventing cognitive issues and fatigue, but not other symptoms of long Covid.[16]

Given these results, if you get Covid, I recommend taking Paxlovid if you are over fifty or otherwise at a higher risk of hospitalization. As for whether it prevents long Covid, the jury is still out.

Boosting the Effectiveness of Your Covid Vaccine

You can make your vaccine "take" better, according to a 2023 study that evaluated the effect of timing on 1.5 million people receiving Covid vaccinations.[17] People who received their vaccine in the morning had lower rates of infections when compared to individuals vaccinated in the evening. This is consistent with results from influenza vaccine and resonates with the importance of optimizing your circadian rhythm, as discussed throughout this book.

If You Suspect Long Covid

If you think you may have long Covid, please see a doctor! This is important for several reasons, including the possibility you actually have a different condition. Your doctor can discern this with a careful history, blood tests, and potentially other types of testing. For example, one of my patients, Evelyn, had shortness of breath several weeks after she recovered from Covid. The cause was in fact a blood clot to the lung. It may or may not have been caused by the initial Covid infection, but in either case, the clot was treatable with blood thinners.

In general, to diagnose long Covid, I recommend several blood tests to first rule out other conditions. These include a complete blood count (CBC) to ensure you are not anemic, ferritin (which checks iron stores), thyroid testing (can cause fatigue), liver-function tests, kidney-function tests, d-dimer (for clotting), HbA1C, vitamin D, and two tests for inflammation: CRP and ESR. In some patients with allergic-like symptoms, a histamine and vitamin B2 level can be useful. If you're experiencing respiratory symptoms, I advise pulmonary-function tests.

One of the principal symptoms of long Covid is extreme fatigue. Regardless of the cause, integrative medicine provides strategies that can boost your recovery. The first, not surprising, is getting restful sleep. (I know, this is easier said than done!) Are you getting at least seven hours? Are you waking up feeling rested? Your goal is to have normal REM and deep sleep. See the "Sleeping Soundly" chapter for detailed advice on getting a good night's sleep. Other foundational recommendations to mitigate long-Covid symptoms and enhance overall well-being include addressing stress (see the "Unwinding Anxiety" chapter), an anti-inflammatory diet (see "Your Rapid Recovery Toolkit"), and pacing,[18] which is a gradual approach to increasing the intensity of exercise.

As many as 14 percent of people with long Covid develop PoTS (postural tachycardia syndrome),[19] in which a person's autonomic nervous system functions abnormally and their heart rate surges upon standing. Symptoms can include fatigue, lightheadedness, palpitations, chest pain, exercise intolerance, and cognitive impairment.[20] If you suspect PoTS, your doctor will assess your blood pressure and pulse while standing and lying down. A diagnosis of PoTS is made when your heart rate increases by at least thirty beats per minute when you move from a horizontal to standing position.

I have seen long-Covid patients with PoTS treated at our clinic respond quickly to allithiamine (also known as thiamine tetrahydrofurfuryl disulfide), which addresses a thiamine deficiency. A forty-five-year-old woman named Yolanda developed PoTS in 2021, two months after being diagnosed with Covid. Whenever she stood up, her heart raced and she felt like she would faint. She was also exhausted and could barely exercise, even though she had been an avid hiker before getting Covid. When Yolanda did push past her fatigue to take a 2 to 3 kilometer (2–3 mile) walk, she experienced postexertional malaise and an abnormally elevated heart rate. She also complained of brain fog, and it was hard for her to get work done. My colleague prescribed for Yolanda 100 mg of allithiamine, a B complex vitamin, and 400 mg of magnesium glycinate. Her PoTS symptoms completely resolved in two weeks, and her fatigue resolved within three. The culprit, it turned out, was a thiamine deficiency. While this dramatic improvement is not the case for all long-Covid patients with PoTS, it can occur when the cause is particular micronutrient deficiencies,[21] so a three-month trial of allithiamine is a low-risk option.

Beyond allithiamine, here is what I recommend for dealing with PoTS:

- Slow down all postural changes, such as from lying to sitting, or sitting to standing.
- Hydrate well by drinking 2 to 2.5 liters (3½–4½ pints) of fluids per day. Increase your salt intake to 3 to 5 grams per day.
- Avoid large meals, which can lower your blood pressure as blood moves to the gut for digestion.
- Elevate the head of your bed by 15 to 25 centimeters (6–10 inches), which can raise circulating blood volume.
- Wear compression stockings, ideally all the way up to the abdomen.

Finally, when exercising, begin with low-intensity horizonal movements such as swimming, rowing, or recumbent cycling for three months. Over time, as you have built up a tolerance for horizontal exercises, you can slowly graduate to upright movements, such as jogging, walking on a treadmill, cycling, or the elliptical machine. A POTS training protocol is available free of charge from the Children's Hospital of Philadelphia,[22] at www.chop.edu.

Long Covid and Your Gut

Fatigue and brain fog are the symptoms most commonly associated with long Covid, but many people experience digestive problems, including loose stools, constipation, and bloating.[23] While the link between GI discomfort and long Covid is not well understood, emerging research suggests that the virus causes distinct changes in gut–brain signaling.

Other studies have shown that the Covid-19 virus harms the microbiome, potentially altering the gut lining and permitting bacteria to enter the bloodstream (a condition known as leaky gut).[24] While research is ongoing, you can improve the health of your microbiome by eating fermented foods, increasing your fiber, and practicing time-restricted eating.

Mind–Body Tools

A recent study carried out in the UK used an inventive strategy to assess the impact of mindfulness on long Covid. The English National Opera (ENO) began a pilot program in partnership with the Imperial College Healthcare NHS Trust. A team of doctors, therapists, and vocal coaches developed a breathing and well-being program for people with long Covid who were still experiencing breathlessness and anxiety.[25] They enrolled 150 such people who met in one-hour zoom sessions for six weeks and taught them to sing culturally diverse lullabies. By the end of the study, breathlessness and overall mental-health well-being improved in the ENO group compared to the control group. ENO Breathe was even described as a "toolbox full of hope" by the participants.[26]

Research supports that practicing mindfulness, especially meditation, improves outcomes in long-Covid patients,[27] possibly by decreasing the amount of inflammatory proteins in the body. Yoga, particularly asana and pranayama, also shows promise as a long-Covid complementary treatment.[28]

Supplements

Supplements can support your recovery reflex and assist in reducing many of the symptoms of long Covid. Here, I discuss the evidence for some of the most commonly recommended supplements.

> **Vitamin D:** Vitamin D has antioxidant, antibacterial, anti-inflammatory, and immunomodulatory properties that can help reduce the severity of acute Covid infections and enhance recovery from long Covid.[29] A meta-analysis of fifty-eight studies comprising fourteen million patients with Covid found that high vitamin-D levels are associated with less severe long-Covid symptoms.[30]
>
> **Zinc:** You may recall from the "Conquering Colds and Vanquishing Viral Infections" chapter that zinc has antiviral and immune-modulating

properties. Zinc deficiency has been correlated with acute and persistent inflammation.[31] I recommend a dose of 25 mg per day.

Turmeric: Often recommended for its anti-inflammatory, antioxidant, antiviral, antibacterial, and neuroprotective properties,[32] turmeric has been used in traditional medicine practices for centuries. Notably, turmeric's active component—curcumin—can cross the blood-brain barrier, making it potentially useful for treating neuroinflammation. A published review of six studies demonstrated that curcumin supplementation reduced common Covid symptoms, length of hospitalization, and mortality rates.[33] I recommend a dose of 1,000 to 2,000 mg per day of curcumin extract, preferably taken with a meal that contains fat. (See "How to Choose a Supplement," appendix 2, for more information about choosing a turmeric supplement.)

Quercetin: Quercetin is a natural mast-cell stabilizer that has anti-allergy, anti-cancer, anti-hypertension, anti-hyperlipidemia, anti-hyperglycemia, antimicrobial, antiviral, neuroprotective, and cardio-protective effects.[34] It has been studied in conjunction with other antiviral medications in acute Covid infections and shown to be helpful. Quercetin has also demonstrated therapeutic effects in mitigating symptoms and shortening duration of long Covid.[35] For long Covid, I recommend a dose of 500 mg twice daily.

Adaptogens: Adaptogens are often used in integrative-medicine practice to alleviate stress, support sleep, and enhance energy. A trial of ninety-nine people with long-Covid symptoms used a supplement combining the adaptogens rhodiola, eleutherococcus, and schisandra for two weeks.[36] The researchers found the adaptogens decreased fatigue and pain levels in 50 percent of participants and improved their ability to work out. They also protected kidney function.

Mitochondrial Support: Another strategy used by many integrative-medicine providers is to support the mitochondria, also known as the cell's "powerhouse." There are many multi-ingredient supplements on the market each containing somewhat different mixes of ingredients designed to support your mitochondria, which play an important role in energizing your recovery reflex.

Medications

Certain medications may help manage your long-Covid symptoms. Here is what I recommend:

Antihistamines: During the pandemic, anecdotal reports suggested that taking over-the-counter antihistamines could reduce the symptoms of long Covid. One case study detailed how two women discovered that taking diphenhydramine for unrelated allergies dramatically reduced their long-Covid symptoms,[37] including fatigue, brain fog, and joint pain. Antihistamines are typically used to treat allergic reactions by blocking the effects of histamine, a chemical the immune system releases during allergic responses. The theory suggests that antihistamines can alleviate long-Covid symptoms by reducing immune-system dysregulation, inflammation, and mast-cell activation.

Continued research supports the use of antihistamines.[38] In particular, a 2024 study identified H1 antagonists (common in several well-known brands) as particularly beneficial.[39] Importantly, the study theorized that H1 antihistamines could also help prevent initial infection and mitigate acute symptoms, as well as reduce long-Covid symptoms. Brand-name and generic H1 antihistamines are available over the counter; I recommend loratadine or desloratadine (available by prescription). If you have insomnia, I suggest cetirizine.

Aspirin: Long-Covid patients are at an increased risk of blood clots,[40] and aspirin is often recommended for its anticoagulant effects. One dosing strategy is to take 325 mg twice daily for two weeks, then half an aspirin a day for six weeks. Please discuss the pros and cons of taking aspirin with your doctor.

Paxlovid: Researchers are now investigating using a longer course of Paxlovid (mentioned above) as a treatment for long Covid. For example, the Yale Paxlovid for Long COVID (PAX LC) trial has enrolled one hundred people and is treating them with a fifteen-day course of Paxlovid or a placebo.[41] A second research protocol prescribes Paxlovid for up to twenty-five days.[42] While persistent virus is only one of the theorized causes of long Covid, in people who continue to have circulating viral particles, this could be an effective strategy.

Mast-Cell Stabilizers: Another theory suggests that long Covid may be triggered in some patients by mast cells, which are immune cells that release histamine and other substances to combat infections.[43] This is especially likely if you have symptoms in a range of organs, such as the skin (hives, and flushing), the gastrointestinal system (nausea, vomiting, diarrhea, and abdominal cramping), the cardiovascular system (rapid heart rate, low blood pressure, and fainting), or the upper and lower respiratory systems (red eyes, itchy nose, stuffiness, wheezing, and shortness of breath). It can be detected through a tryptase blood test to determine if you have mast-cell activation syndrome (which is rare); even if the test comes back normal, discuss a trial of antihistamines, sodium cromoglicate or other mast-cell–stabilizing medications with your doctor to reduce inflammation and stimulate healing.

Alcohol and Long Covid

Since the beginning of the pandemic, anecdotal reports have indicated that alcohol intolerance—characterized by headaches, nausea, fatigue, and feeling hung over—is more prevalent among people with long Covid. While research is ongoing, there is some evidence that suggests alcohol can indeed make long Covid worse.[44]

Alcohol is known to suppress the immune system,[45] making it more difficult for your rapid recovery reflex to eradicate trace amounts of the virus in your system. Alcohol is also proinflammatory,[46] another possible trigger for long Covid. When you are recovering from a Covid infection, I recommend abstaining from drinking alcohol until you feel fully well.

Take it Slow

Dealing with long Covid is understandably frustrating. One in four adults with long Covid report limitations in their daily activity, feeling ashamed, or experiencing isolation. According to the U.S. Centers for Disease Control and Prevention (CDC), more than one million Americans are out of work at any given time due to long Covid.[47] (If you need time off, be aware that long Covid could be considered a disability.[48])

In light of these facts, the temptation to rush back to your normal activities is understandable. But long-Covid researchers are increasingly observing that doing so may prolong symptoms.[49] In one study that enrolled almost five hundred Covid "long haulers," the vast majority reported that physical activity made their symptoms worse.[50] (This is very similar to the experience of people with chronic fatigue syndrome.) Nevertheless, because exercise is incredibly important to your overall health, I recommend pacing, which refers to regulating activity to avoid worsening of symptoms after exercise.[51] In a large international study comprising about three thousand seven hundred people with long Covid, 23 percent reported that pacing was significantly helpful, and 18 percent found it slightly helpful, for symptom management.[52]

Here are some tips for pacing: Focus on your most important tasks first, whether it's work, household chores, or personal care. Let go of nonessential activities to conserve energy. For example, instead of cleaning the house all at once, consider breaking it down into smaller, more manageable steps—say, the bathroom one day and vacuuming another. Take a break when you feel tired, rather than allowing exhaustion to set in. Think ahead and pace your day so that your activities are generously spaced out. Most important, listen to your body. Pay attention to how it responds to your activities and plan accordingly.

We will continue to learn about the varying causes of long Covid and discern who responds best to which treatment. Many different protocols are under investigation, including antivirals, anti-inflammatories, medicinal mushrooms, probiotics, and prebiotics. Anti-inflammatory and ketogenic diets are also being studied. You may also consider low-dose naltrexone (LDN), using traditional Chinese medicine, and quieting your nervous system with a vagus-nerve–toning device (see page 283 in the "Taming Post-Traumatic Stress Disorder" chapter). Seek out long-Covid clinics or the guidance of an integrative or a naturopathic provider for the latest advice.

Your Rapid Recovery Prescription for Overcoming Long Covid

Dealing with long Covid can be frustrating and isolating. Integrative medicine can help your recovery reflex kick into gear to resolve symptoms.

1. Prevent long Covid by getting vaccinated or boosted if you're eligible for a jab. Discuss metformin with your doctor if you have a Covid infection. Paxlovid can help reduce acute symptoms of Covid if you are in a high-risk category and may reduce the risk of getting long Covid.
2. If you suspect you have long Covid, your doctor may request the following tests: complete blood count, ferritin, thyroid, liver function, kidney function, d-dimer, HbA1C, vitamin D, CRP, and ESR.
3. If you have extreme fatigue, see the "Sleeping Soundly" chapter for improving sleep hygiene and consider the supplements listed in point 5, here.
4. Manage emotional symptoms with a mindfulness meditation practice. Yoga can also reduce effects of long Covid.
5. The following supplements can support your recovery reflex as it helps your body return to homeostasis: vitamin D, zinc, turmeric, quercetin, omega-3 fatty acids, adaptogens, and mitochondrial support.
6. Discuss with your healthcare provider the value of antihistamines, aspirin, mast-cell stabilizers, and low-dose naltrexone (LDN) which is available privately.
7. If you have PoTS, I recommend a trial of treatment with allithiamine. Slow down postural changes, stay hydrated, avoid large meals, elevate the head of your bed, and wear waist-high compression support stockings. Begin with low-intensity horizontal movements when exercising.
8. Rushing back to your normal activities can prolong long Covid. Let go of nonessential activities to conserve energy and tune in to the needs of your body.

Part Three

Recovery from Surgery

17

Setting Yourself up for a Successful Surgery

Surgery has a positive intent: It restores the body to homeostasis by repairing a joint or broken bone, removing an infected appendix or gallbladder, repairing a leaky heart valve, or eradicating a cancerous growth, among many other things. But surgery itself is also a major stressor. Incisions through the skin, underlying tissue, muscles, or organs induce an inflammatory response, which can cause pain and crank your metabolism into overdrive.[1] During recovery, the brain releases the stress hormones cortisol and adrenaline, which augment the healing process, but may also make you feel anxious.

In response, your recovery reflex kicks into gear to stimulate healing. Damaged tissues send signals that stimulate the division and proliferation of nearby cells. New blood vessels form at the wound site, ensuring the healing tissues receive ample oxygen and nutrients. Your immune system guards day and night against infection, as white blood cells patrol against pathogens. Discomfort fades with time. Your innate resilience and your drive to recover, aided by the support of family and friends, as well as careful planning and strategies from integrative medicine, will accelerate healing.

One of the most important ingredients for a speedy recovery is a positive mental outlook. It's understandable that many people, when faced with the prospect of surgery, are fearful that something might go wrong.

For instance, staying active was incredibly important to my patient Olivia. In her early seventies, she routinely cycled over a 160 kilometers (100 miles) per week, hiked mountains, and played golf. And she did all this despite the nagging pain in her lower back. For several years she went to physiotherapy, practiced Pilates, had chiropractic adjustments, and received cortisone shots to treat the pain, but nothing really worked. Eventually, the pain began shooting down her leg, causing numbness and tingling in her foot. After she took two bad falls while hiking, she could no longer ignore what had become increasingly apparent: She needed surgery to ease pressure on her pinched spinal nerves.

Olivia was dejected when she came to see me for a consultation. While she had made the decision to have surgery, she was convinced it would fail. "Back surgery never works," she said. "Everyone I know says so."

This attitude, I pointed out, was inconsistent with her absolute determination to resume her athletic passions. I explained that while some back surgeries are not beneficial, her scans pointed to a clear, fixable problem. I agreed with her specialist; it would take time to recover, but with effort, she would likely do well.

I encouraged her to follow specific steps to prepare for surgery, starting with what I call "prehab," or prehabilitation. She began by following my recommendation to listen to author and therapist Peggy Huddleston's *Prepare for Surgery, Heal Faster* audio recordings. I also asked her to work with her physiotherapist on a plan to strengthen her core, back, and leg muscles. Once surgery was scheduled, she recruited her network of friends and family, developing a plan for who would shop for groceries, bring her cooked meals, keep the house tidy, and tag-team living with her after surgery. With everything in place and her body prepared, Olivia felt ready.

The three-hour procedure went well; after the laminectomy, Olivia's surgeon fused together two vertebrae, stabilizing her spine. She would make a full recovery, he vowed, but the inflamed nerves he observed during the procedure meant that her pain would be significant for some time. When Olivia returned home, she could not bend, lift, or twist. She used a grabber tool to pick items off the floor, a humbling experience for a woman used to scaling mountains. Still, she was confident her robust preparation would mean a swift recovery. As the weeks passed, though, the pain did not subside. A month after surgery, she still had an intense burning sensation in her hip. She worried she would never completely recover and that she was becoming a burden on the social support system she spent so long building. "I thought I would be better by now," she told me, clearly frustrated. "I did everything right—why haven't I gotten back to normal?"

I reminded Olivia about the complex nature of her recovery. "Your pelvic muscles and hip joints spent years compensating for the pain," I said, "and now they need to adapt to a new normal. Your body must relearn how to move, and it hasn't been aligned in a long time. It needs time to adjust."

She returned to *guided imagery*, a mind–body practice, in which she imagined the gradual progression of a successful recovery. I suggested hypnotic techniques to numb the pain with her mind; acupuncture; and supplements including fish oil, glutamine, and lion's mane mushroom. Olivia started using hot and cold packs to reduce swelling and manage pain, as well as transcutaneous electrical nerve stimulation (TENS) therapy, which employs low-voltage current to send signals to the brain and provide pain relief. No one thing was a magic bullet, but something magical did eventually happen: Olivia healed. Not overnight, not in a week, not even in a month, but she slowly got better. Within a year of her surgery she had resumed cycling and hiking. She then spent a summer in Scotland, playing golf. It took a full eighteen months for her to heal—but now there is nothing she cannot do.

As Olivia's experience makes clear, the surgical journey does not begin or end at the hospital. To maximize the potential of your rapid recovery reflex, begin preparing as soon as you learn you need surgery. Specifically, I encourage prehabilitation, or prehab, in the weeks and months *before* your procedure. Prehab is multifaceted and includes elements ranging from the physical (a nutritious diet plus targeted exercises to strengthen muscles and improve cardiovascular fitness), to the psychological and emotional (stress-reduction techniques to lower your anxiety and take advantage of the powerful mind–body connection), to the social (activating a robust network so you can feel loved and supported and be able to focus primarily on your recovery). A vigorous prehab regimen will deliver synergistic benefits and will leave your body and spirit strong, nourished, and primed to bounce back after surgery.

As we've seen in this book, your recovery reflex is impacted by your age, overall health, nutritional status, genetics, and supportive relationships. The type of surgery you have also greatly affects how long it takes your recovery reflex to restore your body to homeostasis; laparoscopic gallbladder removal, for instance, takes much less of a toll on the body than coronary artery bypass surgery. In all cases, there are steps you can take to increase your odds of a successful, straightforward procedure and full recovery. In this section, I will walk you through how to prepare and recover from surgery, beginning with prehab through your journey to the operating theatre, and then to your full post-operative recovery.

While I am not trained as a surgeon, for four decades I have counseled patients who are preparing for and recovering from surgery. I have seen firsthand how integrative medicine can accelerate recovery by boosting overall well-being, reducing stress levels, and enhancing the body's innate healing reflex. Every year, the Andrew Weil Center for Integrative Medicine trains more than 160 fellows, including heart surgeons, orthopedic surgeons, surgical oncologists, and general surgeons. I have interviewed many of them for this book, and we will see how they are pioneering integrative approaches in conjunction with conventional surgical care to improve patient outcomes.

If you are approaching surgery, it is quite common to feel anxious. Know that you are not alone. Every year, more than three hundred *million* people worldwide undergo surgery.[2] Still, simply being in the hospital can be anxiety inducing. On top of that, you will be administered anesthetics—in some cases, you'll be intubated and placed on a ventilator—and hooked up to various IV lines. It isn't exactly a picnic. And yet, thanks to advances including laparoscopic and robot-assisted surgery, real-time imaging, and infection control measures, surgery is extremely safe.

This is in part because many hospitals have adopted the Enhanced Recovery After Surgery (ERAS) protocols, which promote a faster recovery and are fully aligned with the principles of integrative medicine. The goals of the ERAS protocols are to minimize postoperative complications and reduce the length of hospital stays. They include guidelines for pre-operative education and counseling; nutrition; standardized anesthetic practices; early mobilization and rehabilitation; and other pre-op and post-op standards that promote a faster recovery. Studies have shown that ERAS practices result in markedly improved patient outcomes in colorectal,[3] orthopedic,[4] gynecologic,[5] and urological surgeries.[6]

Ask your specialist about ERAS protocols, including a personalized care plan for pain management, rehabilitation exercises, and nutrition. Beyond ERAS, I will recommend integrative medicine's broader array of tools and strategies that you can implement to hasten the speed and improve the quality of your recovery.

As you read through the following chapters, you might marvel how your well-designed recovery reflex is activating with ease to heal from surgery and return your body to homeostasis. Keep these affirmations developed by Belleruth Naparstek, a guided-imagery pioneer and clinical social worker, close to heart:

- More and more I can consider the possibility that my body is teaching me something useful—that these circumstances are challenging to learn from, but I can change and grow.
- I call upon intention to heal myself and keep my body well. I engage my powerful will to assist me in doing this.
- The blueprint that I hold in my mind's eye is the picture of a healthy, vital, strong body. I can see it and I can feel it as I hear these words: *healthy, vital, strong.*
- I invite assistance from my friends and loved ones—past, present, and future—to lend me their support and strength.

18

Your Surgical Prehab

For most of my life, I've been very healthy. I never needed surgery—that is, until my mid-fifties, when I noticed some postmenopausal bleeding. It's not exactly a rare condition—around 10 percent of women over fifty-five experience it[1]—but it can indicate a serious underlying issue, namely, endometrial cancer. After an inconclusive workup with an endometrial biopsy and a pelvic ultrasound, I was scheduled for a dilation and curettage, or D&C, a procedure in which the endometrial lining is scraped off and then sent to a pathologist for diagnosis.

A D&C is not a difficult procedure, but I wanted to put myself in the best possible position to heal. My sister offered to fly in a few days before the surgery, and I gratefully accepted. We are close and she is wonderfully supportive. We shared a delicious dinner out together the night before my procedure. Her presence put my mind and heart at rest. Before bed, as I had been doing since I learned I would need the D&C, I listened to Belleruth Naparstek's guided-imagery audio for a successful surgery (guided imagery is described later in this chapter). I listened again on my headphones before entering the operating theatre.

Another part of my prehab was to speak with the anesthesiologist before my procedure. I knew from a prior dental procedure that benzodiazepines (a class of medication given to reduce anxiety) linger in my system for a long time, making me feel zonked. So, he agreed to use an alternative medication. The procedure went well, and I found out that the cause of the bleeding was a benign endometrial polyp—not cancer. I was given a clean bill of health and was even able to take a planned trip to San Francisco a day later!

Your surgery may be more or less complex than mine, but you can similarly activate your recovery reflex and have a successful outcome with a robust prehabilitation, or prehab, regimen. These interventions serve to prepare your body physically and emotionally for surgery. This is true for minor procedures like the one I underwent, and are even more essential for major surgeries that may require extended hospital stays. Your goal is to enter surgery well nourished, well rested, physically strong, and emotionally prepared. Studies have shown that patients who engage in prehab heal faster and have fewer complications after surgery.[2]

Prehab empowers you to assume a central role in your surgical recovery. We'll see in this chapter that by being proactive and prepared, you are setting yourself up for a fast and full recovery.

Frailty and Surgery

Frailty describes a state of increased vulnerability to health complications. It is the opposite of resilience. When you are frail, your body has a much more difficult time bouncing back from stressors—and major surgery, as we discussed, *is* a stressor. Studies routinely show that frailty increases the risk of postoperative complications, or even death.[3]

A frail person—who is usually older—may have loss of appetite, fatigue, weakness, decreased physical reserves, weight loss, a slow or unsteady gait, cognitive decline, or frequent falls. Collectively, these symptoms reduce their ability to recover from surgery. That's why I always recommend that older patients undergo a thorough pre-operative assessment with their healthcare provider to measure health status, nutrition, and muscle strength, which we discuss in this chapter.

Assess Your Nutritional Status Before Surgery

Malnutrition is estimated to be present in 24 to 65 percent of surgical patients.[4] For this reason, a strategy used by doctors involves calculating your body-mass index, assessing the amount of unintentional weight loss over the previous three to six months, counting the number of acute illnesses experienced over the same period, and then combining all these risk factors to create a plan to address any malnutrition.[5]

Ask your doctor or specialist to order blood tests, including an albumin level (albumin is a protein that is produced in the liver and circulates in the bloodstream); vitamins D, B6, and B12 levels; CRP (a measure of inflammation); HbA1C (a measure of your average blood sugar for the past three months); and fasting blood sugar. These tests will help ascertain if you have any risk factors—such as being anemic, having excess inflammation, or diabetes—that could negatively impact your recovery from surgery. With your self-assessment and blood test results in hand, I recommend adjusting your diet to bolster your nutritional status by paying attention to four key factors.

Protein: Protein is the macronutrient that helps build and repair tissue. It is essential in the synthesis of collagen, the primary component of your skin, muscles, bones, tendons, and ligaments. Adequate protein intake is also critical to preserving muscle mass and supporting immune function, making it the single most important nutrient for your recovery. Adults under the age of sixty-five typically need to eat about 0.8 gram of protein per kilogram (0.8 g/kg) of body weight, while those over sixty-five should eat a bit more (1 g/kg). However, you will likely need more protein if you are deficient or when you are recovering from surgery. I recommend protein intake of 20 to 40 grams (¾–1 ½ oz) per meal during prehab and even higher amounts—1.6 to 3 grams per kilogram of body weight per day—when recovering from surgery.[6] I recommend also that you amp up high-quality protein sources in your diet, including cold-water SMASH fish (salmon, mackerel, anchovies, sardines, and herring). Excellent sources of plant-based protein include tofu, tempeh, pulses (legumes), quinoa, almond or peanut butter, nuts, and seeds. Organic cheese, Greek yogurt, poultry, and lean grass-finished organic meat are also healthy protein sources.

Protein Shakes

Note that if you have low albumin, if you don't consume adequate protein, or are frail, I recommend supplementing your diet with protein shakes.[7] Shakes using whey, pea, hemp, or chia seed protein are beneficial. (Shakes containing whey are most easily absorbed by the body, but they are not appropriate for people who don't tolerate dairy.) Read the ingredient label carefully, as many commercial protein shakes are filled with sugars, including frutcose-glucose (high-fructose) corn syrup, cane sugar, maltodextrin, or artificial sweeteners; it is far better to get a protein shake without any added sugars. For sweetness, you can add berries, bananas, peaches, or another fruit, which have the added benefit of boosting the fiber and antioxidant content of your shake. I also recommend avoiding carrageenan, a common emulsifier used to thicken foods, which can trigger inflammation in the bowel.[8]

One shake that has been widely studied, and that I commonly recommend, is Nestlé's Oral IMPACT.[9] When choosing from one of the variety of protein shakes options available, look for a product that provides 30 grams of protein per serving. Buy a single serving to confirm you enjoy the taste before purchasing in bulk.

Micronutrients: Apart from protein, there are many micronutrients that play a specific function in wound healing.[10] Here are some of the most critical:

- *Vitamin A*: Key to immune function and wound healing. Great sources include carrots, sweet potatoes, leafy greens, and eggs.
- *Zinc:* Aids with wound healing, protein synthesis, and immune health. Sources include beans, nuts, red meat, poultry, and dairy products.

- *Vitamin D:* Central to bone and immune health. Primary sources are sunlight (if weather permits, spend at least fifteen minutes outside with your arms and legs exposed to the sun without sunscreen), fatty fish, and fortified dairy products.

Omega-3 Fatty Acids: Surgery induces inflammation as a normal part of the healing response. However, too much underlying inflammation can impede healing. Foods rich in omega-3s can help reduce chronic inflammation, as well as support immune health, promote wound healing, help preserve muscle mass, and enhance mental health.[11] Great dietary sources include SMASH fish, as discussed earlier; omega-3-enriched eggs; purslane; flaxseed; chia seeds; and walnuts.

Fluids: After surgery, the kidneys and liver are responsible for detoxifying your body from anesthesia by breaking down and eliminating these medications. Drinking sufficient (nonalcoholic) beverages is essential for keeping your kidneys and bowels functioning well, while also helping maintain appropriate blood volume and circulation, ensuring that your surgical site is well oxygenated after your procedure. Hydration also contributes to the elasticity and health of tissues, including skin, which can impact how well your wound heals. Women and men should aim for around 2.7 liters (4¾ pints) and 3.7 liters (6½ pints) respectively, of fluids per day from water (sparkling or still) or herbal teas.[12]

Eating and Drinking Right Before Surgery

People used to be advised not to eat or drink anything (including water) eight hours before elective surgery. This short-term fast was recommended to reduce the risk of aspiration, which happens when stomach contents are regurgitated and enter the lungs during anesthesia. But newer research and ERAS guidelines suggest that drinking clear liquids up to two hours before surgery—and solid food up to six hours before—is actually beneficial.[13] It is worth asking your healthcare team, especially if you are scheduled for an afternoon surgery, "How long do I have to fast?"

Additional Nutrition Prehab

Did you know that approximately 30 percent of adults react to stress by skipping meals?[14] As your surgery date approaches, you may find your appetite diminished. But if stress causes you to skip meals, you may not be fully nourished before surgery, which could slow your recovery. This pre-op malnutrition is associated with more infections, worse wound healing, a higher risk of developing pressure ulcers, and higher odds of a prolonged stay in the intensive care unit (ICU) and hospital.

After surgery, your metabolic rate will likely increase by as much as 30 percent.[15] This creates a high demand for nutrients, as your body works overtime to heal and rebuild tissue. Some lean muscle loss is typical during surgery owing to a process called *catabolism*. This is why having a well-nourished body will reduce the likelihood you lose too much muscle, which can impede recovery.

Reviewing Medications and Supplements Before Surgery

Two weeks before surgery, review with your healthcare team all medications and supplements you're taking and discuss those that increase bleeding risk. Certain medications can thin your blood and compromise blood clotting, potentially leading to excessive bleeding during or after surgery. This can complicate the surgical procedure and increase the risk of blood loss.

For instance, both aspirin and nonsteroidal anti-inflammatory drugs, such as ibuprofen and naproxen, are commonly taken for various aches and pains, but they can impair clotting.[16] Herbal medicines and supplements, too, can increase bleeding risk; these include echinacea, ephedra, garlic, ginger, ginkgo, ginseng, green tea, kava, saw palmetto, St. John's wort, valerian, coenzyme Q10, glucosamine, chondroitin sulfate, and fish oil.[17]

Make sure your healthcare team knows all the prescription and nonprescription drugs you are taking, including supplements, so you get guidance on what needs to be stopped in advance of surgery.

Line up Your Social Support

Like anyone preparing for hip-replacement surgery, my friend Caroline was nervous. Even though hip replacements are among the most common and successful surgeries today,[18] she was understandably anxious about having her arthritic hip bone cut into and replaced with a prosthetic. Imagining herself at her most vulnerable, recovering in a hospital bed, she wanted support. So, I agreed to be her "surgical doula." Traditionally, a doula is a professional who provides support and guidance to birthing mothers; in this case, I would be Caroline's surgical doula at the hospital.

What exactly did this role involve? First, in the pre-operative assessment, I advocated with her nurses and anesthesiologist for intravenous medication to help manage her unchecked anxiety. After the procedure, I remained at her bedside in her hospital room. I spoke with her nurses and helped her select medication for pain and nausea. It's important to note that any trusted friend or family member can perform this role; they don't need to be a doctor or nurse to be effective. Essentially, I was there to provide emotional support and advocacy. In the stressful moments before and after surgery, in an unfamiliar and scary environment, Caroline was able to relax in the knowledge she had someone looking out for her.

Dr. Gulshan Sethi is a professor emeritus of surgery at the University of Arizona and the former director of cardio-thoracic surgery. In his half-century of practicing surgery, he has operated on nearly fifteen thousand patients. So, it was a surprise to many of his colleagues when he enrolled in our Integrative Medicine Fellowship in his mid-sixties. But Dr. Sethi is a lifelong learner, and according to him, one of the biggest factors determining how patients recover from surgery is the strength of their social support. "There are many studies demonstrating that patients who do not have a good social support system have worse outcomes compared to those who do," he explains. He encourages a family member or support person to be present for all pre-surgical visits, as he finds companions often better recall his advice than do his patients, who may be too nervous to absorb all the necessary information.

Whether you are arriving for an outpatient laparoscopic procedure or an inpatient coronary bypass surgery, a vital component of your prehab is arranging for someone to bring you to the hospital, stay with you until it is time for surgery, and be there when you wake up. It is incredibly reassuring to have companionship. Numerous studies have shown that patients who have visitors recover faster compared to those who do not.[19] While you may worry about burdening people by asking them to bring you to the hospital or to visit you, remind yourself that feeling supported and cared for when you are at your most vulnerable is critical to your recovery. Choose a surgical companion who will be calm and reassuring to *you*—not someone who will be radiating anxiety. Make a plan for who will be with you in the days and weeks following surgery, particularly if you will need help getting into and out of bed, showering, or preparing meals. If you do not have someone close who can take on this role, perhaps a neighbor, a member of your congregation, or even a paid care worker can be of help.

Finally, a tip on communication: If your surgery is particularly complex, or if you have a wide circle who will want updates, consider enlisting one person to be the point of contact for friends and family. Keeping others informed with constant calls and texts can be challenging, especially when dozens of well-wishers are checking in on your recovery. Directing friends and family to a single source for information will remove a significant burden for you and your caregivers. I often direct my patients to free websites, such as www.caringbridge.co.uk or the Lotsa Helping Hands phone app, which allows you or your caregiver an easy way to provide updates.

Approach Surgery with a Positive Attitude

There is more to prehab than just physical preparation. A large analysis of a wide range of surgeries over three decades found that "the better a patient's expectations about how they would do after surgery or some health procedure, the better they did."[20]

Some trepidation is normal in advance of a major operation, and a relaxation program can help manage these feelings. During pre-op visits, Dr. Sethi teaches his patients either diaphragmatic breathing or the 4-7-8 breathing. (See "Your "Rapid Recovery Toolkit," appendix 1, for more information.) He also encourages pre-operative guided imagery, which he himself used before his own knee and back surgeries. If you are feeling anxious, I encourage you to surround yourself with those who love and support you. You can also improve your mood with physical activity, a favorite hobby, or even something as simple as a crossword puzzle. See the "Unwinding Anxiety" chapter for tips on how to get your relaxation practice started.

I also recommend repeating positive affirmations, which are short, powerful statements used to challenge and overcome self-sabotaging and negative thoughts. When you repeat them over time, they reprogram your thinking patterns and make it easier to behave in more positive ways. They are typically phrased in the present tense and are meant to be specific and relevant to your life goals or situations you wish to change. Studies confirm that repeating positive affirmations before surgery can ultimately reduce anxiety and improve outcomes.[21]

The author Peggy Huddleston has graciously allowed me to reprint the following healing statements from her book, *Prepare for Surgery, Heal Faster*. Before your surgery, Peggy recommends telling your doctor, "There are four statements that I would like you or the anesthesiologist to say to me during my operation."

1. "Following this operation, you will feel comfortable and you will heal very well."
2. "You will have minimal bleeding during surgery." (Repeat five times as surgery begins.)
3. "Following this operation, you will be hungry for (fill in with foods you have told your surgeon or anesthesiologist that you like) _____. You will be thirsty and urinate easily."
4. "Following this operation, _____." (Fill in the blank with the words your surgeon recommends for your recovery. The sentence should

be extremely positive and clearly stated. Ask your doctor to describe your healing process in words and pictures, explaining the physiology of your recovery.)

Guided-imagery pioneer Belleruth Naparstek has also graciously allowed me to share the following healing affirmations, which can be repeated out loud or in your mind beginning one month before surgery:

Immediately after surgery, I see myself recovering quickly and easily, my stomach calm and settled.

I see my body mending quickly and efficiently, healthy new cells weaving into place, old debris washing away in the bloodstream.

Inside my body I sense the rebuilding of new cells—perfect, vital, healthy cells—aligned with the original blueprint.

I see myself surrounded by capable, caring staff during my surgery, working with steady, efficient competence to ensure my well-being.

Melatonin and Licorice Before Surgery

Taking melatonin beginning the night before surgery has been shown in two meta-analyses to reduce the delirium that can sometimes occur postoperatively.[22] Melatonin has also been shown to improve sleep and reduce both pre-op anxiety and post-op pain.[23] I recommend beginning with a dose of 3 mg of sublingual melatonin half an hour before bedtime.

There is one final bit of prehab you can complete before you enter surgery: gargling licorice. In one study, researchers divided patients awaiting back surgery into two groups.[24] The first group gargled with a licorice solution for five minutes before general anesthesia; the other group gargled with plain water. While 72 percent of the water-gargling group had a sore throat following surgery, just 21 percent of those who gargled licorice did.

Practice Guided Imagery Before Surgery

My patient Julie suffered from back pain for many years. She had a large cyst pressing on a spinal nerve, and epidural injections were ineffective. It became clear that a permanent cure would require a discectomy, which is the surgical removal of the damaged portion of a disc within the spinal column. But Julie was reluctant. During a hospitalization years earlier, she had contracted MRSA, a type of bacteria that is resistant to most antibiotics, and the recovery was brutal. She was worried this would happen again.

"This dread is not serving you well," I explained to Julie. "You've become focused on the worst possible result. It's time to envision a positive outcome." In the weeks before her surgery, with coaching, she was able to reframe her attitude. She learned daily breathing practices and positive affirmations to repeat whenever she conjured negative feelings and ideas. Most important, she began a guided-imagery practice, and every day she visualized a successful recovery. She imagined herself hiking, swimming, and cycling without pain. On the day of her surgery, her fears had been replaced with trust in her surgical team and confidence that she would heal. Julie's surgery went seamlessly, and she has been pain free ever since. Now she has her own recommendation for anyone preparing for major surgery: "You have to love your body and remind yourself of all the ways that it serves you."

Guided imagery is a form of focused relaxation in which a person imagines positive outcomes. For instance, one study found that surgery patients who participated in a guided-imagery program as part of their prehab had shorter hospital stays and required less pain medication compared to the control group.[25] Starting a guided-imagery routine in the weeks before surgery can help lower anxiety levels before, during, and after surgery; lower post-surgical pain levels; minimize opioid use; and can even lead to faster recovery.

Peggy Huddleston recommends envisioning three desired end results:

1. **Waking up from Surgery:** Imagine waking up from your surgery with a family member or dear friend holding your hand, smiling, and telling

you the procedure went perfectly. As the grogginess melts away, you feel comfortable, alert, pain-free, and loved.

2. **Midway Through Your Healing:** Envision yourself a few days or weeks after your surgery. You have followed your healthcare team's instructions diligently and they are extremely pleased with your progress. If pain was a reason you needed to have surgery, it has vanished. You are doing something your pain once prevented you from enjoying—maybe it's gardening, lunching with a good friend, or holding your child on your lap. You have come so far, and you are confident that you will make a full recovery.

3. **Far into the Future:** Imagine yourself many years in the future. Perhaps you are at your eightieth birthday party. You are surrounded by dear friends and family. You enjoy the awareness of how good your life is. Your surgery is a distant memory now. If you had a disease like cancer, you have not had a recurrence. Your scars have faded. The pain is gone. You are doing what you love most in the world.

Begin a guided-imagery session by getting physically comfortable; you can lay down or sit up in a chair. You will be guided to imagine a place where you feel safe and peaceful. In this state, offer yourself a vision of a positive surgical outcome.

Preparing Your Home Before Surgery

You can significantly ease your recovery by taking some time before surgery to arrange your home environment so it is conducive to healing. Here's a brief checklist of things you can do to prepare your home. Modify it as needed, depending on the type of surgery you'll be having:

Safety Precautions
- Remove trip hazards like rugs, electrical leads or cords, and clutter.
- Install safety railings or grab bars in the bathroom, especially after surgeries that affect mobility.

- Place nonslip mats in the bathtub or shower.
- Ensure good lighting to prevent accidents.

Accessibility
- Position frequently used items within easy reach, such as any medications, heating pads, or cooling equipment.
- If you'll have mobility limitations, consider relocating your bedroom to the ground floor to avoid stairs.
- Purchase or borrow a shower chair and a raised toilet seat.

Supplies
- Pick up any prescribed post-operative medications, as well as any over-the-counter drugs recommended by your doctor.
- Buy groceries ahead of time. Prep some nourishing meals, such as healthy soups, and freeze them.
- Stock up on essentials like toilet paper and hygiene products.
- Purchase an acupressure wrist band for nausea relief. I recommend Sea-Band or Psi Band.

Recovery Station
- Identify the place you will be spending most of your time after surgery. This could be a spot on your couch or bed, depending on your post-surgical instructions, or a comfortable chair or recliner with armrests.
- Stock a nearby table or stand with essential items like water, tissues, remote controls, phone, charger, books, and snacks.
- Pull out extra blankets and a heating pad. If you've had orthopedic surgery, I recommend picking up a cold-therapy machine. See the "Recovery from Orthopedic Surgery" chapter for more information.

Social Support
- Line up a friend or family member to drive you home from the hospital.
- Prepare a calendar for visitors and for meals. One useful and free online resource is MealTrain.com.
- Consider hiring help or asking friends or family for help with tasks like cleaning, cooking, organizing, or childcare, especially in the initial

recovery days. Having a clean and tidy living space can positively impact your mood.[26]

Pet Care
- If you have pets, be sure their needs will be taken care of, either by prepping supplies or asking someone to assist with their care.
- If you're worried about energetic pets jumping on you, consider temporary arrangements where they might stay with a friend or in a boarding facility.

Post-Operative Instructions
- Get a written copy of your post-operative care instructions. Place them in a common area (e.g., next to the couch or on the refrigerator) so they can be easily referenced by you and your caregivers.

Entertainment
- Set up books, movies, music, or any other entertainment to keep you occupied during recovery.

By thoughtfully preparing your home, you can create a conducive environment for recovery, ensuring that the post-operative period is as smooth and stress free as possible.

What to Take to the Hospital

As you contemplate your hospital stay, consider packing items that will help make your stay more comfortable, especially if you will be staying for a few days or more. While hospitals provide you with the basics, certain personal items can lower stress levels and speed your recovery:

- **Comfortable and Stable Footwear:** For walking around your room or down the hall, choose slippers, walking shoes, or trainers or sneakers that are stable yet easy to take on and off.

- **Eye Mask and Earplugs:** Hospitals are often loud and bright, which can challenge sleep.
- **Aromatherapy:** Choose essential oils you find relaxing. Research supports lavender and bergamot.[27] There are also many "calming" blends. For more information about using aromatherapy, see the following chapter, "Your Post-Op Experience."
- **Glasses and Glasses Case:** If you wear glasses, bring them. Avoid wearing contact lenses in the hospital.
- **Toiletries:** If you are staying overnight, bring a toothbrush and toothpaste, comb or brush, deodorant, lip balm, and moisturizer. (Hospitals can be very dry.)
- **Books and Magazines:** You may want something to occupy and distract you if you are waiting or have an extended stay.
- **Electronic Devices and Chargers:** Bring your phone, tablet, e-reader, or other device to take notes; keep in touch with loved ones; listen to music or audiobooks; watch shows; or read.
- **Headphones or Ear Buds:** These are especially important if you will be sharing a room.
- **Mind–Body Apps:** I recommend downloading an app such as Insight Timer, Calm, or Headspace, all of which provide thousands of relaxation tracks.
- **Loose, Comfortable Clothing:** Consider items that are easy to put on and take off, especially if you're having surgery on your abdomen or anywhere that will inhibit your range of motion.

Your Rapid Recovery Prescription for Surgical Prehab

I recommend beginning a prehab regimen in the weeks or months before your procedure. Here is how to get started:

1. Eat an anti-inflammatory diet rich in healthy proteins, including nuts, beans, eggs, fish, or organic lean poultry or meat; get physically

stronger with the help of a physiotherapist (if necessary); and take steps to manage stress. Be sure you are getting enough protein, micronutrients, omega-3 fatty acids, and fluids.

2. Check your blood test results, including an albumin level, before surgery. If your albumin is low, add higher-protein meals and shakes to raise your level to a healthy range.
3. Line up your social support before surgery. Who is bringing you to the hospital? Who will be there when you wake up? Who will drive you home and who will help prepare meals, if necessary? Choose a companion who will be calm and reassuring.
4. Approach surgery with a positive attitude. Make sure you get all your questions answered by your healthcare team. Practice breathing exercises and repeat positive affirmations to help yourself relax.
5. Use guided imagery to visualize three positive outcomes: waking up feeling comfortable after surgery, making steady progress, and your completely healed body far in the future.
6. Prepare your home before surgery and make it conducive to healing. Take all necessary safety precautions, ensure your living spaces are easily accessible, stock up on supplies, identify and prepare a recovery station where you will be spending most of your time after surgery, and if necessary, ensure your pets will receive good care.

19

Your Post-Op Experience

When the operating lights dim and the anesthetics slowly dissipate from your body, your surgery is complete. Now begins your recovery, which, depending on your procedure, may take days, weeks, or months. Most of my patients tell me they feel well within days after a laparoscopic gallbladder or appendix removal. In contrast, many are surprised by how long it takes to recover from cardiac surgery or a joint replacement. For some, it takes a full year until they feel themselves again. Setting appropriate expectations for your recovery will put your progress in context; it helps to know your body is hard at work healing and making incremental progress. Fortunately, you can influence the recovery process, and there are many steps you can take to shepherd your body toward healing.

Recovering from Anesthesia

Anesthesia is a part of almost every surgery, and everyone responds to it a bit differently, depending on the medications administered, overall health, and the length and type of particular surgery. Genetic differences between us—sometimes referred to as SNPs (single nucleotide polymorphisms), or "snips," determine the speed at which we metabolize anesthetics. Age also impacts how long the effects of anesthesia linger.

General anesthesia is the term used when you are "put to sleep." With this broad kind of anesthesia, you are typically intubated and placed on a ventilator to support your breathing. (General anesthesia works in part by paralyzing muscles, including the respiratory muscles.) When you wake up, you may experience a sore throat, nausea, fatigue, fogginess, or muscle aches. Anesthesia can also be regional, usually in the form of a nerve block (such as the type used when your dentist fills a cavity), or local, such as lidocaine numbing before a cut is stitched. Regional and local anesthesia usually have a shorter recovery period than general anesthesia, which we will be covering in this section.

To optimally recover from the effects of general anesthesia, I recommend people have a plan ready. The following steps are useful in the days and weeks after your procedure to help you to recover faster:

- **Stay Hydrated:** Drinking lots of water will help your kidneys flush the anesthetic drugs from your system, while also reducing symptoms of nausea and muscle aches.
- **Practice Sleep Hygiene:** Quickly returning to a consistent sleep schedule can help reduce lingering effects of anesthesia. If you are staying in the hospital overnight, come prepared with earplugs, eye masks, and your favorite sleep app.
- **Walk:** Movement can enhance circulation and reduce the risk of post-operative complications like blood clots. Your nurses or a physiotherapist will encourage walking when you are in the hospital. Once you return home, continuing to get up and move will speed your recovery. I recommend three ten-minute walks per day as a good early strategy (unless you receive different instructions from your doctor).
- **Do Breathing Exercises:** Deep-breathing exercises help to fully expand your lungs, which is especially important if you were intubated during general anesthesia. See "Your Rapid Recovery Toolkit" (appendix 1) for more information.

Recovering from anesthesia can vary, depending on the type of medication used, your response, and the length and type of the procedure. Here are the most common side effects you may experience.

Nausea and Vomiting: These are some of the most common side effects of general anesthesia; roughly a third of all patients experience them after surgery.[1] One simple and inexpensive approach is to use an acupressure wrist band;[2] I recommend using Sea-Band or Psi Band, which are easy to find and wear.

Aromatherapy can also help. Peppermint is one of the most popular essential oils for nausea relief. Inhaling the aroma can reduce queasiness and is valuable after surgery. In fact, inhaling peppermint often outperforms drugs used to treat nausea. In one study, people felt the onset of relief with inhaled peppermint after an average of only two minutes, compared to forty-four minutes with ondansetron, a commonly used anti-nausea medication.[3] Ginger is also known for its anti-nausea properties and can reduce post-operative nausea and vomiting.[4] There are many effective forms of ginger for nausea, including ginger tea (made with freshly grated ginger and some honey), chews, essential oils, capsules, and even ginger ale (but only if there is real ginger in it, and not just artificial flavors).

Sore Throat: More than 60 percent of patients experience sore throat after anesthesia, especially if they required intubation.[5] To ease post-op throat pain, I suggest gargling with a licorice product. My patient Diana had lung surgery to remove a benign tumor. She happily emailed me after her surgery, "I used licorice tea for post-intubation sore throat and had minimal to no discomfort." Post-operative coughing, another troublesome side effect of intubation, was also reduced by the licorice gargle.

The following are several supplements I often suggest taking after surgery to mitigate the negative effects of anesthesia. People often ask me, "Should I take one of these? Or all of these?" The answer depends on several factors. Personal experience can help you discern; if you know you have had trouble feeling normal after anesthesia in the past, you may want to take the first two on the list: milk thistle and NAC. If you are young, healthy, and have never had any trouble after anesthesia, you may not need any. Ask your doctor about these supplements:

- **Milk Thistle:** Scientifically known as *Silybum marianum*, milk thistle is a plant traditionally used to treat liver and gallbladder disorders.

Your liver plays a central role in detoxifying drugs, including anesthetics. The active component, silymarin, has demonstrated antioxidant, anti-inflammatory, and liver-protecting properties. Milk thistle at a dose of 140 mg three times a day can help detoxify anesthetic chemicals from the body and speed recovery.[6]

- **N-acetyl cysteine (NAC):** NAC is used by the NHS in the treatment of paracetamol overdoses, which can shut down the liver. As a supplement, NAC has been shown to help with detoxification and support of the liver.[7] A dose of 600 mg twice daily works well in conjunction with milk thistle. Joan, a patient of mine, was scheduled for a hip replacement. She had previously experienced mental fogginess when recovering from anesthesia. This time around, she avoided brain fog entirely after I recommended milk thistle and NAC.
- **Vitamin C:** I recommend asking your healthcare team for intravenous vitamin C. Multiple studies reveal that vitamin C administered intravenously reduces post-operative pain and the need for opioids.[8] (Taken orally, vitamin C does not seem to work better than a placebo.) It has been known for more than two hundred years that vitamin C plays a role in wound healing, when it was found to be a cure for scurvy. It also has been shown to prevent complex pain after foot and ankle surgery at an oral dose of at least 500 mg a day.[9] Food sources include citrus fruits, strawberries, bell peppers (capsicums), and tomatoes.
- **B Vitamins:** Certain B vitamins, like B1 (thiamine), may play a role in reducing the negative cognitive effects of anesthesia. In one study, patients undergoing abdominal surgery were administered 200 mg of IV thiamine or a placebo.[10] Those who received the thiamine had significantly lower rates of post-operative delirium while in the ICU. As with receiving IV vitamin C, this will require your healthcare team's assent. I especially recommend it if you are malnourished.

Preventing Infection

Our skin is covered with bacteria, viruses, and fungi, which collectively make up the skin microbiome.[11] Normally, the skin functions as a physical barrier, preventing microbes in the outside world from entering the body. A surgical incision, like any cut or scrape, disrupts that barrier. A surgical site infection (SSI) is an infection that occurs after surgery in the part of the body where the surgery took place. The infection can occur on or near the surgical incision, or in the deeper tissues and organs involved in the procedure. SSIs can range from a superficial skin infection to sepsis, a systemic infection that affects your entire body and can be life threatening.

Your risk of a SSI is higher if you go in for surgery malnourished, overweight, immunosuppressed, or with high blood sugar.[12] Any infection can delay your recovery, which is why surgeons commonly administer antibiotics intravenously before your operation. Antibiotic prophylaxis, as this practice is called, is intended to minimize the chance of post-operative infection; still, there are steps you can take to prevent SSIs. After surgery, you will be instructed in how to care for your wound. Usually this consists of keeping the surgical site clean, dry, and bandaged. Wash your hands well before applying new dressings. Keep an eye out for signs of infection, which include increased redness, swelling, warmth at the site, pus, discharge, and fever.

Finally, after surgery, your gut's microbiome may be out of whack, especially if you were given antibiotics. Studies show that taking probiotics (beneficial bacteria in supplement form) can help prevent SSIs, particularly when combined with prebiotics,[13] which are nondigestible compounds that help healthy bacteria proliferate. Ask your healthcare team about synbiotics, which are capsules combining prebiotics and probiotics. I recommend *Lactobacillus* spp. and *Bifidobacteria,* which are the most commonly studied organisms.

Feeling Tired After Surgery Is Normal

After you emerge from anesthesia, it is normal to experience some fatigue. How long this lasts will depend on the length, type, and extent of your surgery, as well as the type of anesthetic you were administered.

In the hours after your procedure, you can expect to feel drowsy as the anesthetic medications leave your system. General tiredness can persist for a few days as your body increases its metabolism to heal. It may even be normal to have significant fatigue for several weeks. As one study in the *British Journal of Surgery* noted, even "uncomplicated abdominal surgery is followed by a pronounced feeling of fatigue, which may persist one month after surgery in about one-third of patients."[14]

Post-Surgical Anxiety

After surgery, I hope that you will feel a strong sense of relief. The scariest part is behind you! Still, it's also normal to feel post-op anxiety. Anesthetics and pain medications can cause stressful feelings, restlessness, or confusion. If you must stay in the hospital for a period of time, or if you are dependent on others for care while you are recovering, you may feel particularly vulnerable.

In addition to aromatherapy's impact on reducing nausea after anesthesia, it can also be beneficial in managing post-surgical anxiety. One study among patients who underwent a breast biopsy, for instance, found significant reduction in self-reported anxiety when using lavender-sandalwood aromatherapy.[15] Chamomile, fennel, spearmint, lemon balm, linalool, geranium, lemongrass, and rose have also been shown to be helpful for reducing anxiety.[16] I advise my patients to bring a small vial with them to the hospital. You can find many blends on the market, and stores often let you test them before buying. Different scents appeal to different people.

Music is also a potent therapeutic tool, and it has been used for centuries to evoke emotions, memories, and physiological responses. Calming music has been shown to decrease blood pressure, reduce heart rate, and lower stress-hormone levels.[17] In contrast, upbeat music can elevate your mood by stimulating the release of neurotransmitters like dopamine, which are associated with pleasure. Data from more than seventy trials including some seven thousand participants found that "patients were significantly less anxious after surgery . . . and reported significantly more satisfaction after listening to music."[18] In another study, live, spontaneous harp music was played in the ICU rooms of patients after cardiac surgery.[19] A 27 percent reduction in pain was found in the patients who listened to the harp music compared to those who did not. What music will you put on your recovery playlist?

Guided Imagery for Relaxation

One of the best ways to reduce post-operative anxiety is to adopt a regular guided-imagery practice, in which you focus on positive mental images to promote relaxation and reduce stress. Studies have long shown that guided imagery can lower pain while potentially reducing hospital stays.[20] For best results, listen to a professionally recorded script; I often recommend recordings by Belleruth Naparstek, Emmett Miller, and—following here—that of Martin L. Rossman, MD.

> Now that your surgery is completed, you can focus on thoughts and images that can help make your recovery more comfortable and continue to encourage the healing ability of your body and mind. Your body is always actively involved in the healing and recovery process. And this is a time when you can support that healing by relaxing, getting the rest you need, eating well and using the same ability to relax and imagine that has helped you before. Remember, your body knows how to heal as it has many times before. And you may want to recall all the times you may have suffered a cut or a bruise or a burn or a cold or other illness or injury that you recovered from and how amazing it is that your body knew just what to do to repair the injury or wound or to eradicate the infection or to heal from the illness so it knows what to do. And it has already begun that natural process of healing. Your blood is constantly circulating, bringing fresh oxygen and nutrients, immune cells and other special repair cells that know exactly where to go and exactly what to do in order to help you heal completely and well.
>
> Take a few moments each day to focus on the areas of your body actively healing, repairing, and strengthening themselves. As the body brings itself back into wholeness, it brings special attention to any area needing repair, healing itself in such a way that it becomes even stronger in that

> area than it was before. And as your body heals, imagine yourself having a full and complete recovery, working with your body and mind to build strength and resiliency.

Reducing Post-Operative Pain

As advanced as modern surgical techniques are, some post-operative pain is normal. While many patients fly through recovery with no discomfort, others require a course of pain medication.

One effective pain-reduction strategy is acupuncture. Researchers have found that acupuncture needles may have an anti-inflammatory effect, improve blood flow, or stimulate the central nervous system.[21] In one study among post-op surgical patients, an acupuncture program resulted in a 21 percent reduction in the need for opioids after eight hours, a 23 percent reduction after twenty-four hours, and a 29 percent reduction after seventy-two hours.[22] These patients also experienced fewer opioid-related side effects, like nausea, dizziness, mental fog, itching, and urinary retention. Acupuncture is available in some NHS surgeries and hospitals, so ask your healthcare team if this safe and effective strategy is suitable. Note that acupuncturists may also offer electroacupuncture, which may amplify the benefits of traditional acupuncture by sending a continuous electrical current between pairs of needles.

I also recommend self-hypnosis. My patient Sam had terrible memories of vomiting repeatedly when he took an opioid painkiller after his wisdom-teeth extraction; not wanting to repeat that unpleasant experience, he used self-hypnosis to recover from gallbladder surgery without the use of painkillers.

There are many other integrative methods for managing pain after surgery. Here are some of the most effective:

- **Cold and Heat Therapy:** Applying cold packs can reduce inflammation and numb the surgical site. Heat, on the other hand, can improve blood flow and soothe muscular pain. I recommend using both (though cold is more commonly used in the first few days post-op to reduce swelling). Always use a cloth barrier between your skin and the cold/heat source. You can purchase heating pads or cold packs at most pharmacies. I also recommend vibrating cold packs, which work by interrupting pain signals traveling up the spinal cord.[23]

- **Massage:** A gentle massage can promote circulation, reduce muscle tension, reduce pain, and has also been shown to reduce excessive scar tissue formation.[24] Massage can be provided by a healthcare provider, a family member (think foot massage), or a professional massage practitioner.
- **TENS (Transcutaneous Electrical Nerve Stimulation):** This device sends small electrical pulses to the body, which can reduce the pain signals being sent to the brain. One meta-analysis involving five randomized controlled trials with 472 patients explored the use of a TENS unit after knee-replacement surgery.[25] People receiving TENS had less pain and used less opioid medication at twelve, twenty-four, and forty-eight hours after surgery. As a side benefit, people using TENS units also had less post-op nausea and vomiting. TENS units are available online.
- **Electrical Nerve Stimulator:** A new set of devices is being developed that stimulates nerves to reduce pain. In the U.S., one type of nerve stimulator which is used on the ear, has been shown to reduce post-operative need for opioid medication. In a study of patients undergoing kidney surgery, use of a nerve stimulator led to a near 42 percent reduction in pain and a 75 percent reduction in opioids at twenty-four hours.[26] Electrical nerve stimulators are available online; ask your healthcare provider about their recommendations.
- **Virtual Reality:** Really! The newest tool on the shelf uses a virtual 3D environment viewable with goggles that provides a 360-degree immersion. Evidence supports the use of VR in post-op pain relief.[27] Virtual scenes include everything from alpine forests to lush prairies, to cobalt blue skies with chirping birds.[28] In the background, you may hear a narrator guiding you through a relaxation exercise.
- **Auditory Stimulation:** This is another tool shown to reduce the need for post-operative opioids.[29] The headphones play two auditory impulses

(sometimes called *binaural sounds*) with different frequencies simultaneously in each ear, creating the perception of a single beat. This reduces post-op pain and can lead to an effect called *hemispheric synchronization of the brain*, which corresponds to the states of focused alertness that occurs with meditating or doing creative work. My patients have had good results downloading audio tracks by Hemi-Sync (www.hemi-sync.com).
- **Sleep:** Sleep matters when it comes to healing. During deep sleep, your body produces growth hormone that helps repair organs and tissue.[30] Sleep also reboots your immune system, which helps prevent post-surgical infections. For more information about developing healthy sleep habits, see the "Sleeping Soundly" chapter.

Minimizing the Risk of Opioids

Opioids are considered one of the most powerful painkillers, but given the risks of dependency, you may be understandably wary of taking them. Opioids work by binding to opioid receptors in the brain, spinal cord, and GI tract, blocking the transmission of pain messages. Over time, the brain can become reliant on the drug, leading to tolerance and dependency—a central reason why ERAS protocols have shifted to implementing multimodal pain-management strategies as early as possible.

Oftentimes we assume we'll need opioids because well-meaning doctors or nurses predict we will have pain, a phenomenon called *hexing*. For example, they may say, "You'll probably have some pain, so when it begins . . . " (rather than *if* it begins). Or, they may say, "We'll try to limit your suffering." (*Try* can imply failure.) Ideally, your doctor will say something like, "Some people have pain, though I think you will do well. If it should happen, we will be able to effectively treat you." If you feel you have been hexed, you can tell yourself: "This doctor has experience with other patients, but they can't predict with certainty what will happen to me." To avoid hexing, my colleague Steve Bierman, MD, author of the provocative book *Healing: Beyond Pills & Potions,* recommends asking your anesthesiologist or surgeon to recite the following statement before your procedure: "When you wake, you will wake with delightful comfort that persists—so much so that when you hear the word pain, it will act as a trigger to make you even more comfortable."

Before your surgery, ask about the typical timeline for needing opioid medication and when you can expect to begin tapering down your dose. If you have a history of dependency, be sure to discuss an alternative pain-management regimen with your healthcare team. For instance, I recently had a patient who had a history of opioid addiction and wanted to avoid opioid painkillers after his knee replacement. He was able to effectively manage his pain using paracetamol and a vibrating ice pack.

Whether or not my patients have a history of addiction, I typically suggest they ask about using a combination of pain-relief methods, including over-the-counter drugs such as paracetamol or nonsteroidal anti-inflammatories (NSAIDs), cold and heat treatments, acupuncture, and physiotherapy. As recovery progresses, you may be surprised to discover how quickly you no longer need medication for pain. Substituting heat, ice, rest, a virtual reality device, or a TENS unit may do the trick.

Finally, if you do take opioids for pain, avoid alcohol and other sedatives. Combining opioids with alcohol or sedative medications increases the risk of respiratory depression and overdose.

Ramping up Your Digestive System

Surgery tends to put the GI track to sleep, making it hard to pass wind or gas or have a bowel movement in the days following a procedure. (This is especially true after abdominal surgery.) After you wake up, eating may be the last thing on your mind, but it's important to get your intestinal track working again. Dr. Elizabeth Raskin, the surgical director for inflammatory bowel disease at Hoag Memorial Hospital in Southern California, and a fellowship graduate of the Andrew Weil Center for Integrative Medicine, recommends chewing gum or sucking on boiled sweets or hard candies to jump-start the gut–brain connection and regain your appetite. Once you are cleared by your surgeon to eat full meals, focus on nourishing foods that are easy on the stomach. Soups and stews with cooked vegetables are my go-to, as they are highly nourishing and easy to digest.

Physical activity will help get your bowels going, and you can start with something as simple as getting up and walking after surgery. Acupuncture or acupressure can be extremely helpful, too.[31] I recommend stimulating the acupressure point called *large intestine 4* (LI4), which is known for its effectiveness in treating everything from digestive issues to headaches, neck pain, stress, and fever.[32] You can stimulate LI4 on your own by making an "L" with your thumb and index finger. Then, with your other hand, squeeze the muscular webbed space at the base of the "L." Gradually increase the pressure on the point and hold for three minutes. You can do this every three to four hours for several days.

Your Post-Surgical Diet

After ramping up your digestive system, it's time to nourish it! The nutrients in your diet are the building blocks of a speedy recovery, aiding everything from rebuilding tissue, reducing inflammation, warding off infection, and regaining strength. As I have described elsewhere, I recommend an anti-inflammatory diet rich in vegetables, fruits, whole grains, and lean proteins (especially from fish). Early in recovery, I recommend cooked rather than raw foods, and you may find soups especially nourishing. As you liberalize your diet, I suggest prioritizing protein and fiber-rich foods.

> **Protein:** After your surgery—especially if it was a major one—you might experience a breakdown of lean body mass; this is called *catabolism*. To offset this loss, you will need to consume more protein than usual. When recovering from surgery, I recommend you boost your daily protein intake to 1.5 g/kg or more.[33] For example, suppose you are a 70 kilogram (11 stone/154 lb) person; you would need to consume about 105 grams (3¾ oz) of protein daily. (The following protein amounts are approximated.) This protein total can be accomplished by eating two eggs (12 grams protein) for breakfast with two slices of rye bread (5 to 6 grams).

You could also add 30 grams (1 oz) of Cheddar cheese (6.5 grams). For lunch, a can of tuna fish (27 grams) atop of a salad (raw spinach has 2 grams protein per 30 grams/1 oz)) sprinkled with 30 grams (1 oz) of walnuts (4.5 grams) and 1.5 tablespoon of chia seeds (7.5 grams). At dinner, 100 grams (3½ oz) of organic chicken (31 grams) with 90 grams (3¼ oz) of cooked quinoa (4 grams) and 75 grams (2½ oz) broccoli (2.5 grams). You can see why if your appetite is not fully back, eating this much can be a challenge. Alternatively, continuing to drink a protein shake, as described in the previous chapter, may be a good idea. Here are some additional healthy protein sources:

- Pulses (legumes), such as lentils 100 grams/3½ oz = 9 grams protein) or chickpeas, kidney beans, and black beans (75 grams (2½ oz) of all beans = 8 grams).
- Seafood, particularly omega-3-rich SMASH fish (salmon, mackerel, anchovies, sardines, and herring; between 30 and 40 grams protein per 85 to 175 gram/3–6 oz serving).
- Plain full fat Greek yogurt 140 gram/5 oz serving has 12 to 18 grams protein, but check the label, as amounts vary). You can add to the flavor profile with berries, which contain healthy antioxidants.
- Organic poultry or meat. I recommend eating grass-finished meats and antibiotic-free sources (about 9 grams protein per 30 grams/1 oz chicken or meat).
- Organic tofu (about 3 grams protein per 30 grams/1 oz), tempeh (about 5 grams per 30 grams/1 oz), and edamame (8 to 9 grams per 85 grams/3 oz).
- Cooked whole grains, including quinoa (about 8 grams protein per 185 grams/6½ oz), oats (10 grams per 235 grams/8¼ oz), buckwheat (between 5 and 6 grams per 170 grams/6 oz), barley (between 3 and 4 grams per 160 grams/5½ oz), and brown rice (about 5 grams per 200 grams/7 oz).

Fiber: Fiber plays an essential role in your diet, yet many people following a Western-style diet do not consume sufficient amounts.[34] It's particularly important in your recovery, for several reasons. As discussed, surgery can disrupt normal bowel function, and this is especially true for abdominal procedures. Moreover, opioids—whether taken post-operatively or administered as part of general anesthesia—can lead to constipation, which will be eased by consuming adequate fiber. A high-fiber diet also promotes healthy gut microbiota, which is important for immune function and overall recovery. To increase your fiber intake, focus on vegetables and fruits; mushrooms; beans; whole grains like oats, millet, brown rice, and quinoa; pulses (legumes); and nuts and seeds. If you struggle with constipation, be sure you are drinking sufficient water, and consider adding daily prunes, kiwifruit, or an over-the-counter psyllium supplement. Choose a product with no added sugar or artificial sweeteners. (Stevia, a sugar substitute derived from plants, is fine and may increase the diversity of the microbiome.[35])

Exercising After Surgery

Getting active after surgery plays a vital role in your recovery, though how much you can exercise depends on your specific procedure. No matter what surgery you have had, remember that some degree of movement is critical in the early days and weeks of your recovery. Even walking around the house can improve circulation and decrease the risk of blood clots and pneumonia. Movement also stimulates bowel activity, reducing the chance of post-operative constipation.

Post-operative scar tissue can also restrict your movement. I've had breast-cancer patients develop shoulder or back pain because their mastectomy scars led them to alter their posture. As soon as you have your doctor's sign-off, begin stretching exercises that gently mobilize the scars that form at the incision. Several minutes each day of stretching can improve your range of motion at the wound site. And, don't be afraid to gently massage the surgical scar once the stitches are out and the skin has healed.

Your Rapid Recovery Prescription to Optimize Your Post-Op Experience

Your body is built to heal. Still, after surgery, it may take some time until you feel your normal self again. Fortunately, you can influence this process. Here is how to set yourself on track to make a full recovery:

1. Have a plan in place to recover from the lingering effects of anesthesia, including staying hydrated, getting enough sleep, moving around, and practicing breathing exercises. Licorice gargle or tea, milk thistle, NAC, and aromatherapy can all help with the side effects of anesthesia.
2. Ask your anesthesiologist or surgeon to recite the following statement before your procedure: "When you wake, you will wake with delightful comfort that persists—so much so that when you hear the word pain, it will act as a trigger to make you even more comfortable."
3. Lower your risk of a surgical-site infection by keeping your wound clean, dry, and bandaged. Taking probiotics—I recommend *Lactobacillus* spp. and *Bifidobacteria*—can help reset your microbiome and fight infection.
4. Manage any lingering post-op anxiety with aromatherapy, breathing exercises, music, and guided imagery.
5. Reduce post-op pain with one or more of the following: acupuncture, cold and heat therapy, massage, a TENS unit, an electrical nerve stimulator, virtual reality, auditory stimulation, and proper sleep hygiene.
6. If you need opioid medicines, ask your surgical team about putting together a tapering plan. Consider a combination of pain-relief methods, including the mentioned therapies, paracetamol, or NSAIDs.
7. Ramp up your digestive system after surgery with light physical activity and nourish it with soups and stews rich with cooked vegetables.
8. Eat an anti-inflammatory diet rich in vegetables, fruits, whole grains, and sufficient protein. Add high-fiber foods to minimize constipation.

20

Recovery from Orthopedic Surgery

By the age of age fifty-seven, my patient Aaron knew a knee replacement was inevitable. Decades of running and basketball had taken their toll, and when his knees were swollen—which was often—Aaron was unable to hike, an activity he was especially fond of, as he lived in the mountains near Tucson, Arizona. Arthritis ran in his family, and both his mother and brother had undergone knee-replacement surgery. His specialist recommended a bilateral (both left and right knee) replacement.

Aaron was fit and ate a healthy diet, but the arthritis had affected his gait and he had developed some muscle atrophy. I recommended prehab with a physiotherapist to strengthen his muscles and to develop a plan for post-op strength-training exercises. He set up a gym in his house and was diligent at practicing prehab stretches with dynamic bands and using light weights to strengthen the muscles around his knees in the weeks leading up to his surgery.

Aaron's surgeon performed the procedure using robotic technology to perfectly align his knees. The first days of recovery were tough, which surprised him, as he thought of himself as resilient when it came to pain. We discussed self-hypnosis techniques, as well as using an ice machine he had rented. Happily, his pain quickly diminished, and with twice-a-week, in-person physiotherapist sessions, Aaron made a swift recovery. Within six months he was able to start hiking again. A year out, he is thrilled with his new knees!

Orthopedic surgeons are dedicated to the diagnosis and treatment of injuries of the musculoskeletal system. This is a complex network of bones, muscles, joints, ligaments, tendons, fascia, and other connective tissues that work together to provide structure, support, and movement for the body. Bones form the framework, muscles generate the force to move the bones, ligaments and tendons provide stability and allow smooth movement at the joints, and cartilage cushions the joints to prevent bone-on-bone contact. It's a beautiful system, but when an injury or an imbalance early in life—say, being slightly bowlegged or knock-kneed—alters this harmony, it increases the risk of an arthritic joint years later. In other words, it's not only active individuals like Aaron who need orthopedic surgery. In fact, orthopedic procedures are among the most routine surgeries performed in the U.K. as they are in the United States.[1]

In this chapter, we'll discuss three of the most common types of orthopedic procedures: hip replacements, knee replacements, and back surgery (which is also performed by neurosurgeons). While the suggestions from the previous two chapters apply, here I offer specifics for orthopedic surgery.

Your Hip or Knee Replacement Surgery Prehab

Joints can wear down over time and cause pain. The most common cause is osteoarthritis, which occurs when the protective cartilage that cushions the ends of the bones gradually deteriorates, leading to inflammation, painful bone-on-bone contact, bone breakdown, and diminished mobility. Repeated stress from running, heavy lifting, excess weight, malalignment, or prior injury can in particular wear down the hip and knee joints. Surgeons perform almost 550,000 hip replacements and nearly 800,000 total knee replacements every year in the United States,[2] figures that continue to grow as the population ages.

During a hip-replacement surgery—also known as an *arthroplasty*—the surgeon removes the damaged hip joint and replaces it with an artificial one made from metal or plastic compounds. The procedure takes about two hours and is typically successful, allowing the patient to resume activities they previously had set aside. Once fully recovered from surgery, most of my patients have had high satisfaction from their hip replacement and happily returned to favorite activities like golf, dancing, hiking, and playing on the floor with grandchildren. They often remark how natural their new hip feels. In fact, most of my patients lament they didn't do it sooner!

In a knee replacement—also typically a two-hour procedure—the surgeon removes damaged cartilage and bone between the femur and tibia and replaces it with synthetic components to make up the joint, along with spacers to create a smooth gliding surface that mimics the functions of your natural knee. A "new" knee, however, is a bit less likely to feel like the real thing, compared to a "new" hip, and your overall post-surgery satisfaction may not be quite as high. For this reason, one of my patients, Cynthia, an avid runner and cyclist, has avoided having knee surgery. Instead, she sees an orthopedic surgeon every four to five months for hyaluronic acid and PRP (platelet-rich plasma) injections. These treatments have allowed her to continue to compete, at age sixty-nine, in mountain bike races, although she has mostly given up running.

Treatments like hyaluronic acid and PRP are not for everyone, owing to their high cost, and sometimes surgery is the best option. As we saw with my patient Aaron, with diligent physiotherapy, knee replacement can produce great results. Dr. William DeVault, an orthopedic surgeon based in South Carolina and a graduate of the Integrative Medicine Fellowship at the Andrew Weil Center, notes that about 90 percent of his patients who have knee or hip replacements do well, thanks to modern practices and materials. He explains that new surgical techniques are less invasive, requiring smaller incisions and causing less damage to surrounding tissue. Additionally, the latest prosthetics are made from incredibly wear-resistant materials, and advanced imaging allows him to have a detailed understanding of each person's particular anatomy before surgery, resulting in a customized artificial joint fit.

That said, Dr. DeVault stresses that his most successful patients have a robust prehab regimen, which includes these steps.

Attend Physiotherapy Before Surgery: Like Aaron, you may have some muscle atrophy from disuse. Each surgery comes with some limitations that might affect your ability to carry out basic functions, such as getting out of bed or off the toilet. A physiotherapist can help you prepare you for these changes. To improve your strength and endurance, and put you in the best possible position for a full recovery, aim to strengthen the muscles surrounding your hip, knee, and core prior to surgery. You might need to use crutches or a Zimmer frame for a few weeks following surgery. Although these are essential tools for balance and support, they can be hard on the shoulders and back. Have a physiotherapist teach you how to use them prior to surgery; acclimating yourself now will reduce your stress after surgery and lower your risk of injury.

Use the Mind–Body Connection: A meta-analysis examining a variety of interventions, including relaxation, cognitive behavioral therapy, hypnosis, and emotional counseling, also revealed improved post-operative recovery with less pain and anxiety in people undergoing orthopedic surgery.[3] In a separate literature review, guided imagery was shown to reduce pain after orthopedic surgery.[4]

Get Diabetes Under Control: An hbA1c test measures your average blood sugar over the past three months. Research shows the risk of complications, particularly infection, from joint-replacement surgery is higher among people with hbA1c levels greater than 42. If you have diabetes or prediabetes, work to get your blood sugar under better control. See the "Reversing Type 2 Diabetes" chapter for my recommendations to better manage (or potentially reverse!) your diabetes.

Recovery from Hip or Knee Replacement

Full recovery for hip replacements takes an average of six months, while knee replacements can take as long as a year, since the joint is less stable. Immediately after surgery, you'll typically stay in the hospital for one or two days. There, you'll begin physiotherapy and start moving around with the help of a Zimmer frame or crutches. You may be surprised that initially you feel little or no pain; this can be due to medication injected directly into your knee or hip at the time of the replacement.[5] If you wish to avoid opioids, which can lead to nausea, vomiting, and constipation.

Dr. DeVault, mentioned earlier, notes that intravenous paracetamol, or the nonsteroidal anti-inflammatory drug ketorolac, has been shown to be effective post-surgery.

Here are my additional recommendations for recovering after your surgery.

Cold Therapy: For both knee and hip replacements, cold therapy—also known as *cryotherapy*—can reduce pain, swelling, and inflammation after surgery.[6] You can use ice or gel packs or, even better, rent a cold therapy system that automatically circulates cold water around the surgical site. Dr. DeVault recommends applying cold therapy every hour while awake for at least three to five days following surgery, with the skin protected from direct contact by an ACE bandage wrap or small towel. Afterwards, the cold therapy can be used intermittently following physiotherapy or exercise. Most people find the cold extremely helpful; I recommend you have a rental unit delivered to your home in time for your discharge.

Physiotherapy: A physiotherapist will guide you through exercises to strengthen the muscles around your hip or knee and improve flexibility. This will progress in stages from your hospital stay to around eight weeks after you go home. I can't emphasize enough how important it is to keep up with your physiotherapy program to achieve the best possible outcome. Sadly, I have seen patients who have not put in the work and have ended up in a wheelchair for many weeks after a surgery that was supposed to increase mobility! Walking without an assistive device, climbing stairs, and regaining range of motion of the hip and knee are important goals.

Acupuncture: Many of my patients laud the benefits of acupuncture, which can help reduce post-surgical pain and decrease the reliance on opioids. Acupuncture can stimulate blood flow, which may speed up the healing process and improve mobility. A meta-analysis of acupuncture after total knee replacement found it decreased pain and delayed the need for opioid medication.[7] This is a great option, especially if you know someone who will come to your home.

Lifestyle Adjustments: To protect your new joint, you may need to alter some characteristics of the way you live and move. If you've had a hip replacement from the back of your hip (posterior approach), for instance, during the first six weeks (but possibly up to six months), you will be warned not to cross your legs, walk pigeon-toed, or flex your hip more than 90 degrees, so as to prevent the risk of a hip dislocation.[8] When it comes to knee replacement, some surgeons advocate limiting weight bearing initially, especially with porous-coated implants, which need bone ingrowth for more stability, as opposed to cemented implants, which are stable at the time of surgery. Make sure to ask your healthcare team about specific restrictions.

When a Joint Becomes Toxic

A few years ago, my seventy-five-year-old patient Dianne began complaining of two seemingly unrelated problems. She had been pain-free for a decade following successful hip-replacement surgery, routinely completing vigorous hikes throughout the world. Now, the artificial hip was causing her pain. She was also having trouble retrieving words during conversation—extremely disconcerting for Dianne, a former English teacher. Blood tests revealed elevated levels of both cobalt and chromium, which suggested that Dianne's artificial hip was leaking metals into her blood.

Hoping to avoid another surgery at age seventy-five, Dianne came to see me eager to try chelation, a process that uses medicines and supplements to remove harmful metals from your blood. She diligently followed an oral chelation protocol and supportive diet, and she regularly used a sauna to aid in detoxification. While her cobalt and chromium levels dropped a bit, her artificial joint continued to degrade. To fully recover, she needed to stop the metals from leaching from her hip into her body. She reluctantly agreed to a revision total hip replacement. Thankfully, this second procedure was successful; not only did Dianne's pain disappear, but her cognition returned to normal.

Dianne's story is an example of a lesser-known side effect of joint replacements: cobalt poisoning. Your symptoms may be cognitive, similar to Dianne's, or you could experience skin rash, hearing loss, vision problems, mood changes, fatigue, and nerve pain.

If you've had a metal joint replacement in the past fifteen years, the FDA and the UK's Medicines and Healthcare Products Regulatory Agency both recommend that you have your blood checked for elevated levels of cobalt and chromium.[9] How often you get these blood tests depends on whether you have symptoms and if you have impaired kidney function.

What About Stem Cells?

Patients who have significant degeneration of their hips and knees and want to avoid surgery often ask me about stem cells. I believe stem cells will play a prominent role in orthopedic care of the future. At present, they are not approved for orthopedic surgery. Still, they are available "off label" for osteoarthritis of the knee.[10] The most commonly used kind of stem cells for arthritis are mesenchymal cells, which are thought to reduce inflammation and alter immunity, rather than acting as a true stem cell (which can directly differentiate into cartilage or other structural tissues).[11] These two mechanisms serve to create a regenerative environment that helps heal the injured knee.[12]

If you decide to go this route, I highly recommend that you get *autologous* mesenchymal stem cells, meaning your own stem cells and not a donor's. Another person's stem cells injected into your body may be interpreted by your immune system as a foreign invader and attacked. Autologous stem cells are usually derived from fat (using liposuction) or from bone marrow. Future possibilities for stem cells are exciting, as they are being investigated in conditions that are especially challenging to treat,[13] such as tendinopathies (inflammation of the tendon) and fractures that do not heal.

Recovery from Back Surgery

Every year, hundreds of thousands of people undergo surgery to treat herniated or ruptured disks, vertebral fractures, degenerative disk disease, spinal stenosis, and countless other problems that cause chronic pain.[14] Still, the decision to have back surgery is a difficult one. Why?

In some cases, spinal surgery has a high success rate; studies show that about three-fourths of patients are satisfied with the results of their laminectomy, or removal of the vertebra.[15] But other procedures are less successful, and research indicates that up to 40 percent of patients continue to have pain after back surgery, a phenomenon known as *failed back surgery syndrome*.[16]

Some indications for urgent back surgery are clear-cut, such as numbness or weakness in a limb, which can be signs of nerve impingement. Similarly, a tumor, infection, and certain injuries are also reasons to move forward right away. And, as we saw in the introduction to surgery section with my patient Olivia, back surgery may be necessary for permanent pain relief. But if you have chronic back pain without an identifiable cause, I encourage you to read the "Deactivating Pain Signals" chapter. In many cases, back pain is not caused by a physical problem but, rather, by central sensitization syndrome, in which the nervous system is in a perpetual state of high alert, resulting in an exaggerated pain response. Before you explore surgical options, make certain the cause of your back pain has been carefully diagnosed.

I want to briefly stress the importance of staying active. This may not be easy, as back pain is extremely difficult to live with. As someone who suffered from chronic back pain, I understand how difficult just getting through the day can be. But by remaining active, you are conditioning and strengthening the muscles that support your back as well as your core. You will be relying on them in the weeks and months following your surgery.

You will need to practice patience as your body heals from back surgery. After the procedure, your surgeon will provide you with a list of specific instructions about what you can and cannot do. Follow these directions closely. A physiotherapist can guide you through exercises to improve your mobility, strength, and flexibility, all while ensuring you don't overdo it. Your body heals during rest, so get plenty of sleep and take breaks throughout the day. Recovery may be slow going. Don't rush your body's healing process by doing too much, too soon. With your PT's guidance, gradually resume your regular activities as your strength and mobility improve.

Finally, many people find significant stress reduction and sleep improvements after back surgery by starting regular acupuncture. Find a licensed practitioner with experience in treating people who have undergone back surgery.

Your Rapid Recovery Prescription After Orthopedic Surgery

Your musculoskeletal system is a mechanical marvel; still, injuries and arthritis increase the possibility of needing surgery. Orthopedic procedures such as hip or knee replacements and back surgery are among the most routine surgeries performed and often make it possible to return to beloved activities. These steps can speed recovery:

1. Build a robust prehab regimen, including physiotherapy before surgery, strength training, and learning what to expect post-op (including the use of mobility aids).
2. Get your hbA1c level to 42 or under. Review the "Your Surgical Prehab" chapter for tips on what to eat before surgery to optimize your overall nutritional fitness, which can speed recovery and minimize complications.
3. Prepare your home and develop a stable of relaxation techniques.
4. Cold therapy and acupuncture can help you manage pain. For other pain-management tools, see the "Your Post-Op Experience: chapter.
5. Commit to a post-operative physiotherapy program to speed up and maximize recovery.
6. If you've had a joint replacement in the past fifteen years, request blood tests to assess levels of cobalt and chromium.

21

Recovery from Heart Surgery

For most of her adult life, my patient Robin lived with a mitral valve prolapse, a small defect in one of the four heart valves that allows blood to leak backwards from the ventricle into the atrium. It's generally not life threatening, but over time Robin had become more symptomatic, suffering occasional bouts of dizziness and shortness of breath, as well as bothersome fatigue. At age forty-four, she decided it was time for surgery to fix the valve. She was operated on by a cardiac surgeon who was trained to perform her procedure using a minimally invasive, robotic procedure. Then, together, we planned a prehab routine. Her procedure went well, with no complications.

A few days after Robin went home, I called to check on her. To my surprise, she was miserable: She felt bloated and nauseous, had no appetite, and most distressing, was severely constipated—a likely side effect of her opioid pain medications. She described the pain at her incision as "really bad." Her surgeon could do nothing but provide more pain medications, which only made her constipation worse.

I suggested she try acupuncture, which has been shown to improve pain and anxiety, as well as relieve stomach issues among patients recovering from heart surgery.[1] At first, she was resistant; after surgery, the last thing she wanted was to be punctured by *more* needles. But given her misery, she relented and booked an appointment with an acupuncturist. A few days later she called me, barely able to contain herself.

"You saved my life!" she exclaimed. The acupuncture had reduced her pain from an 8 to a 4 out of 10. She finally had a bowel movement, and her nausea was almost gone. Yes, Robin had a twenty-first-century surgery—but it took a three-thousand-year-old remedy to fully activate her recovery reflex.

Coronary bypass surgery is one of the most common heart procedure in the world—for example, in the United States alone it is performed on some 350,000 patients each year.[2] When the coronary arteries are clean, blood easily passes from your heart to your muscles and organs. Over time, however, fatty deposits called *plaque* can build up on the walls of your arteries, restricting blood flow and making your heart work harder. This is called *coronary artery disease* (CAD), one of the most common types of heart disease.[3] (I discuss how to prevent, manage, and potentially reverse CAD without surgery in the "Healing Heart Disease" chapter.) Significant blockages can increase your risk of a heart attack, and your doctor may recommend bypass surgery, in which case a healthy blood vessel is taken from elsewhere in your body and grafted around the blockage. Blood then bypasses the damaged artery to reach your heart muscle.

While you may feel like recovery from something as complex as heart surgery is out of your control, this is not true. If you haven't yet, I encourage you to read the "Assess Your Nutritional Status Before Surgery" (page 308) in the surgical prehab chapter. Being well-nourished is particularly important before heart surgery: One study found[4] that the three- and eight-year survival rates for people who were properly nourished before heart surgery were 93 percent and 77 percent, respectively. For patients who were malnourished, those figures dropped to 83 percent and 68 percent, respectively. Beyond diet, this chapter covers the essential steps you can take in the days and weeks prior to and after surgery to strengthen your body, minimize complications, and ensure a complete recovery.

Banking Your Own Blood

If you have enough time (five days to six weeks before heart surgery), talk to your healthcare team about the possibility of banking your own blood, a process called

Pre-operative Autologous Donation (PAD). The benefit of using your own blood is less risk of allergic reactions, transmitted infections, and other complications associated with mismatched blood. Stored blood may also undergo biochemical changes over time, so having a fresh supply of your own blood will maximize the efficacy of a transfusion.

Exercising Before Heart Surgery

If you are facing cardiac surgery, you might be worried that exercise will take too great a toll on your heart. But unless your cardiologist or healthcare team tells you to avoid it, moderate exercise before your procedure can strengthen your heart, lungs, muscles, and immune system, increasing your resiliency and the speed of a full recovery.

In one study out of McMaster University in Canada, patients scheduled for bypass surgery exercised twice a week, including a warm-up, thirty minutes of brisk walking, and a cool down.[5] After surgery, these patients spent an average of one day less in the hospital, compared to the control group, and six months later reported a better quality of life. Even minor strength-training exercises work. In a study run by King's College Hospital, London, people over sixty-five waiting for valve replacement or bypass surgery did simple at-home balance and strengthening exercises in the months before their procedure.[6] During recovery, they were significantly fitter and less frail compared to the people who did not follow the protocol.

Stopping Supplements and Medications Two Weeks Prior to Heart Surgery

Your surgeon will provide a detailed list of instructions before your bypass, including what medications to stop taking. As discussed earlier, I often recommend that my patients cut out most dietary supplements two weeks before surgery, especially those that have an anticoagulant effect, including garlic, ginger, ginkgo, ginseng, and omega-3 fatty acids.[7] Some people forget or prefer not to tell their doctors about supplement use. When you are having cardiac surgery, this is a serious mistake. As an example, published studies have documented the rejection of heart transplants in recipients taking the botanical St John's wort,[8] which revs up liver metabolism and reduces the effectiveness of ciclosporin, the medicine used to block rejection of a transplant.

When approaching surgery, your body may already be in a heightened sympathetic nervous system state—the fight-or-flight mode—due to stress. If you add sympathomimetics (drugs that, as the name suggests, mimic the stimulation of the sympathetic nervous system), you may increase your risk of cardiac events like heart attack and stroke during surgery. This category includes supplements such as licorice (the deglycyrrhizinated form is safe), and ephedra (sometimes used in weight-loss supplements).

I also recommend not taking sedatives, also called "nervines" by herbalists. Sedatives are herbs and supplements that relax your nervous system. There have been case reports of people who took kava kava or valerian at home before receiving sedatives at the hospital before surgery.[9] When these compounds were combined, some patients found it more difficult to wake up following surgery.

In addition to the above supplements, be sure to ask about cutting out the following:

- **Aspirin:** Aspirin acts as a blood thinner and is often used to help prevent a heart attack or stroke. However, this very blood-thinning property also increases the risk of post-operative bleeding.
- **Beta Blockers:** Beta blockers are used to control heart rhythms, treat angina, and lower blood pressure. Check with your doctors about stopping in advance of surgery, typically forty-eight hours before your procedure.

Supplements to Take Before the Two-Week Window

As discussed, you should stop taking most supplements two weeks prior to your surgery. In the months before, however, certain supplements can help prepare your body for surgery. A study of 117 patients who were planning to have elective coronary bypass surgery found that supplementation with CoQ10, magnesium, alpha lipoic acid, omega-3 fatty acids, and selenium before surgery was associated with less cardiac damage and a shorter post-operative hospital course.[10] I encourage taking the following for one to two months leading up to that two-week period:

- **Coenzyme Q10:** Also known as CoQ10, this antioxidant protects cells from damage and plays an important role in metabolism. Taking CoQ10 is especially important if you are on a statin, which can reduce CoQ10 levels in the body. In the study just mentioned, the dose was 300 mg per day.[11] Note that CoQ10 been shown to improve symptoms of congestive heart failure and may help improve cognition after surgery, so you may be able to continue taking it up until the day of surgery. Still, CoQ10 carries a slight risk of increased post-operative bleeding, so confirm with your healthcare team that it's okay for you to take it.
- **Omega-3 Fatty Acids:** These have a potent anti-inflammatory effect. I recommend taking 1,000 mg of EPA and DHA daily. For more information about omega-3 fatty acids, see "Your Rapid Recovery Toolkit" (appendix 1).
- **Vitamin D:** If you are vitamin D deficient, taking a supplement may prevent the occurrence of atrial fibrillation after bypass surgery.[12] Take enough to reach a blood level of 40 to 50 ng/ml. (A good starting dose is 1000 IU daily.)
- **Once-Daily Multivitamin-Multimineral Supplement:** Check the label to be sure it includes vitamins A (as mixed carotenoids), E (as tocopherols) and C, and the minerals selenium (200 mg) and zinc (15 to 25 mg).
- **Alpha Lipoic Acid:** This is an antioxidant that reduces inflammation and helps control blood sugar. Take 300 mg twice a day.
- **Magnesium:** Magnesium can help to reduce arrhythmias after coronary bypass surgery.[13] I recommend that you take 400 mg of magnesium citrate at bedtime.

Staying Positive

In the "Your Surgical Prehab" chapter, we discussed the importance of staying positive before surgery. I have a sad personal experience with the converse. Many years ago, my grandmother needed aortic valve surgery. While it was clearly indicated—she was passing out and injuring herself—she did not want to have the procedure. She was in her mid-eighties at the time, and while she was otherwise in good health, she arrived at the hospital believing she would not survive. Sadly, that's what happened; the surgery went forward as scheduled, and she died hours later.

I tell this story to encourage you to assess your emotional state before surgery. While blood work and other objective data reveal a great deal, numbers alone don't paint the whole picture. If you are not *feeling* ready—and if your surgery is not an emergency—you can consider postponing, giving yourself time to ask more questions, bolstering your social support system, or finding another way to manage your health. Dr. Sethi, the former director of cardio-thoracic surgery at the University of Arizona whom I mentioned in the "Your Surgical Prehab" chapter, will not operate on a patient who is in a negative mental state. He told me, "In my surgical experience, when a patient tells me before surgery that they are going to die, or if they tell a loved one that they are going to die, they usually end up dying. That's why if a patient tells me they are not ready, I tell them to go home and wait until they feel better."

I agree with Dr. Sethi. If you feel reluctant to proceed with elective surgery, I suggest that you put it off until you feel ready. Consider talking with your family or a therapist, journal about your concerns, or practice guided imagery to prepare for a successful outcome.

Post-Operative Course

You will almost certainly be in the ICU for several hours or days after your cardiac surgery. The less time you spend there, the better. When you wake up, you will likely have an endotracheal tube in your throat, a chest tube protruding from your chest, a catheter in your bladder, and numerous IV lines in your arm. You will probably be surrounded by many people. While it can be frightening—both for you and for your loved ones—you will do better if you have visitors in the ICU. Ask someone to be there when you wake up, and warn them about the tubes and drains, which while scary looking are normal and necessary.

While you are in the ICU, bear in mind that simple touch can be healing. After all, the touch of a loved one conveys warmth and caring, and studies show that touch reduces anxiety in cardiac patients.[14] A study[15] published in 2012, in which 152 patients received massage therapy revealed reduction in pain, anxiety, and muscular tension, and an increase in relaxation compared to the control group who rested. Similar results were seen in another study that found patients had less pain and anxiety when nurses performed a ten-minute foot massage after cardiac surgery.[16] This is a role that your family can play. You don't need a professional masseuse; a gentle foot rub will do.

Unless you had a minimally invasive procedure, metal wires will be holding your sternum together, and it will take several weeks for the stitches in your skin to dissolve. Common post-operative symptoms include swelling, redness around your wound, loss of appetite, difficulty sleeping, and constipation. Depression is also a possibility, and we'll discuss later in this chapter how to manage it during your recovery.

Your surgeon will provide you with a detailed cardiac recovery regimen, including appropriate medications. Ideally, you will be referred for cardiac rehab, a medically supervised exercise and lifestyle education program designed to enhance your heart health. (If you aren't, please request it.) While cardiac rehab has been shown in studies to reduce mortality and depression, doctors rarely prescribe it, and only one in five patients complete it, despite the fact that the NHS and most private insurance carriers provide it.[17]

Cardiac rehab is more than just exercise; the socialization component may have equal importance. You will meet people in rehab who have been through a similar ordeal. Some may be a bit ahead of you in their recovery, and you will witness them getting better. Use them as your inspiration and proof that your pain will subside, your activity level will improve, your stamina will increase, and you will heal.

The recovery time for valve-replacement surgery is generally shorter than bypass surgery, especially if your procedure was minimally invasive. Expect a four- to eight-week recovery period,[18] although it can take a few months before you feel like your old self. A full recovery from bypass surgery can take as long as twelve months. This is one reason prehab is so important: The fitter and more resilient you are going into surgery, the faster your recovery will be. As your body heals, you may frequently feel tired, and some days may be more challenging than others. Regardless of which type of surgery you had, after approximately six weeks you will likely be able to resume normal activities. The strategies that follow will supplement your cardiac rehab and help you recover faster.

Warding off Depression

Even patients who prepare well and have a terrific social-support system can struggle with depression after heart surgery, which occurs in about 20 percent of cases. Why? Between going under general anesthesia, having your chest cut open, and spending long hours on a heart-lung machine and a ventilator, your body chemistry can be significantly altered. Every person is different, and it's difficult to predict precisely how you will cope.

On top of that, the lengthy recovery process can be a downer, notes Dr. Rosie Sheinberg, a cardiac anesthesiologist at the University of Washington and a graduate of our Integrative Medicine Fellowship. In the specific case of bypass surgery, she says that her patients "are always surprised that they don't bounce back within a couple of months. It's six months to a year before they feel they have their baseline exercise tolerance back." When the recovery does not go as quickly or as smoothly as you might like or expect, depression is a real possibility.

Other patients become depressed because they believe their body has failed them. Dr. Benjamin Remo, a cardiologist, electrophysiologist, and Integrative Medicine Fellowship graduate, explains that many of his patients believe their heart will never be the same. Their self-image changes. They begin seeing themselves as fragile, and they fear a slide toward the end of life. In such cases, Dr. Remo advises, "Don't focus on what happened; focus on where you're going and what you have left to do." This partially explains why cardiac rehab can be so transformative. In one major study, depressed patients who participated in cardiac rehab experienced a 63 percent decrease in depression compared to those who did not participate.[19] And notably, depressed patients who completed cardiac rehab had a 73 percent reduction in cardiovascular mortality over a three and a half-year period.

Whether or not you attend cardiac rehab, it's vital after surgery to attend to your mental health by setting realistic goals and expectations while celebrating incremental progress. One surprising exercise shown to be beneficial for heart patients is laughter therapy.[20] This consists of deep breathing, stretching, meditation, and simulated laughter exercises. Dr. Sethi, mentioned earlier, is such a believer in the power of laughter that he teaches laughter yoga sessions in his spare time to patients and hospital staff alike. "Laughter activates the body's natural relaxation response," he explains. "It's like internal jogging. It provides a good massage to all the internal organs while toning the abdominal muscles."

Indeed, a study by researchers at the University of Maryland Medical Center in Baltimore found that people who had previously had a heart attack or had undergone coronary artery bypass surgery "generally laughed less, even in positive situations, and they displayed more anger and hostility."[21] While researchers aren't entirely sure why laughter is so potent, they suspect it may be because it releases endorphins, which in turn release the molecule nitric oxide, a chemical compound that has been shown to relax arteries.[22]

During your recovery from heart surgery, find as many ways as possible to laugh. Put on your favorite comedy or, better yet, surround yourself with people who make you smile. Because when it comes to your heart, as the old saying goes, laughter truly is the best medicine.

Maintaining a Sharp Brain

Research shows that up to 70 percent of all cardiac bypass patients experience memory loss or other cognitive issues following surgery.[23] Usually the brain regains its sharpness relatively quickly, but for some people, brain fog and forgetfulness can linger for many months. A number of theories have been put forth to explain the link between heart surgery and cognitive decline, including microvascular "mini" strokes;[24] the use of potent anesthetics;[25] or adverse side effects from the heart-lung machine.[26]

Fortunately, your lifestyle can go a long way toward reducing or even eliminating memory issues after heart surgery. Eating a Mediterranean-style diet, avoiding smoking, controlling blood pressure, and minimizing alcohol consumption all contribute to a faster recovery and can also positively affect cognition after surgery. Additionally, certain supplements may help to restore the post-operative brain in the domains of thinking, learning, and remembering.[27] These include lion's mane mushroom (*Hericium erinaceus*), ginseng, bacopa (water hyssop), ginkgo, or the adaptogens schisandra (*Schisandra chinensis*), ashwagandha, and rhodiola rosea. Finally, N-acetyl cysteine (NAC) is a supplement thought to improve cognition by reducing inflammation and oxidative stress.

Getting Active

After you have heart surgery, the last thing you may want to do is exercise. Check with your doctor, but you'll likely be advised that exercise is not only safe after valve replacement or bypass surgery but also an integral component of your cardiac rehab program. Regular exercise has been shown to improve long-term outcomes after many types of heart surgery, particularly bypass.[28] As you begin, focus on time, not distance, and integrate warm-up and cool-down periods.

An integrative cardiac rehab routine—consisting of one-hour sessions two or three times per week for three months—involves prescribed exercise training, risk-factor modification, extensive nutrition education, and other strategies to build up your health and strength post-surgery. Engage in the program fully for the best outcome and reach out to your healthcare team with questions.

Your rehab program will include a progressive home-exercise program. Cardiac rehab ranks exercise intensity with a unit called METs (metabolic equivalent of tasks). For context, 1 MET is about the same as sitting quietly; walking slowly is a light intensity activity with a range from 1.6 to 3 METs; brisk walking or raking leaves is considered moderate activity at 3 to 6 METs; while vigorous activity like running or taking an aerobics class is 6 or more METs.[29] Cardiac rehab aims to help people achieve at least 4 METs,[30] such as by walking at a moderate pace of 6.4 kilometers per hour (4 mph). Depending on your progress, by week 6, you may be advised to do higher-MET exercises such as cycling, weight training, and flexibility training. Your cardiac rehab team will develop an individualized plan for onsite and at-home exercises that should be reviewed and updated by your supervising physician every thirty days.

What to Eat After Heart Surgery

Immediately after surgery, you may notice your appetite is diminished, and eating may not be particularly enjoyable. Nevertheless, proper nourishment is critical to recovery, especially if your ICU stay is prolonged. This was confirmed by a post-op study of 787 people who had cardiac surgery, which found that 40 percent of those with an ICU stay longer than three days received no nutrition support.[31] Nutrition therapy (NT) can be delivered intravenously, through a nasogastric tube, or best of all, by eating. A 2018 study evaluated the effect of NT in 351 patients who had bypass or aortic-valve surgery and were not consuming 60 percent of their caloric need.[32] They were followed for a full year after surgery. There was less arrythmia in male patients who received the nutrition support, while female patients receiving NT had less pneumonia and higher survival rates overall.

    I often recommend soup as an ideal food in the first days following surgery, as it is easy to digest and can be highly nutritious. In the weeks and months following heart surgery, I suggest a Mediterranean-style diet, which is further described in "Your Rapid Recovery Toolkit" (appendix 1). One way to make life easier is to prepare and freeze meals ahead of surgery, so you can simply reheat later. Alternatively, provide recipes to your support team at home and ask that they prepare these healthy meals for you early in your recovery. Beginning a heart-healthy diet immediately after surgery will help your body recover faster, reduce your risk of complications, and protect you for the long haul.

Your Rapid Recovery Prescription After Heart Surgery

Recovering from heart surgery may seem daunting. I hope this chapter has revealed the significant amount of control you have over your progress. These steps can strengthen your heart, minimize complications, support your recovery reflex, and enhance your return to normal activities:

1. In the months leading up to surgery, consider taking these supplements: CoQ10, omega-3s, vitamin D, a once-daily multivitamin-multimineral, alpha lipoic acid, and magnesium. Discontinue all supplements two weeks before surgery or as directed by your doctor.
2. If you are scheduled for bypass surgery, ask your doctor about discontinuing the following medications two weeks before surgery: aspirin, beta blockers, anticoagulants, sympathomimetic drugs, and sedatives.
3. Unless your cardiologist directs you otherwise, exercise moderately before surgery to strengthen your heart, muscles, and immune system.
4. Check your attitude. If you feel reluctant to proceed with elective surgery, delay it until you are comfortable.
5. Request cardiac rehab after your surgery to speed your recovery and reduce the risk of complications.
6. Pay attention to your food intake and push yourself to eat, even if you don't feel like it. Soup is an ideal food in the first few days after surgery, as it is easy to digest and can be highly nutritious.
7. Attend to your mental health by setting realistic goals and expectations while celebrating incremental progress.
8. To avoid the lingering cognitive effects of bypass surgery, eat a

Mediterranean-style diet, avoid smoking, and minimize alcohol consumption.
9. Begin a moderate exercise regimen as soon as you are cleared by your doctor. Exercise is an integral part of your cardiac rehab and will strengthen your heart.

22

Recovery from Breast Cancer and Its Surgery

A few years ago, a seventy-two-year-old woman named Catherine visited my office after being diagnosed with breast cancer. A biopsy had recently confirmed she would need a lumpectomy and, like any of the hundreds of thousands of women who are diagnosed with breast cancer annually,[1] Catherine was scared. She had been healthy her entire life, and all at once her world was turned upside down. The positive news was that her form of cancer—invasive ductal carcinoma—was highly treatable, and it was discovered early. Even though her prognosis was excellent, Catherine couldn't shake her unwelcome new identity: cancer patient. She was concerned about how the lumpectomy would affect her breasts, her body image, her sense of herself as a woman. She felt fundamentally off.

Her husband accompanied her to my office, and at one point in our conversation she grabbed his hand. "Honey," she said with great distress. "I'm a woman with *cancer*."

He smiled at her and without missing a beat, said, "Honey, you're also a woman who dances."

It was like someone flipped a switch in her brain. Catherine wasn't a cancer patient; she was a dancer, a wife, a mother, a world traveler, and a chef. She was many, many things, and being a woman with a cancer diagnosis was far down on the list. I've spent over twenty-five years providing integrative-medicine consults to women with breast cancer, some with aggressive forms that had spread throughout the body and others with highly treatable varieties like Catherine's. Just about all of them struggle with the fear, shock, anger, disbelief, depression, and numbness that follows those four words: "You have breast cancer." For some, though, it becomes an identity, despite the fact that breast cancer is now a highly treatable disease.

If you have been diagnosed with breast cancer, you likely have become informed about your particular cancer, so I won't cover the significant differences between ductal carcinoma in situ and invasive ductal carcinoma. Your medical team has put together a specific treatment and recovery plan for your cancer. What you'll find in this chapter are recovery strategies you can use to complement your conventional treatment, whether that's surgery, chemotherapy, radiation, hormone therapy, immune therapy, or a combination. Although this section is focused on surgery, surgery is rarely a solo treatment for breast cancer. So, you'll also find integrative approaches to help activate your recovery system not just from the surgical procedure but also from the full array of treatments.

When surgery is necessary to remove part or all of the breast, women often feel they are losing a fundamental part of themselves. Because of this, recovering from breast-cancer surgery may necessitate more than physical healing alone. It may require gaining a new self-image and renewed confidence to shed feelings of isolation and reconnect emotionally and sexually with a partner.

As you read this chapter, remember that breast cancer is a highly treatable condition. Localized breast cancer, which my patient Catherine had, has a five-year relative survival rate of more than 99 percent; women with breast cancer that has spread regionally have an 87 percent five-year survival; and for those for whom it has spread distantly, the survival rate is 32 percent.[2] Overall, new therapies have led to a 44 percent drop in breast cancer deaths in the past twenty-five years.[3] Because modern breast-cancer treatment is specifically targeted based on the diagnosis, no matter what form of breast cancer you may have, you likely have many promising treatment options at your disposal.

Your Surgery Options

Most women with breast cancer will have some sort of surgery. You and your oncologist will choose between removing the tumor and radiating the remaining breast tissue, known as a lumpectomy plus radiation, or removing the breast entirely, called a *mastectomy*. While surgery was once the first-line treatment after a breast-cancer diagnosis, this is no longer true; women now sometimes have chemotherapy or hormone therapy first to shrink the tumor and make the surgery less extensive.

Lumpectomies are typically performed as outpatient procedures with general anesthesia. Your surgeon will remove the tumor and a small amount of healthy surrounding tissue to ensure there are no lingering cancer cells. Your surgeon may also remove and analyze the sentinel nodes, which are typically the first place cancer cells spread from a primary tumor and help to indicate whether your cancer has spread beyond the breast.

The breast tissue obtained during a biopsy will be analyzed for hormone-receptor status and genetic markers. Typically, your doctor will also order an Oncotype DX test, which can predict the likelihood of your cancer returning. Your recurrence score, which ranges from 0 (minimal chance of recurrence) to 100 (very high risk of recurrence), will help your oncologist determine whether you should have chemotherapy. Recurrence scores are interpreted in conjunction with age and menopausal status, as well as lymph-node involvement; they are most relevant for women with estrogen receptor-positive cancer. As an example, it may be advisable for a forty-year-old with, say, a 30 recurrence score to have chemo, while a seventy-year-old with the very same score may be told chemo is unnecessary. Your oncologist will help put your score into context. When there is a lack of clarity about the best treatment, consider having a second opinion with a specialist who generally has expertise in treating your particular cancer. While the Oncotype DX is the most commonly administered test, other emerging scoring systems can also calculate your cancer's aggressiveness.

When to Consider a Mastectomy

Some years ago, my thirty-six-year-old patient Helen was forced to make a heart-wrenching decision. She had learned that, like her mother and grandmother before her, she carried a genetic mutation in the BRCA1 (breast cancer gene 1) gene that greatly increased her risk of developing breast cancer in her lifetime. In fact, her mother and grandmother both had died of the disease in their forties. Given her family history, Helen decided to have a prophylactic (preventive) double mastectomy after she weaned her third baby. You may remember when Hollywood actress Angelina Jolie announced in a *New York Times* op-ed in May 2013 that she was having both breasts removed even though she didn't have cancer. She, too, had a mutation in the BRCA1 gene.[4]

For the vast majority of women with breast cancer, there is no survival benefit to opting for a mastectomy over a lumpectomy. However, women like Helen and Jolie, who have inherited a harmful mutation in the BRCA1 or BRCA2 (breast cancer gene 2), may have a greater than 60 percent chance of developing breast cancer over their lifetimes.[5] In this particular situation, studies do show a survival benefit to having a prophylactic double mastectomy. (Other cases where mastectomy may be warranted include when there is an exceptionally large tumor, when the tumor is very close to the chest wall, when there are multiple areas of breast cancer, or if there is a recurrence of cancer after a previous lumpectomy.)

The good news is that the BRCA gene mutations are exceptionally rare, affecting, for example, just 0.2 percent of the U.S. population.[6] While testing is not recommended for most people, having a BRCA genetic test may be indicated if you have a family history of breast or ovarian cancer. A geneticist can help determine whether you should have your DNA tested.

Create a Healing Ceremony Before Surgery

Some of my patients have found comfort and a bolstered sense of resilience by creating a ceremony, either before their breast surgery or as an adjunct to chemotherapy. Dr. Ann Marie Chiasson, fellowship director at the Andrew Weil Center for Integrative Medicine, teaches how to develop a ceremony. She advocates for simplicity: "A ceremony requires a beginning, middle, and end."

The beginning of a ceremony can be as simple as lighting a candle. Next, choose a ritual that is significant to you. For instance, over the years, women I have cared for have made plaster molds of their breasts, written letters of gratitude for the pleasure they derived from them in lovemaking, or spoken of their time breast-feeding a baby. Other women pray over their chemotherapy infusion bag, turning the intravenous medication into a source of sacred healing. The end of a ceremony is intended to help with the transition back to ordinary reality. Symmetry works well for closing. In other words, if you lit a candle to begin, you can extinguish it at the end. If you open with a poem or a prayer, you can recite another one to close.

I have also seen amazing tattoos on the skin where a breast was once present—imagine flowers and vines weaving their way around the chest wall. One patient who lost her hair during chemo even tattooed her scalp. These actions challenge conventional ideas about beauty and femininity and place power in the hands of women.

Recovery Immediately Following Lumpectomy or Mastectomy

Your surgical team will provide a detailed list of instructions for recovery after your lumpectomy or mastectomy. During the first two weeks, take care to reduce your chance of lymphedema, which is swelling caused by a buildup of lymph fluid in the tissues. If sentinel nodes or others were removed during your surgery, you are at increased risk for lymphedema. In this case, be sure not to exercise the affected arm for at least two weeks following surgery.

While suturing your incision, the surgeon will take care to preserve your breast's appearance. You may find the scar tissue that forms around your incision site is hard at first, but it will soften over the months following your surgery. Dr. Doreen Wiggins, an associate professor of surgery at Brown University and a graduate of our Integrative Medicine Fellowship, notes that many women are reluctant or afraid to touch that area, so she shows them how to gently massage their scars to bring movement to the stiff tissue and aid with healing. She recommends lightly massaging around the scar and surgical area using a gentle sweeping motion, beginning one week after surgery.

Once your surgical wound fully heals—usually in three to four weeks—you will likely begin radiotherapy, which deploys high-energy rays to destroy any cancer cells that may still be present in your breast. This will minimize the risk of a recurrence in the years ahead. While it was once common practice to have radiation five days per week for up to six weeks, radiation oncologists are increasingly opting for accelerated schedules of just three to four weeks. Modern radiation treatments largely avoid harming healthy cells, however, damage can still occur, resulting in side effects that include fatigue; skin breakdown; changes in the size, shape, or feeling of the breast; and difficulty moving your shoulder.

Dietary Recommendations for Post-Surgery

Breast cancer is considered a systemic disease rather than a localized one, meaning that a lumpectomy or mastectomy may not remove every cancer cell from the body. Even if your surgeon discovered only a small tumor, there is still a risk that undetected cancer cells have spread elsewhere. The good news is you can exert a level of control over how effectively your body fights off these stray cells. In addition to chemotherapy and hormone-blocking therapy, such as tamoxifen or an aromatase inhibitor (both used to dramatically decrease estrogen levels), variables that include your diet, exercise, stress-management practices, and environmental exposures can reduce the risk of a recurrence.

Nationwide trials of diet in women with breast cancer provide valuable data regarding the important link between diet and cancer recurrence. Here are the most powerful choices you can make.

Prioritize Anti-Inflammatory Foods: Over time, chronic inflammation can damage healthy cells and increase cell mutations, including in the breast.[7] Eating an anti-inflammatory diet has been shown to reduce overall mortality after a diagnosis of breast cancer by reducing risk of death from cardiovascular disease.[8] (This is important because survivors are ultimately more likely to die of heart disease than cancer![9])

Eat an Abundance of Vegetables and Fruits (Seven to Nine Servings Daily): Data from a Harvard University study that followed nearly nine thousand women with breast cancer for up to thirty years concluded that "Those who consumed higher amounts of fruits and vegetables after their diagnosis were less likely to die during the study period than those with lower amounts of fruits and vegetables in their diets."[10] I encourage you to "eat the rainbow" daily, meaning eating vegetables and fruits of varying colors, each offering unique phytonutrients. In particular, load up on cruciferous vegetables like broccoli, kale, cauliflower, cabbage, and leafy greens.[11] (I often remind my patients who tell me that they do not like cruciferous veggies that coleslaw counts!) Research also shows that while all survivors benefit from eating vegetables, those who take tamoxifen may benefit most, with the greatest reduction in a recurrence of breast cancer.[12]

Eat Soy Foods: There is a common misconception that eating soy foods can increase your risk of developing breast cancer or having a recurrence. This theory began because soy contains plant estrogens called *isoflavones*. Since some cancers, including hormone receptor–positive breast cancer, are fueled by human estrogen, it was widely believed that plant-based estrogens were equally dangerous. In fact, two large studies have demonstrated that a diet rich in soy foods can actually *reduce* a woman's risk of having a recurrence of breast cancer.[13] Note that it is *whole* soy foods, such as tofu, edamame, tempeh, and miso, that have been shown to be safe, and not soy or isoflavone supplements (which I do not recommend).

Eat Only Organic Dairy: Dairy may have an inverse relationship to breast cancer, meaning the more dairy you consume, the lower your risk.[14] But not all dairy is alike, and I recommend consuming only organic dairy. Minimally processed yogurt and cheese are considered better to consume than milk, as they are partially fermented and therefore contain helpful probiotics. Full-fat products are also a good choice because they are typically less processed than low- or nonfat varieties. For more information, check out www.soilassociation.org a UK-based organization whose website is full of details on a range of organic practices.

Avoid Beef: Eating red meat has been linked to higher rates of multiple cancers, including breast cancer.[15] For this reason, I recommend either avoiding red meat entirely or eating it rarely. Processed meats such as sliced ham or pastrami, hotdogs, and bacon typically contain nitrates and have the highest cancer-causing risk of all.[16]

Prioritize Complex Carbohydrates: All carbs are not created equal, especially when it comes to reducing your risk of breast-cancer recurrence. Refined carbohydrates like those found in white (and even wholemeal or whole wheat) bread, breakfast cereals, crackers, white rice, and many other processed foods can boost your levels of insulin-like growth factor-1 (IGF-1), a hormone that stimulates cell proliferation.[17] On the other hand, complex carbohydrates—found in whole foods including vegetables, fruits, brown rice, quinoa, pulses (legumes), nuts, and seeds—are associated with a *decreased* risk of breast cancer.[18]

Incorporate a Prolonged Overnight Fast: Time-restricted eating—a form of intermittent fasting—has been shown to reduce the risk of breast-cancer recurrence.[19] The key is to have a thirteen-hour or longer overnight fast. (For example, stop eating and drinking anything with calories by 6 or 7 p.m., then don't begin eating again until 7 or 8 a.m.) Black coffee, tea, or water are all fine to consume during your fasting period.

Why Fasting During Chemo Makes Good Sense

Recent studies have shown that for women who have chemo following breast surgery, a forty-eight hour fast—twenty-four hours before chemo and twenty-four hours after—can significantly improve treatment tolerance.[20] This is a fast solely from food; it's fine to drink water, herbal teas, clear broth, and black, unsweetened coffee. While cancer cells continuously divide no matter how much (or little) you eat, healthy cell division dramatically slows down when you fast.

Because chemotherapy cannot differentiate between cancer cells and normal cells, the latter are spared during fasting, as they effectively go dormant until you eat again, reducing harmful side effects. This fast may sound difficult, but the research shows that fasting is usually well tolerated and reduces nausea, fatigue, and headaches.[21] Speak to your doctor about how best to incorporate this strategy into your care.

Eat Linseeds (Flaxseed): Include 1 tablespoon of freshly ground linseeds in your daily diet. Linseeds contain lignans, which can bind to estrogen receptors and decrease cell growth. Studies have shown that consuming 25 grams (1 oz) of linseeds a day may reduce tumor growth in breast cancer, and they may enhance the effectiveness of tamoxifen, a hormone therapy commonly prescribed to prevent breast cancer recurrence.[22] Side benefits include less constipation and lower blood pressure. Linseeds should be eaten ground; otherwise they pass through you undigested. You can mix the ground linseeds into yogurt, include them in a smoothie, or sprinkle them onto cereal or porridge. I recommend freshly grinding them yourself in a coffee grinder or buying store-ground and keeping them in the freezer. (Ground linseeds go bad quickly.) If the linseeds smell like paint thinner, throw them out; they have become rancid through oxidization and are no longer safe to eat.

Drink Green Tea: EGCG, the primary polyphenol in green tea, has been shown in studies to limit the growth of breast cancer cells.[23] In one study of 472 women with breast cancer, pre-menopausal women with early-stage breast cancers who drank the most green tea had the least spread of cancer. Moreover, women who drank at least five cups of green tea daily were less likely to have a recurrence.[24]

Avoid Alcohol: Many apologies to my wine-loving friends, but research shows that drinking alcohol increases women's risk of hormone receptor-positive breast cancer by boosting estrogen levels in the body and damaging DNA in cells. The relationship is linear: The risk of breast cancer increases by 10 percent for every additional drink you consume daily.[25] For survivors, even three to four drinks per week can increase the risk of recurrence. Although it is not available everywhere, and it is banned in the U.K., kava tea, which is made from the *Piper methysticum* plant is used as a drink to promote relaxation.[26] For more information about reducing anxiety, see the "Unwinding Anxiety" chapter.

Supplements for Breast Cancer Recovery

There is evidence that taking a multivitamin-multimineral can help prevent the recurrence of breast cancer. During the early 1990s, researchers put together a huge prospective study—meaning one that enrolls a group of people and then observes events as they happen—called the Women's Health Initiative (WHI).[27] Of the 160,000 postmenopausal women enrolled in the study, about eight thousand were diagnosed with breast cancer and followed for an average of seven years after their diagnosis. Those who were taking a multivitamin-multimineral supplement upon enrolling in the trial were 30 percent less likely to die of breast cancer.

I also recommend adding an omega-3 fatty acid supplement. These have two components: eicosapentaenoic acid (EPA) and docosahexaenoic acid (DHA). The combined amounts of EPA and DHA should be a minimum of 1 gram daily, or 2 grams if you suffer from anxiety. One big advantage of a high-quality fish oil supplement over eating actual fish is that the former is molecularly distilled to remove PCBs and mercury.[28]

Sleep and Breast Cancer

Your sleep habits may affect your risk of breast cancer. Research suggests that women who live in areas with high levels of external light at night, including street lights, may have a higher risk of breast cancer.[29] For this reason, I recommend avoiding bright lights close to bedtime. Turn off overhead lights and turn on dimmer lamps, use blackout curtains, and reduce screen time (or use blue-blocking glasses[30]) for at least an hour before bedtime.

People who work outside of typical business hours have been shown to have a higher risk of breast cancer.[31] Millions of people work night shifts, which can influence their risk of cancer, diabetes, heart disease, and more. There are ways to mitigate risk even when you must work shifts. As discussed on page 206, eating within a ten-hour window can improve blood sugar and blood pressure. Additionally, be sure to get adequate sleep (seven to eight hours), and see circadian-rhythm information in the chapter "Sleeping Soundly."

Exercising After Breast Surgery

After surgery, push yourself to begin gentle exercise, such as walking or yoga. Exercise has been shown to play a major role in improving patient outcomes after breast surgery;[32] it modulates immune function, inflammation, angiogenesis (the formation of new blood vessels), sex hormone production, antioxidant production, mood, and autonomic function (your body's involuntary physiologic processes like heart rate, blood pressure, and breathing[33]). One exception: If any of your lymph nodes were removed during your surgery, as noted earlier, you are at increased risk for lymphedema. Restrain from exercising the affected arm for at least two weeks following your procedure.

Exercise is linked to improved survival rates after a breast-cancer diagnosis, no matter how extensive your surgery. A recent review of data from the Nurses' Health Study, one of the largest and longest-running investigations into the risk factors for major chronic illnesses in women, concluded simply that "Physical activity was associated with lower risk of death following diagnosis."[34] Even one to three hours of walking each week was associated with improved outcomes. Studies also suggest that exercise during chemotherapy can lead to a reduced likelihood of cancer recurrence.[35] Many patients experience fatigue as a side effect of chemotherapy, and regular physical activity has been shown to increase energy while preserving muscle mass and bone density.[36]

As in other areas of integrative medicine, there is synergism between exercise and eating well, and the best outcomes occur in women with breast cancer who exercise regularly and eat a diet rich in fruit and vegetables.[37] In one recent study from the Yale Cancer Center, 53 percent of women receiving chemotherapy treatments for breast cancer who exercised regularly and increased their vegetable and fruit intake saw a disappearance of all invasive cancer cells in the breast, compared to just 28 percent of women in the control group.[38] I like the straightforward advice offered by researchers from the National Cancer Institute's Division of Cancer Control and Population Sciences: "Move as often as you can, when you can."[39]

Regaining Sexual Desire

One difficult side effect of breast-cancer surgery and recovery is rarely discussed: loss of sexual desire. This deserves attention, as studies reveal significant associations between sexual health and improved quality of life, less depression, and reduced anxiety. I believe a healthy sex life is one more way to support your recovery reflex. As many as 75 percent of women report a lower libido after a breast cancer diagnosis.[40] Hormonal therapies can cause constipation; nausea; fatigue; hot flushes; mood swings; and vaginal dryness, burning, or pain—all of which can lower sexual desire.[41] Vaginal dryness in particular can lead to pain before, during, or after intercourse. This condition, known as *dyspareunia*, is common, but you might feel uncomfortable talking about it with your doctor or specialist. (If you think your surgeon's bedside manner needs a little work, just try talking about the *bedroom*!) There are, however, many effective treatments for dyspareunia, and I encourage you to bring this up with your medical team.

For vaginal dryness, you can find lubricants that are water based, oil based, or silicone based. Water-based lubricants rinse off easily from skin and fabric and are safe to use with a condom, but they are absorbed quickly into the body and may require reapplication. Oil-based lubricants are long-lasting but difficult to wash off fabric and skin, and should not be used with condoms since they can damage the latex. A silicone-based lubricant may offer the best of both worlds, as they last almost as long as oil-based lubricants while being safe for condoms. (However, do not use silicone lubricants with silicone sex toys, as it can cause them to degrade over time.)

If you have tried a lubricant and are still having discomfort during sexual intercourse, ask your doctor about vaginal estrogen, which can be delivered as a cream, tablet, or thin circular tube inserted into the vagina, known as a *pessary*. This can help restore the normal vaginal tissue and promote natural lubrication.

Whenever I bring up vaginal estrogen with breast-cancer survivors, their first question is: Shouldn't I be *avoiding* estrogen? Won't it increase my risk of recurrence? This is an understandable question, but rest assured: Vaginal estrogen is a localized treatment, and research indicates that using it does not increase overall levels of estrogen in the body. The Women's Health Initiative Observational Study tracked more than 160,000 postmenopausal women for fifteen years and found no increase in breast-cancer risk among women using vaginal estrogen.[42] And in 2016, the American College of Obstetricians and Gynecologists officially recommended vaginal estrogen for breast-cancer survivors who were having pain during sexual intercourse and did not find benefit from moisturizers or lubricants.[43] Vaginal estrogen is available by prescription only, so consult with your doctor if you think you need it.

While physical discomfort and pain are common reasons for loss of desire, they are certainly not the only ones. Change in body image after breast surgery can contribute, as can stress or fatigue related to cancer treatment. Sometimes a partner fears touching a surgically scarred breast area, which can interfere with lovemaking.

For ten years I taught at a retreat for women with cancer. Its Tibetan Buddhist founders dubbed it Courageous Women Fearless Living, and it incorporated teaching in meditation, yoga, and expressive arts (such as playing music, dancing, painting, theater, and creative writing). I led workshops on diet, supplements, environmental exposures, and sexuality after a cancer diagnosis. I heard many poignant stories from women about loss, including loss of pleasure from breast stimulation, loss of self-image, and loss of confidence in showing their body, even to longtime partners.

One activity that helped restore women's sensual and playful sides was 5Rhythms, a form of dance created by the American dancer Gabrielle Roth. I will never forget the wonderful energy of seventy women dancing freely to Marvin Gaye's "Let's Get it On" and Gloria Gaynor's "I Will Survive." The women felt strong and sensual as they finally let loose after a stressful journey. One woman in particular stood out. She had undergone a bilateral mastectomy, but that didn't stop her from making playful and suggestive movements, carried out in rhythm with the music. She radiated joy, and boy was she sexy on the dance floor!

You don't need to go to a retreat or join a group to tap into your sensual side, however. Consider dancing at home to music that makes you feel alive. Or, think about other activities that make you feel vibrant and sexy. If you're not one for dancing, you might take a bath with aromatic essential oils or read an erotic novel. If you are not coming up with much, there are sexual wellness apps available online and on your phone.

Environmental Health Recommendations

Reducing estrogen is the goal of much of breast-cancer treatment, so it might be disturbing to learn that we are routinely exposed to estrogens in multiple ways. Xenoestrogens are the estrogens in industrial chemicals,[44] and they show up in things like plastics, pesticides, receipts (when they're coated with Bisphenol A, or BPA), phthalates (found in personal-care products and cosmetics), flame retardants, and just about everything that says "fragrance" on the label. We can reduce our exposure to xenoestrogens by eating organic food, minimizing the use of plastic for food and beverage storage, avoiding microwaving anything in plastic (use glass or ceramic instead), and steering clear of these chemicals in our personal products. There are several smartphone apps to help you check food and cosmetic products by allowing you to scan barcodes and get a readout on a product's safety, including its allergenic, carcinogenic, and reproductive toxicant risks. You can also learn more by visiting www.chemtrust.org; this organization provides helpful information for avoiding endocrine disruptors in food, food packaging, and when cooking or consulting the Yuka app.

You might be wondering whether changing your personal-care routine to avoid risky ingredients actually makes a difference when it comes to preventing breast cancer. Several studies suggest the answer is a resounding yes! A recent, innovative study asked healthy volunteers without breast cancer to undergo two biopsies of their breast tissue four weeks apart.[45] The first biopsy was done when the participants used their regular personal-care products (think shampoo, conditioner, makeup and moisturizers). The second was twenty-eight days after switching to personal-care products free of phthalates, parabens, and fragrance. By reducing their use of these products for just one month, they had fewer cancer-associated changes in follow-up biopsies!

The Spiritual Challenge of Breast Cancer

Many of the women I care for see breast cancer as an existential threat. Despite an often-good prognosis, they fear death will be the outcome. For some women, this leads to a deepening of their religious or spiritual life. I will never forget one patient, Nan, who told me, "I have never felt as close to God as when I had my cancer." Another one of my patients reported to me that throughout her breast-cancer treatment she found comfort in Psalm 57: "Be merciful to me, O God, be merciful to me, for in you my soul takes refuge; in the shadow of your wings I will take refuge, till the storms of destruction pass by."

Your Rapid Recovery Prescription After Breast Cancer Treatment

Most breast cancer is highly treatable, thanks to modern therapies. No matter what form of breast cancer you have, there are many promising options at your disposal, and integrative-medicine strategies can supplement your treatment to improve your odds of a full and speedy recovery and a reduced risk of recurrence:

1. Ask for an Oncotype DX test, if you have not had one yet. This score is interpreted in conjunction with your age. When there is a lack of clarity for treatment, ask for a second opinion from a specialist.
2. Lumpectomy-plus-radiotherapy is as effective as mastectomy and may lead to fewer side effects. The exceptions are women with large tumors or those who have inherited the BRCA1 or BRCA2 genes.
3. If you have had lymph nodes removed during surgery, avoid exercising the affected arm for at least two weeks to reduce the risk of lymphedema.
4. After surgery, eat seven to nine servings of vegetables and fruit daily, a tablespoon of ground linseeds, and green tea. Prioritize organic products and include soy foods in your diet.
5. Adopt a thirteen-hour or longer overnight fast to reduce the risk of cancer recurrence. If you are having chemotherapy, a forty-eight–hour fast (twenty-four hours before chemo and twenty-four hours after) can significantly improve treatment tolerance.
6. Take a multivitamin-multimineral and omega-3 supplements to lower the risk of cancer recurrence.
7. Push yourself to begin gentle exercise, such as walking, immediately after surgery (except if you've had lymph nodes removed).
8. If you are experiencing vaginal dryness, a lubricant or moisturizer can help. If that doesn't do the trick, ask your doctor about vaginal estrogen. If you've had a loss of sexual desire, seek out activities such as dancing that help restore your sensual and playful side.
9. Reduce your environmental exposure to estrogen by avoiding xenoestrogens and anything that says "fragrance" on the label. Additionally, minimize the use of plastic containers for food and beverages.
10. Create a healing ceremony either before your surgery or as an adjunct to radiation or chemo to help with the transition back to ordinary life.

23

Recovery from Minimally Invasive Surgery

On September 13, 1980, Dr. Kurt Semm attempted a surgery so controversial that it nearly cost him his career. The president of the German Surgical Society recommended Semm permanently lose his license, while his colleagues at Germany's University of Kiel forced him to undergo a brain scan because, as one put it, "only a person with brain damage" would try such a dangerous procedure.[1]

What was this scandalous surgery that caused such an uproar? Semm had made several incisions near his patient's belly button, and into one, had inserted a thin tube with a camera at the tip. He then sliced off the patient's appendix and removed it through another incision. The procedure took less than an hour and the patient went home a few days later. Dr. Kurt Semm had performed the world's first laparoscopic appendectomy.

Five years later, another German surgeon, Erich Mühe, realized the same minimally invasive procedure could remove gallstones. Instead of making a 15-centimetre (6-inch)-long incision across his patient's right upper abdomen just below the ribcage, he made a few tiny slits, inserted a fiberoptic camera, and removed the gallstones using tiny surgical tools and a TV monitor. After conducting nearly one hundred such procedures, he announced his research at the Congress of the German Surgical Society in 1986. Like Semm before him, Mühe faced withering criticism and was ultimately censured by the courts.[2]

Fast-forward forty years and today, minimally invasive surgery is considered the standard of care. More than thirteen million minimally invasive procedures are performed worldwide every year. In the United States alone, 750,000 laparoscopic cholecystectomies (gallbladder removals) are performed yearly,[3] and a large proportion of the three hundred thousand appendectomies performed each year in the United States are also done laparoscopically,[4] as are almost half of the country's six hundred thousand annual hysterectomies.[5] Before the work of pioneers like Kurt Semm and Erich Mühe, these surgeries involved a large incision, which often resulted in more pain, larger scars, and a higher risk of complications, like bleeding and infection. In contrast, minimally invasive surgery requires only a few small incisions. Laparoscopic procedures result in less scarring, increased accuracy, less blood loss, less pain, and shorter hospital stays.

Increasingly, minimally invasive surgery is performed with the assistance of robotic technology. Similar to laparoscopic surgery, robotic surgery begins with the surgeon making a few incisions, then inserting surgical instruments and a tiny camera. However, instead of manipulating the surgical tools by hand, the surgeon sits at a computer console displaying a magnified three-dimensional image of your body. Using the controls, the doctor can direct the robotic arms with extreme precision, eliminating minute hand tremors while allowing for greater range of motion. The most popular robotic method—the da Vinci Surgical System—has been used on more than 750,000 patients worldwide undergoing urologic, cardiac, prostate, and gynecologic procedures.

While minimally invasive surgery takes much less of a toll on your body compared to an open surgery, the principles of prehab (see the "Your Surgical Prehab" chapter) still apply for the fastest recovery. This chapter will focus on specific recovery routines for some of the most common minimally invasive procedures.

Recovery from Gynecologic Surgeries: Fibroids and Hysterectomy

A hysterectomy is performed to remove the uterus and sometimes the ovaries. They are the second-most common surgical procedure for women in the United States after C-sections.[6] A hysterectomy may be carried out for many reasons, including abnormal bleeding, fibroids, painful menses, endometriosis, gynecologic cancers (uterine, ovarian, cervical, or endometrial), and gender-affirming care. Nearly 90 percent of hysterectomies are performed for benign conditions, and research shows that one-third of all women will have the procedure by age sixty.[7]

For instance, a few years ago, a forty-five-year-old woman named Megan came to see Dr. Anne Kennard, gynecologist and graduate of our Integrative Medicine Fellowship in Central California, owing to bouts of very heavy menstrual bleeding. She had a ten-day cycle every twenty-eight days, which necessitated multiple changes of clothes and super-absorbency tampons and maxi pads. She was also anemic, had frequent headaches, and was constantly fatigued. Megan was diagnosed with fibroids, and she and Dr. Kennard agreed that an ovary-sparing hysterectomy was the right course of action. In pre-menopausal women, sparing the ovaries means they will continue to produce the hormones estrogen and progesterone until the age of menopause, thereby helping prevent the onset of osteoporosis and cardiovascular disease.[8] (For more information about menopause, see the "Mastering Menopause" chapter.) After an extensive prehab that included eating a rainbow of veggies and fruits, pulling together a robust social support network, practicing guided imagery, doing pelvic floor exercises, and taking iron supplements, Megan underwent a successful laparoscopic hysterectomy. She had minimal pain and very few side effects, largely thanks to her effective prehab work.

A hysterectomy may be recommended if you have fibroids that cause heavy menstrual bleeding. Fibroids are benign tumors formed from muscle cells and fibrous connective tissue that develop in the uterus. (Fibroids tend to shrink with menopause, so often women choose to wait rather than having surgery.) With the exception of a hysterectomy performed for uterine cancer, most hysterectomies are performed laparoscopically or vaginally. Afterward, your incisions will be closed with stitches or glue, which usually dissolve on their own in a few weeks. Forty-eight hours later, you should be able to remove any bandages and shower. Both laparoscopic and vaginal procedures may seem fully healed after only a few weeks. However, complete internal healing is an average of three months, as it takes some time for your abdominal and pelvic organs to shift into the space once occupied by your uterus. Most surgeons recommend avoiding sexual intercourse and strenuous physical activity for six weeks.

One common hysterectomy side effect is constipation. I recommend eating high-fiber foods to promote regular bowel movements, including fruits, especially berries; green leafy vegetables; starchy vegetables like squash and sweet potatoes; ground linseeds; and pulses (legumes). If fiber-rich foods are new to you, build up your tolerance slowly to avoid uncomfortable bloating.

Work to strengthen your pelvic muscles beginning four to six weeks after your hysterectomy. This can help to prevent pelvic organ prolapse, a condition in which the bladder or rectum collapses into the vagina. Ideally, you will be guided by a pelvic-floor physiotherapist who will customize a plan for you, based on an exam. Sometimes the pelvic muscles need strengthening, which the exercises that follow can help with, but other times they are too tight and you may need to learn to relax them. Your physiotherapist will help guide you through the best course of action.

If you don't have a pelvic-floor physiotherapist available, here are post-surgery exercises that are frequently recommended:

- **Pelvic floor (Kegel) exercises:** These exercises specifically work your pelvic-floor muscles. Here's the procedure: Squeeze your pelvic muscles as if you are holding back the flow of urine. You will feel an upward pulling or lifting sensation in your rectal or vaginal area. Squeeze for three seconds, relax, and repeat five to ten times. Perform two or three times daily. You can also practice these exercises while sitting on the toilet to urinate. Begin the flow of urine and then pull up on your muscles to stop. Do this several times and you will master the technique.
- **TA Holds:** Your transversus abdominus (TA) muscle is in your lower abdomen and wraps around your pelvis to help stabilize your core and lower back. Strengthening the TA is important after a hysterectomy. Target it by lying on your back with your knees bent and your feet flat on the floor and shoulder-width apart. Pull your navel down

toward the floor, feeling your lower spine flatten against the floor. Hold for ten seconds and then relax. Repeat five to ten times. Begin with one set a day, and over the next four weeks, increase to three times daily.
- **Walking Backwards:** A surprisingly effective way to lift your pelvic floor that I learned from pain specialist Esther Gokhale, L.Ac, is to walk backwards, holding on to a rail or wall, for ten to twenty steps. You will notice a lift and a realignment of your posture. (Check out www.gokhalemethod.com/europe for more information.)

Treating Fibroids without a Hysterectomy

Fibroids are not always treated with hysterectomies. Hormones and directed embolization (cutting off blood flow to the uterus to shrink fibroid tumors) are options, as is a lesser surgical procedure called *myomectomy* (removal of the fibroid tumor alone, thereby preserving the remainder of the uterus). Dr. Suzanne Bartlett Hackenmiller, gynecologist and integrative-medicine fellowship graduate, told me about one of her patients, Julia, who was diagnosed with a very large fibroid when she was in her early forties; it caused heavy bleeding, cramping, and anemia severe enough to require repeated IV iron and blood transfusions.

Julia did not intend to have more children, so her gynecologist recommended a hysterectomy. Julia resisted; she had been sexually assaulted as a young woman and could not come to terms with losing her uterus. Psychologically, it felt to her like another instance of someone else taking control of her body. She found a gynecologist willing to perform a laparoscopic myomectomy. Exerting control over the treatment for her fibroid felt validating and empowering. Dr. Hackenmiller explained that Julia described it like a symbolic and life-changing triumph to eradicate the tumor and keep her uterus intact. Her experience demonstrates the value of finding a doctor who listens to and honors your preferences, even if you have to seek out a second or third opinion. Dr. Hackenmiller's takeaway is that she often sees patients who need salves and balms for the soul, not the physical wound.

Recovery from Abdominal Surgery

Dr. Elizabeth Raskin, surgical director at the Margolis Family Inflammatory Bowel Disease Program at Hoag Hospital in Southern California and a graduate of the Andrew Weil Center for Integrative Medicine fellowship program, recommends all patients have their albumin levels checked prior to major surgery. Albumin is a protein produced by the liver that serves as a marker of your overall nutritional status. If you have not been eating enough—a common problem among people with inflammatory bowel disease—your body may be less effective at healing after your procedure. Patients who have a low albumin have a significantly increased risk of postoperative infectious complications,[9] she explains. A diet high in healthy proteins, including nuts, beans, eggs, fish, and even organic poultry or grass-fed lean meat, can help boost your albumin levels.[10]

Dr. Raskin describes one former patient, Jacob, who arrived for emergency treatment at a hospital with multiple partial bowel obstructions due to his Crohn's disease. Obstructions can be resolved laparoscopically, but when she saw that Jacob's albumin level was very low and that he was anemic, she postponed his surgery. "We needed to prehabilitate him on a nutritional level," she explained. Dr. Raskin used intravenous protein sources since it was difficult for Joseph to eat. After a few weeks, his albumin level was restored to normal, and then she proceeded with the surgery. His improved nutritional status meant she was able to spare all his bowel (rather than having to remove multiple sections), as well as widen the strictures instead of performing a more invasive surgery. Jacob made a full recovery.

With regard to your diet, advance slowly if you are recovering from surgery for inflammatory bowel disease (IBD). Some people who suffer from IBD greatly limit their diets due to pain, diarrhea, or a fistula (an abnormal connection between two body parts, such as your bowel and your skin). After surgery, they may be able to eat a much wider selection of foods, including foods loaded with fiber. But high-fiber foods can also cause bloating or, worse, an obstruction, especially for those with a history of Crohn's disease who have narrowing in parts of their intestines. Also note that some people with inflammatory diseases don't tolerate gluten or dairy, so do be careful as you reintroduce food groups into the diet.

Gallbladder Surgery

The gallbladder is a pear-shaped organ that sits just below the liver. When healthy, the gallbladder collects bile, a thick fluid produced by the liver that aids in the digestion of fat. If the delicate chemical balance of bile gets thrown off, one of its components, cholesterol, can crystallize and form into gallstones, which can block bile ducts and cause intense pain. In some cases, the gallbladder can become inflamed or even infected. One in ten people in the U.K. will get gallstones, and they affect nearly 25 million Americans,[11] of whom about 1.2 million per year require a cholecystectomy, or the removal of the gallbladder.[12]

While removing the gallbladder used to require a wide incision across the abdomen that made recovery challenging, laparoscopic surgery has improved matters dramatically. In fact, most patients go home the same day and healing is rapid. Pay close attention to your diet: I recommend avoiding fatty, greasy, or spicy foods, which could lead to diarrhea, for three weeks following your surgery. Gradually increase your fiber intake and drink six to eight glasses of water daily to promote regular bowel movements.

Your Rapid Recovery Prescription After Minimally Invasive Surgery

Today, minimally invasive surgery is considered the standard of care. Seek it out whenever possible, as it takes much less of a toll on your body compared to open surgery. These steps will enhance your recovery:

1. If you've had a hysterectomy, avoid sexual intercourse and strenuous physical activity for six weeks. Complete healing takes an average of three months, as your pelvic organs shift into the space once occupied by your uterus.

2. If you are constipated following a hysterectomy, drink lots of fluids and include high-fiber foods. Be careful to increase fiber slowly if these foods are new to you.
3. Ideally, work with a pelvic-floor physiotherapist after hysterectomy, particularly if you are struggling with the exercises or if your recovery seems to be progressing slowly. If you do not have access to a physiotherapist, strengthen your pelvis with pelvic floor exercises, TA holds, and by walking backwards.
4. Ensure your albumin level is in a normal range before major surgery. A diet high in healthy proteins including nuts, beans, eggs, fish, organic poultry, or grass-finished lean meat can help boost your albumin levels.
5. After gallbladder surgery, avoid fatty, greasy, or spicy foods for three weeks. Gradually increase your fiber intake, and be sure to drink six to eight glasses of water each day to promote regular bowel movements.

24

Final Considerations

I sincerely hope you have found answers within these pages to improve your health. Whether you're healing from surgery, a short-lived condition, or a longstanding one, my goal has been to provide inspiration and direction to stimulate and support your recovery reflex.

Each person's path to recovery may look a bit different: Some traverse a straight path, while others experience twists and turns before discovering what works for them. When we think about recovery, it's easy to focus on the material, such as medications, physiotherapy, surgery, or supplements. I want to reiterate the power of less visible variables that may also be influencing your recovery. The food you eat, the air you breathe, the chemicals in your household products, the stress you carry, and the quality of your sleep—all these unseen forces can play a role in how quickly and fully your recovery reflex activates, and thus how well your body repairs and rebuilds. As discussed in these pages, the invisible influences are alterable, whether it's by purchasing organic food, using a HEPA filter, assessing household products for harmful chemicals by scanning their barcodes with an app, adopting a mindfulness practice, or practicing sleep hygiene. By addressing these unseen elements, you set yourself up with the best possible foundation for long-term wellness and resilience.

I also want to address another "invisible" impact on your health you may not think about: who your doctor is. Your doctor does more than prescribe treatments; they understand your history, listen to your concerns, and tailor their approach to your specific needs. The doctor treats *you* as an individual, not a disease or a list of symptoms.

I cannot overstate how important this relationship is. One study, for instance, found that *who* a patient's psychiatrist was had a greater treatment effect on their recovery from depression than antidepressant medication.[1] The researchers concluded that "the health care community would be wise to consider the psychiatrist not only as a provider of treatment, but also as a means of treatment."

This isn't only the case for mental health. Another study examined the impact of empathy on the duration and severity of the common cold.[2] Three hundred and fifty patients aged twelve and older were randomly assigned to receive either a standard medical visit or an enhanced visit emphasizing empathy from a doctor. The conclusion? Clinician empathy "significantly predicts" the duration and severity of illness and is even associated with positive immune system changes. Finally, a review of clinical trials found that a doctor's bedside manner can impact everything from obesity to asthma, blood pressure, blood sugar, and overall pain levels.[3]

Remember that *homeostasis* is defined as a return to a similar, but not identical, status. In other words, a new normal. In my practice, I take care of many women with breast cancer whose diagnoses and subsequent treatment change their bodies, and often their priorities. As part of their healing journey, some decide to leave a job, a relationship, or an environment that has not suited them for a long time. Similarly, dietary change is a common factor for my patients who are reversing diabetes or heart disease. Some dramatically reduce carbs, others adopt a practice of time-restricted eating, and all commit to daily (or near daily) exercise. My most successful patients, no matter what they are recovering from, embrace healthy lifestyles that often produce surprising side benefits.

Lifestyle changes can be made more palatable and more potent when you have support. Many organizations (such as WeightWatchers, Alcoholics Anonymous, and local community running groups) have shown that the greatest success often comes when you commit to another person or group who holds you accountable.[4] Other studies have found that the presence of a doula during childbirth reduced the C-section rate by 25 percent.[5]

If you have not yet found your path to recovery, ask for another opinion. New eyes may offer new treatments or pick up a misdiagnosis. We live in a time of breathtaking medical progress. But I encourage you to look beyond the realm of conventional Western medicine. I have pointed out the power of traditional Chinese medicine, yoga, guided imagery, and hypnotherapy. I have provided in this book several examples of the profound effect that an elimination diet can have when you identify foods that are negatively impacting your microbiome, as well as the power of diversifying your microbiome with plant foods, fermented foods, and fiber. We've seen how the mind–body connection can quiet the nervous system. Much of the power of integrative medicine lies in the synergism of approaching a problem from multiple angles. I hope you will consider addressing your food choices, stress, sleep, light exposure, environmental chemical exposure, and any other triggers that may be impeding your recovery reflex. Remember, you have profound control over your health and your recovery.

I acknowledge that there is a lot of *doing* in this book. Remember, as well, to take the time to rest. Sit in the sunshine, watch a sunset (as I do), listen to the birds—do whatever makes your heart sing! When you breathe, take note of the brief pause between the in and the out breath. Minute by minute, hour by hour, your body is creating opportunities to rest. While you may feel like nothing is happening, your recovery reflex is hard at work.

For now, take time to celebrate every bit of care you've given yourself, every bite of healthy food, every moment of centering and relaxation, and every stride of your daily walk. Your actions have added to the foundation of your recovery and to the resilience of your body and spirit. And, please do email me at info@drvictoriamaizes.com and tell me about your recovery journey! I want to learn so that I can share your struggles and triumphs with others.

Throughout this book I have shared healing affirmations to recite when your journey becomes difficult. As you put this book down, I encourage you to write your own centering words. I leave you with a final affirmation I have written for you as you begin your journey to rapid recovery:

May you find your way to healing.
May you trust in your capacity to recover.
May you activate your innate healing responses.
May you discover your path to health and happiness.

Your Rapid Recovery Toolkit

When it comes to being prepared for life's health hiccups, a well-stocked recovery toolkit is your go-to resource. A key to rapid recovery is quickly responding to whatever ails you. For example, if you develop a cold or the flu, you can minimize symptoms and recover faster if you immediately begin taking garlic, zinc, or an antiviral botanical. Similarly, for an ankle sprain or headache, having the right supplies on hand will activate your recovery reflex faster and can save you a trip to the pharmacy.

This section begins with items I recommend everyone have on hand, as they provide relief from a wide range of conditions. Then we move to items that are a good idea for people with inflammation or pain to keep stocked. Finally, I end with three conceptual items that don't exactly fit into a medicine cabinet, but are still vital components of your toolkit: the Mediterranean diet, the elimination diet, and deep-breathing exercises. I frequently recommend them in my integrative practice to promote optimal health and assist with recovery.

Essential Toolkit Items

Anxiety

L-theanine supplements: Derived from tea, the amino acid L-theanine can help promote relaxation without causing drowsiness, making it a valuable supplement to take when you're feeling particularly anxious.

It can be useful during the day or taken before bed if a restless mind keeps you from falling asleep. The usual dose is 200–400 mg per day.

Essential Oils: Essential oils are most commonly employed in aromatherapy using an atomizer or diluted and used on the skin or added to a bath. I also like placing a drop on my wrist. For anxiety, I recommend lavender essential oil. Diffusing or inhaling the oil directly can have immediate calming effects on the central nervous system; it can also be taken orally in a specific formulation called Silexan. I recommend blends of essential oils as well; look for products that include chamomile, ylang-ylang, or bergamot.

Heartburn

Deglycyrrhizinated licorice (DGL): A form of licorice root from which the compound glycyrrhizin has been removed. Available in chewable tablets, capsules, and powders. DGL can minimize symptoms of GORD by soothing the stomach lining, reducing inflammation, and supporting mucous production, and is a safe and effective alternative to medications. I recommend chewing one or two 380 mg tablets as needed for symptom relief.

Cold and Flu

I use a combination of the following items to shorten the duration of viral respiratory infections. You do not need to have all these products in your toolkit, but I do recommend the first five—honey, a head of garlic, throat coat tea, a sinus rinse, zinc lozenges—and at least one of the botanical antivirals.

Honey: Honey forms a protective coating on the mucous membranes of the throat, reducing irritation and calming that tickling sensation that triggers coughing. One to 2 teaspoons can be consumed two or three times a day, especially before bedtime or added to a cup of tea.

Raw Garlic: Crushing or chopping a head of garlic releases allicin, a sulfur-containing compound that can inhibit the growth of bacteria, viruses, and fungi. After chopping, let the garlic sit for 10 minutes to maximize potency. Add it to dressings, dips, spreads, or your morning toast.

Throat Coat Tea: I am a big fan of medicinal teas and keep a variety in my cupboard for cold and flu symptoms. I also stick them in my suitcase when I travel. Throat coat tea contains ingredients such as licorice root, marshmallow, or slippery elm, which soothe sore throats. I recommend blends from the brands Yogi and Traditional Medicinals, which favor organic ingredients.

Sinus Rinse: A nasal irrigation system is designed to cleanse your nasal passages by flushing out mucus, allergens, and irritants. I recommend that you look for one that consists of a squeeze bottle and pre-measured salt packets. My patients sometimes need a bit of encouragement to initiate use—"You want me to shoot salt water up my nose!?" they exclaim—but then are amazed and delighted by how effective it is. See page 20 for more information.

Zinc Lozenges: I recommend sucking on a low-dose zinc lozenge at the first hint of a cold, then every two to three hours while awake until symptoms subside. You can find them at pharmacies, health and wellness shops, and sold online.

Vitamin C: While researchers continue to debate just how effective vitamin C supplements are for cold and flu, I recommend adding them at the first sign of a cold. They are inexpensive and rarely cause any side effects. I personally recommend an effervescent vitamin C supplement that can be added to water and has a pleasant fizzy taste.

Echinacea: A perennial plant native to North America thought to stimulate the activity of white blood cells, such as macrophages and natural killer, which are crucial for fighting infections.[2]

Andrographis: As discussed in the chapter "Conquering Colds and Vanquishing Viral Infections," Andrographis is an herb that treats respiratory infections and digestive issues and can improve immune health. I recommend purchasing in powdered form.

Medicinal Mushrooms: Fungi containing bioactive compounds that may support the immune system, reduce inflammation, and enhance brain function. Reishi, shiitake, maitake, turkey tail, lion's mane, and *Cordyceps* mushrooms are associated with immune-boosting benefits. You can add them to soups, stews, and stir-fries, or brew them into teas. Another easy way to take mushrooms is as an extract or capsule.

Allergic Reactions

Cetirizine: Used for treating common allergy symptoms like sneezing, runny nose, itchy eyes, and skin rashes. It is helpful to have on hand should you have a reaction to an insect bite or develop hives as a result of an allergic reaction. The typical dose of cetirizine for adults is 10 mg once daily. Some people do find that it makes them drowsy.

Hydrocortisone Cream: An over-the-counter topical steroid that works by reducing inflammation pain, itching, redness, and swelling. One percent hydrocortisone is widely available, but for anything stronger you will need a prescription.

Burns and Sunburns

Aloe: Aloe is a succulent plant, with *Aloe vera* being the most well-known species. Aloe gel has a natural cooling sensation, which soothes burns and sunburns. I keep aloe growing in my garden; it's easy to cut off a stalk, slice it open, and apply the mucilaginous gel that is excreted directly onto a burn. (Do avoid the yellowish sap called *aloin*, which can irritate your skin.)

Tummy Trouble

Yogi Egyptian Licorice Tea or Stomach Ease Tea: A cup of either tea can dramatically soothe all kinds of digestive symptoms. I recommend infusing the tea bag in hot water with a lid over the cup for 5 to 10 minutes before drinking.

Acupressure wrist band: A wrist band that can help reduce nausea and vomiting. The band works by applying pressure to the P6 acupressure point, which is located on the inner wrist about three finger-widths distal to the base of your palm. Studies show that acupressure wrist bands like Sea-Bands are effective at reducing nausea.[3] I recommend using for nausea related to motion sickness, surgical recovery, or pregnancy.

Crystallized Ginger: Ginger root that has been boiled and coated in sugar, making it sweet and chewy. The compounds in ginger, including gingerols and shogaols, help reduce nausea and vomiting, and improve digestion.

Musculoskeletal Injuries

Sprains, strains, and cramps happen, but how you choose to recover can make the difference between spending the weekend on the couch and quickly resuming your normal activities. I recommend having the following items in your home.

Foam Roller: A column-shaped roll of dense foam used for self-massage and myofascial release. You can get the rolls in various sizes, densities, and textures. Foam rollers allow you to apply pressure to the connective tissue surrounding muscles, known as the fascia. Foam rolling helps to relieve tight spots, known as trigger points or knots, while improving range of motion and flexibility. When getting started, begin with soft foam rollers.

Heating Pads: Therapeutic devices that apply heat to sore or tense muscles. They come in various forms, including electric pads, microwavable packs, and even adhesive patches that can stick directly onto the skin. If you purchase an electric pad, choose a product with an automatic shut-off feature to prevent overheating and reduce the risk of burns. I also recommend products filled with buckwheat, which are warmed in the microwave before use.

Ice Pack: Use ice acutely for swelling, ligament sprains, and muscle strains.

ACE Bandages wrap: Wrap the injury site with an elastic ACE bandage wrap, overlapping the bandage by half its width on each wrap to ensure even support.

Pain-Relief Lotion: Pain-relief lotions interrupt the transmission of pain signals to the brain, reduce inflammation, and create a cooling or warming sensation depending on the active ingredient. (Generally speaking, menthol for cooling and camphor or capsaicin for warming.) I recommend pain-relief lotions that are for muscle, joint, back, and neuropathic pain.

Optional Toolkit Items

Omega-3 Fatty Acids

As I have described in this book, Omega-3s reduce inflammation, helping to relieve conditions in which inflammation pays a key role, including arthritis, mental health, and heart disease.

You can obtain omega-3s through diet or supplements. Which is better? I generally recommend opting for whole-food sources of omega-3s. Studies suggest that eating seafood is more effective at reducing the risk of heart disease when compared to omega-3 supplements.[4] If you regularly eat SMASH fish, you likely do not need to take an omega-3 supplement. When people ask me if they should take a supplement, I ask about their diet and then order a blood test that measures the amount of EPA and DHA in the cell membranes; a desirable omega-3 index is 8 percent or higher.[5]

If you are struggling to reach this level through diet alone, don't like the taste of fish, or are vegetarian or vegan, choose an omega-3 supplement that is molecularly distilled to remove mercury and other environmental contaminants. (Vegetarians and vegans can purchase omega-3s made from algae rather than fish.) Read the back of label, as you want to be sure it contains a minimum of 1 gram of EPA plus DHA. Be discerning: many products may claim 1 gram of fish oil, but it may be predominantly ALA and therefore not what you ultimately want.[6] I recommend a dose of 1 gram daily for people who do not eat fish regularly, 2 grams daily for anyone with anxiety, and even higher doses (3 grams or more) for people using it to treat arthritis. Some people prefer bottles of liquid fish oil, which also tends to be less expensive than capsules.

Note that fish oil can go bad, which is a big reason I don't recommend everyone buy it for their toolkit. To help prevent oxidizing, which causes rancidity, keep the bottle in the fridge or freezer. Likewise, if the capsules smell rancid, it's time to toss them. Some people do complain of fish burps when taking fish oil capsules. You can reduce this effect by taking your capsules with your largest meal of the day and in between bites of food. You can also limit fish burps by putting the capsules in the freezer and taking them frozen.

Vitamin D

While you can obtain small amounts of vitamin D from fatty fish, such as trout or salmon, mushrooms, and fortified foods like milks and cereals, your primary source is sunlight. Exposing yourself to sunlight each morning will help regulate your circadian rhythms (read more about this in the "Sleeping Soundly" chapter), improve your sleep, and generally promote a healthy equilibrium. The amount of sun exposure you need depends on many factors, including your age, skin color, and geographic location; studies suggest that people living above the thirty-seventh parallel are unable to synthesize vitamin D from autumn until spring.[7] More than a third of American adults are believed to have vitamin D deficiency, and the U.K. government advice is that everyone should take a vitamin D supplement during these months.[8]

I recommend getting your vitamin D level checked with a blood test. If it is low, supplement with vitamin D3. They are widely available online, at your local pharmacy, or at health food stores in liquid, chewable, and pill forms. A good starting dose for most adults is 1,000 (25 micrograms) to 2,000 IU daily. Depending on your blood test, your doctor may recommend a larger dose (4,000 IU per day or more). For optimal absorption, take vitamin D3 with a meal that contains fat.

Turmeric

Turmeric: Turmeric can inhibit the activity of molecules and enzymes that are involved in inflammation, helping to reduce joint pain and swelling. Choose your product carefully. Specific products (Meriva,

Indena, and Theracurmin) have been studied at a dose of 90 to 100 mg of curcumin twice daily. Alternatively, certain turmeric extracts (Turmacin by Natural Remedies and Curcugen by DolCas Biotech) have been shown to reduce pain and the need for analgesics, as well as improve function when dosed at 500 mg twice daily. Side benefits of turmeric includes improvement in nonalcoholic fatty liver disease, less GERD, and less depression! Note it can take six to twelve weeks for turmeric to show effects.

The Mediterranean Diet

The Mediterranean diet is a heart-healthy way of eating inspired by the traditional dietary habits of people living in countries bordering the Mediterranean Sea, such as Greece, Italy, and Spain. It emphasizes whole-plant foods, healthy fats, fish, high-quality dairy products, and small amounts of meat.

Studies show that people with existing heart disease who follow the Mediterranean diet have a 50 to 70 percent lower risk of recurrent heart disease, compared to those who follow the American Heart Association's Step-I Diet, which involves limiting total fat intake, saturated fat, and dietary cholesterol.[9] A study of about twenty-six thousand women found that a Mediterranean diet reduced the risk of heart disease by 25 percent, while a meta-analysis analyzing twenty-two thousand people followed for over twelve years found the diet led to a 23 percent lower risk of premature death.[10] As I've described, the Mediterranean diet can also reduce your risk of everything from type 2 diabetes to obesity, gut health, skin conditions, and depression. Unsurprisingly, *U.S. News and World Report* perennially ranks the Mediterranean diet as number-one in its annual best-diet rankings.[11]

There are several variations on the Mediterranean diet, including an anti-inflammatory version advocated by Dr. Andrew Weil, the father of integrative medicine. (More about this following.) Here are the basics for getting started.

Prioritize Plant-Based Foods: Strive to fill half your plate with colorful vegetables and fruit, either fresh or frozen. Organic is preferred if your budget allows it. Opt for whole grains, such brown rice, quinoa, and barley, over refined grains, like white rice or pasta.

Emphasize Olive Oil: Olive oil is a central component of the Mediterranean diet, as it is rich in healthy monounsaturated fats. Choose extra-virgin olive oil at the grocery store, which means it is minimally processed and rich in antioxidants.[12]

Choose Omega-3-Rich Fish: Opt for *s*almon, *m*ackerel, *a*nchovies, *s*ardines, and *h*erring (SMASH). These cold-water fatty fish are rich in omega-3 fatty acids, which support heart and brain health; are an excellent source of lean protein; and tend to be low in mercury and other toxins, compared to larger fish like tuna, shark, or swordfish. Other good sources of omega-3s include wild rainbow trout, halibut, and striped bass, as well as walnuts, ground linseeds, and purslane.[13] Include fish in your diet at least twice a week.

Enjoy Dairy and Eggs in Moderation: Fermented high-quality dairy products, like Greek yogurt and kefir, as well as minimally processed cheeses, like parmesan, feta, and ricotta, are regularly consumed in the Mediterranean diet. Full-fat (whole) milk, low-fat milk, or nonfat cow's milk are rarely consumed.

Limit Processed Foods and Meat: Minimize processed foods like sugary beverages, crisps (chips), cereals, pastries, or any product that has a laundry list of ingredients. While you can eat meat on occasion, enjoy it sparingly. Remember, the foundation of the Mediterranean diet is vegetables, fruits, olive oil, beans, whole grains, and fish.

The anti-inflammatory diet includes the staple foods of the Mediterranean diet, but goes a step further by emphasizing foods that reduce inflammation. This includes the use of spices with anti-inflammatory properties, such as turmeric, ginger, garlic, and cinnamon. The anti-inflammatory diet also includes medicinal mushrooms, such as reishi, shiitake, lion's mane, chaga, and turkey tail, owing to their anti-inflammatory and immune-supporting properties. Notably, dark chocolate with cocoa content greater than 70 percent is considered anti-inflammatory due to its high antioxidant levels.[14]

> ### Sample Mediterranean Diet Meal Plan
>
> - **Breakfast:** Greek yogurt or kefir topped with organic berries, walnuts, and ground linseeds or chia seeds.
> - **Lunch:** Large salad with mixed greens, cherry tomatoes, cucumbers, red peppers (capsicums), olives, chickpeas, feta cheese, and toasted pumpkin seeds. Use olive oil and lemon juice or vinegar for dressing.
> - **Snack:** Hummus with carrots, cucumbers, and peppers (capsicums) or a handful of nuts.
> - **Dinner:** Grilled salmon with roasted courgette (zucchini), peppers (capsicums), and aubergine (eggplant) over a bed of quinoa.

Elimination Diets

An elimination diet is a tool I commonly use in my practice to identify and treat food intolerances, sensitivities, allergies, and other longstanding conditions. There are many different elimination diets to choose from, depending on your medical condition or history. In the "Soothing the Gut" chapter, I discuss specific elimination diets for GORD and IBS. There are also common food eliminations for migraine headaches. I sometimes have people remove just one food group, such as dairy or gluten, if they have a strong suspicion they are reacting to it.

Another common approach that I use is the six-food-group elimination diet.[15] In this trial, you eliminate the six most common food allergens: milk, eggs, soy, wheat, nuts (including tree nuts and peanuts), and fish (including shellfish). I also recommend removing pro-inflammatory foods, including meat, sugar, and alcohol. The trial generally lasts four to six weeks. Here is what you should eliminate:

- All dairy products including milk, cream, cheese, cottage cheese, yogurt, butter, ice cream, and frozen yogurt. (Read labels for hidden sources, including casein and whey.)

- Beef, pork, and veal.
- Gluten and any foods that contain wheat, such as spelt, khorasan, oats, rye, barley, or malt.
- All corn products (including tortilla chips).
- Eggs and egg substitutes.
- Soy foods and the many processed foods that include soy.
- Alcohol.
- Caffeine, such as sodas, cold brews, energy drinks, and herbal tinctures.
- Processed foods, refined sugars, commercially prepared condiments, and vinegar.
- Margarine, vegetable fat, and butter.
- Peanuts, pistachios, and peanut butter.
- Brown sugar, honey, glucose-fructose syrup, molasses, and corn syrup.

I know what you're thinking—that's *a lot* to give up. Yes, it is. However, if you can stick to the plan, this is the fastest and most efficient way to identify food intolerances. Ideally, after about eight weeks, you'll know exactly what is causing your symptoms and you can go back to eating your (nontriggering) favorite foods.

Now, here are the foods that are fine to eat during the elimination phase:

- Chicken, turkey, and lamb.
- Brown rice, millet, buckwheat, quinoa, gluten-free flour products, or potato, tapioca, and arrowroot products.
- Beans and lentils.
- Any vegetables (organic preferred).
- All fruits except citrus and strawberries.
- Breads made from rice, quinoa, amaranth, buckwheat, millet, potato flour, or arrowroot.
- Cold- or expeller-pressed unrefined olive oil, as well as pumpkin and sesame oils.
- Herbal teas, rice and nut milks, vegetable juices, non-citrus fruit juice (fresh or unsweetened).
- Brown rice syrup and fruit sweeteners.
- Six to eight glasses of water per day.

> ## Sample Elimination Meal Plan
>
> **Breakfasts**
> - **Chia Seed Pudding:** Made with coconut milk, chia seeds, and a sweetener such as maple syrup or fruit puree. It can be topped with blueberries, raspberries, and banana slices.
> - **Gluten-Free Toast:** Prepare with avocado or a sunflower seed butter.
> - **Sweet Potato Hash:** Dice sweet potatoes, sauté with olive oil, and add spinach and bell peppers (capsicums). You can add cooked minced (ground) turkey or chicken for protein. Season with salt, pepper, and spices.
>
> **Lunches or Dinners**
> - **Grilled Chicken Breast:** Add slices to a bed of mixed greens. Include sliced cucumber, shredded carrots, and avocado. Dress with olive oil, lemon juice, and a pinch of salt.
> - **Quinoa and Vegetable Bowl:** Add roasted vegetables such as courgettes (zucchini), bell peppers (capsicums), and aubergine (eggplant). Include chickpeas or lentils for protein. Drizzle with tahini or olive oil and lemon juice.
> - **Baked Sweet Potatoes:** Stuff with sautéed black beans, diced tomatoes, and fresh coriander (cilantro). Top with avocado and a drizzle of lime juice.
> - **Stuffed Bell Peppers (capsicums):** Fill with cooked minced (ground) turkey, mixed with diced courgettes (zucchini), tomatoes, and rice.

During the elimination phase, keep a close record of how you are feeling. Create a table and make columns for the date, time, foods eaten, symptoms noticed, and how long they lasted. (See page 30 for a simple table to help you track symptoms.) You can track everything from a skin rash to a headache or an upset tummy. At the end of four weeks, notice if you have fewer of the symptoms that led you to begin the trial elimination. If this is the case, you may have discovered a link between a particular food and your symptoms.

Remember, the goal is not to maintain the elimination diet indefinitely;

it is to discover which specific food or foods caused your symptoms so you can return to eating a wider range of foods. After four to six weeks, reintroduce an eliminated food to your diet every two days. Look for any recurrence of symptoms. Begin with a small amount of the eliminated food and gradually increase the amount. At some point, you may have a return of symptoms, typically within hours after the culprit has been reintroduced. Continue to gradually reintroduce foods in case more than one caused your symptoms.

Breathing Exercises

Breathing exercises are easy and free practices that usually have you slow, deepen, and make your breath more regular. They can help reduce stress, increase oxygen flow, and promote mental clarity and calmness. You can deploy them whenever you are feeling stressed. Here are my favorites.

> **Box Breathing:** Box breathing, also known as square breathing, is a simple exercise that involves breathing steadily with equal counts for each step. You can do it in any position. Imagine the dimensions of a box and use the four sides to direct your breathing as follows: Inhale through the nose for four counts, hold for four counts, exhale through the nose for four counts, and hold again for four counts. Build up until you can continue box breathing for five minutes at a stretch. While this may seem rudimentary, don't underestimate its power; indeed, U.S. Navy Seals are taught box breathing to help manage high-stress situations.[16]
>
> **4-7-8 Breathing:** Popularized by Dr. Andrew Weil, this breathing practice originates from yoga, which includes an array of breathing practices called Pranayama. Place your tongue on the roof of your mouth, on the ridge behind your upper front teeth, and keep it there through the entire practice. Breathe in quietly through the nose for 4 seconds, hold your breath for 7 seconds, and exhale forcefully through your mouth (and around your tongue) for 8 seconds. Repeat these three steps four times. The prolonged exhalation is key to relaxation. By practicing this daily, you will gradually tone your parasympathetic nervous system.

My patient Diane, who complained of unbearable anxiety, committed to practice the 4-7-8 breath three times a day. At our follow-up visit two months later, she couldn't stop gushing about how much it was helping her!

Five-Finger (Starfish) Breathing: This is an effective mindfulness exercise that combines controlled breathing with tactile sensations; I find it especially helpful with children. Extend one hand in front of you and spread your fingers wide like a starfish. Use the index finger on your other hand to slowly trace the outline of your extended hand, beginning at the base of your thumb. Inhale slowly through your nose as you trace up the side of one finger, and exhale through your mouth as you trace downward. When you reach your pinky, reverse the pattern. You'll find the physical act of tracing your fingers helps distract you from anxious or racing thoughts.

For more resources, I recommend using one of the free apps available on your smartphone.

How to Choose a Supplement

Supplements are regulated in the U.S. by the Food and Drug Administration, but in a different way from how medications are handled. This is due to the Dietary Supplement Health Education Act, which was passed into law in 1994. This act defines dietary supplements as vitamins, minerals, botanicals, amino acids, and other substances intended to supplement the diet—and therefore are a subset of foods.

Supplement manufacturers must follow good manufacturing practices for purity, strength and composition. Still, picking a reputable brand is important. Ask your healthacare provider for their recommendations; the Food Standards Agency in the U.K. has raised concerns about internet purchases, where customers may be sold counterfeit products (an indication is prices cheaper than their competitors) or ones that are nearing their use-by date. You certainly do not need to use a single manufacturer for all your products; different companies have expertise in different product areas.

If a supplement is from a US supplier, a sign of quality and safety on the supplement label is the term "USP-verified" or the NSF certification mark. USP is the abbreviation for United States Pharmacopeia, a nonprofit agency that confirms, among other things, that products contain the ingredients listed on the label and do not contain harmful levels of specified contaminants.[1] NSF International is an independent organization that similarly tests and certifies many common products.

Beyond the brand, there are details you should inspect on the label. For example, with botanicals (supplements derived from plant sources), you want to see the common plant name as well as the scientific binomial; this is because sometimes more than one plant can share a common name. For some plants, you will also want to know which part of the plant was used, as different parts have different properties.

You will also want to know the dose. For instance, for a multivitamin, it could take six capsules to reach the specified dose; that's a lot of pills to swallow, and you may prefer a more concentrated product from a different brand. Throughout this book, I have given my recommended dosages for many supplements, and when appropriate, what the supplement should be standardized to. Standardization is your way of ensuring a product contains a consistent and measurable amounts of particular compounds that have been shown to have therapeutic value. (Take turmeric, for example, which may be standardized to 95 percent curcuminoids.)

If you are taking medications, you will want to know about any potential interactions with supplements. Ask your pharmacist to assess how your prescriptions may interact with each other and with any supplements you're taking to assess how your prescriptions may interact with each other and with any supplements you're taking.

There are online resources you can use to learn more about herbal medicines and supplements The NIH Herbs at a Glance is a series of fact sheets available free of charge at https://nccih.nih.gov/health.

Acknowledgments

I am profoundly grateful to my mentors, teachers, colleagues, fellows, students, and most of all, my patients. I have learned so much from all of you!

Thank you to Andy Weil for our (almost) thirty-year conversation about integrative medicine. Thank you to my wonderful colleagues at the University of Arizona, Andrew Weil Center for Integrative Medicine: Randy Horwitz, MD, PhD; Ann Marie Chiasson, MD, MPH; Mari Ricker, MD; Patricia Lebensohn, MD; Lise Alschuler, ND; Stephen Dahmer, MD; Esther Sternberg, MD; Vivian Kominos, MD; Devorah Coryell; Molly Burke, MFA; Paula Cook; Kevin Ryan; Kayla Espinoza; Matt Gates Stoner, MA; Robert Rhodes, PhD; Ray Runyon, PhD; Fred Craigie, PhD; Steve Gurgevich, PhD; and Rubin Naiman, PhD. It has been the gift of a lifetime to work and learn together with you. I am also truly grateful to former Center faculty Rocky Crocker, MD; Tieraona Low Dog, MD; Dan Shapiro, PhD; Sally Dodds, PhD; Audrey Brooks, PhD; Iris Bell, MD, PhD; David Rychener, PhD; Howard Silverman, MD; Hilary McClafferty, MD; and Bob Lutz, MD.

I am deeply grateful to the many Center fellowship graduates I interviewed for this book, including Drs. Apple Bodemer, David Cannon, William DeVault, Suzanne Bartlett Hackenmiller, Randy Horwitz, Annie Kennard, Vivian Kominos, Naomi Lamm, Elizabeth Raskin, Manoj Reddy, Ben Remo, Gulshan Sethi, Saloni Sharma, Rosie Sheinberg, Jill Weintraub, and Doreen Wiggins. Their integrative medicine expertise across a wide range of specialties fortifies the content. Thank you as well to my colleagues Naresh Rao, DO; Carla Kuon, MD; Peggy Huddleston, MTS; Mary Marian, RD; and Kathie Swift, RD, whom I also interviewed for this book. I am so grateful to Belleruth Naparstek, MSW, and Marty

Rossman, MD, for giving me permission to print their guided imagery exercises in this book. I am especially grateful for the many long conversations with colleagues Myles Spar, MD, and Karen Koffler, MD, which have enriched and shaped my thinking over the years. I want to express my sincerest appreciation for my assistant, Becky Perry, who pulled hundreds of scientific articles for me!

Thanks to the awesome team at Inkwell Management, including Kristin van Ogtrop and Lyndsey Blessing! Words cannot adequately express my appreciation for my agent, Richard Pine. Thank you, Richard, for seeing me and being an amazing and steadfast supporter.

A huge thank you to Nick Bromley for your masterful help with the craft of writing this book. Together we wrangled my ideas and a tremendous volume of content into a readable book!

Thank you to my editor at Simon & Schuster, Ian Straus, who took this project to heart and gave wonderful edits and encouragement. Thanks to Priscilla Painton, Phil Metcalf, Julia Prosser, and Carole Berglie, as well as the rest of the team at S&S.

Thank you to the fabulous team at AARP, who embraced and helped shape this book with their wisdom and insights, including Jodi Lipson and Leah Miller. Thank you to Stephanie Abramson and Jamie Gold for their meticulous fact checking, and to all those who took the time to offer feedback and support from across the organization.

Massive thanks go to my sister, Rachel Maizes, who is always willing to read my work and offer her thoughtful feedback and expert editorial input. Similarly, my wonderful friend and thought partner Tara Lemmey offered invaluable advice, resources, and honest feedback. Thank you to Jim Donat for listening to me talk, reflect, and process while holding me through it all!

I am deeply grateful to Rachel Naomi Remen, Jon Kabat-Zinn, and Belleruth Naparstek—all pioneers in the field of Integrative Medicine and mentors who inspired me and paved the way for this book. Thank you for your life's work, which has so enriched my own.

I will end with eternal gratitude for my parents, Hannah and Isaac Maizes, of blessed memory, who gave me the priceless gifts of education and support. And finally to my children, Gabrielle, Aaron, and Zoe; son-in-law Ran; and my grandchildren Lev, Emma, and Naia, who enrich my life.

Index

abdominal obesity, 155
abdominal surgery recovery, 380–81
Abraham, Rebecca, 72
A1C, 153, 201, 206, 209, 212–13, 340
accessibility, in-home, 318
ACE bandages, 391
acid reflux, 218
acne, 97–103
action plans for asthma, 223–24
acupressure, 333
acupuncture
    for gut health, 39
    for headaches, 179
    heart surgery and, 346–47
    for menopause, 143
    for musculoskeletal pain, 86
    for nerve pain, 185
    for PTSD, 272
    surgery and, 329, 341, 345
acyclovir, 22, 24–26
adaptogens, 18, 70, 294
advanced glycolic end products (AGEs), 163–64
affirmation for recovery, 386
age, bone health and, 231
Agency for Health Care Policy and Research, 87
air pollution, 167, 179, 217
albumin, 308, 309, 321, 380, 382
alcohol
    abstention from, 5, 8–9
    bone health and, 232, 240
    breast cancer and, 367–68
    long Covid and, 296
    PMS and urogenital health, 121
    sleep and, 46–48
Alexander method, 95, 172, 177
alignment, musculoskeletal, 77–78

allergic reactions, Your Rapid Recovery Toolkit for, 390
allergies, elimination diet for, 29–31, 36–37, 396–99
allithiamine, 291
aloe, 390
alopecia areata (autoimmune disease), 110–12
alopecia (hair loss), 109–13
alpha-lipoic acid (ALA), 184, 209–10, 350
Alpha-Stim, 71
alternative therapies, defined, 6
American Academy of Family Physicians, 55
American Cannabis Nurses Association, 72
American College of Cardiology, 157, 168
American College of Gastroenterology, 36
American College of Obstetricians and Gynecologists, 121, 371
Americans with Disabilities Act, 297
Ames, Bruce, 255–56
amino acids, 23, 401
Amish people, asthma and, 215
AMMEND trial, 254
Andrew Weil Center for Integrative Medicine, 2, 6, 8, 106, 158, 192, 217, 280, 304, 312, 332, 339, 353, 363, 364, 377, 379, 380
androgens, 97
andrographis, 18, 389
anesthesia recovery, 322–25
animals, 215–16, 217–18, 284, 319
ankle sprains, 78–81
antacids, 32
anthocyanins, 18
antihistamines, 54, 295
anti-inflammatory foods, 365
anxiety, 57–76
    benefits of stress, 57–59
    breath work for, 64–65

anxiety (cont.)
  cannabis for, 72
  cognitive behavioral therapy (CBT) for, 61–63
  community and, 59–60
  as excitement, 60–61
  exercise for, 66–67
  medications for, 73–74
  post-op surgery and, 327–28
  remedies for, 71
  sleep and, 49–50
  spiritual practices for, 65–66
  supplements for, 67–70
  triggers of, 63–64
  Your Rapid Recovery Toolkit, 387–88
apolipoproteins A-I and B, 154
apps and trackers
  for anxiety, 71
  breast cancer and, 372
  for breathing exercises, 220
  for cosmetics, 108
  for exercise, 165
  for sleep, 50, 51
arginine, 23
aromatherapy, 320, 324, 327
arthritis, 90
arthroplasty, 338–42
Ascension Providence Hospital, 170
ashwagandha, 70
aspartame, 64
aspirin, 210, 295, 349
Aspirin in Reducing Events in the Elderly (ASPREE) trial, 210
asthma, 215–29
  action plans for, 223–24
  anxiety and, 64
  biologics for, 228
  breathing exercises for, 220–21
  diet and, 221–22
  intermittent/persistent categories of, 216
  lungs, healing of, 4
  managing symptoms of, 216–17
  medications for, 64, 216, 226–27
  microbiome and, 215–16
  mind-body connection for, 224–25
  moderate/severe categories of, 216
  nasal breathing and, 219–20
  supplements for, 222–23
  triggers of, 217–19, 225
astragalus root, 16, 18
Atherosclerotic Cardiovascular Disease (ASCVD) Risk Estimator, 157, 168
atopic dermatitis (eczema), 103–9, 114
atorvastatin (Lipitor), 157–58

attention-deficit/hyperactivity disorder (ADHD), 64
auditory stimulation, 330–31
augmentation, 263
autoimmune conditions, 29, 110–12, 191, 193–94, 288
autologous blood donation, 347–48
autonomic nervous system, 58, 291
The Awakened Brain (Miller), 249–50
Ayahuasca, 279, 282, 283
Ayurveda, 18

back pain, 172–77
back surgery, 343–45
bacterial vaginosis (BV), 126, 129–31
balance exercises, 244
bathing and showering, 49, 107, 263
Beckham, David, 217
bedrest for pain, 78, 84, 91
Be Fruitful (Maizes), 122
benzodiazepines, 73
benzoyl peroxide, 102–3
berberine, 210
Berceli, David, 273–74
beta blockers, 73–74, 349
β-hexachlorocyclohexane, 146
The Better Brain (Kaplan), 255
Bierman, Steve, 331–32
Bifidobacterium, 258
big T events, 268
biochemical individuality, 7
biofeedback, 100
bioidentical hormone therapy, 125, 138, 141
biologics, 228
biomechanics, 187
birth control pills, 122, 257
bisphenol A (BPA), 167
bisphosphonates, 230, 233–36
black cohosh, 141–42
black pepper, 3
black tea compress, 106
blood pressure, 153. *see also* heart health
blood tests. *see* testing
blood transfusion, 347–48
B9 (methylfolate), 259
Bodemer, Apple, 106
The Body Keeps the Score (Van der Kolk), 272
body weight. *see* weight
Bone, Estrogen, Strength Training (BEST) study, 244
bone health, 230–45
  bone remodeling and bone mineral density (BMD), 230–31
  calcium supplements for, 241–42

INDEX

diet and nutrition for, 236–40
exercise for, 242–44
fracture risk and, 232–33
medication and, 230, 232, 233–36
menopause and, 137, 144
osteoporosis risk and, 231–32
bone resorption inhibitory food items (BRIFI), 237
boric acid, 129, 131
boswellia, 195
botanical medicines. *see* herbal medicines
Botox, 180
bowel movement, post-op, 333, 346–47, 378
box breathing, 399
brain. *see also* anxiety; depression; pain signals, deactivating
   asthma triggers and, 225
   central sensitization, 169–70, 174, 178
   glucose for, 253
   gut-brain axis, 255
   heart surgery and cognitive issues, 354–55
   hormone therapy and, 137
   joint toxicity and, 342–43
   neural circuit pain, 170–71
   neuroplasticity of, 171
   neurotransmitters, 28, 117–20, 170, 180, 279, 280, 327
BRCA gene mutations, 362
breast surgery and breast cancer, 359–74
   BRCA gene mutations, 362
   chemo and, 366–67
   diet and, 364–68, 370
   environmental health and, 372–73
   exercise post-surgery, 369–70
   healing ceremony prior to surgery, 362–63
   hormone therapy and, 140
   identity and diagnosis of, 359–60
   lumpectomy, 359–64, 374
   mastectomy, 361–64, 372
   sexual desire and, 370–72
   sleep and, 368–69
   spirituality and, 373
   supplements post-surgery, 368
   surgery options for, 361–62
   surgery recovery, 363–64
Breath Ball app, 220
breathing exercises
   for anxiety, 64–65
   for asthma, 219–21
   post-op surgery, 323
   pranayama, 65, 220, 293, 399
   for PTSD, 276
   Your Rapid Recovery Toolkit, 399–400
Breath (Nestor), 220

Breathwork app, 220
Brewer, Jud, 71
Brigham and Women's Hospital, 116
British Medical Association, 134
broken bones, 90–91
bronchodilators, 216, 226. *see also* asthma
Brooks, Alison Wood, 60–61
Brown University, 364
burns, 390
Buteyko, Konstantin, 221
Buteyko Breathing Technique (BBT), 220–21
butterbur extract, 182, 223
bypass surgery (heart), 347–48, 350, 353–56

caffeine, 46–48, 49, 63, 240
calcium, 118, 236–40, 241–42
calcium score, 154
Calhoun, Lawrence, 277
Calm app, 51
calorie counting, time-restricted eating vs., 207
camping, 55
cancer, breast. *see* breast surgery and breast cancer
cancer, uterine, 377
Candida, 126–28
cannabis, 72, 184–85
Cannon, David, 212–13
capsaicin, 88, 95, 182–83, 189, 197, 392
capsicum, 88
carbohydrates, complex, 366
carbohydrates, diabetes and, 202–3, 204–5. *see also* glycemic index (GI)
cardiac rehab, 352–53, 355–56
caregivers, for surgery, 312–13, 318–19
CaringBridge, 313
carminatives, 39
cartilage, 186
catabolism, 311
CDC (Centers for Disease Control), 165, 297
central sensitization (CS), 169–70, 174, 178. *see also* pain signals, deactivating
cetirizine (Zyrtec), 390
chamomile, 39
Change Your Diet, Change Your Mind (Ede), 256
chasteberry, 119–20
chelation, 342
chemical imbalance theory of depression, 248–49, 251
chemotherapy, breast cancer and, 366–67
Chiasson, Ann Marie, 363
chicken soup, 16
Childhood Asthma Management Program Study, 227
Children's Hospital of Philadelphia, 292

INDEX

chiropractic, 86–87
cholesterol
  abnormal lipids, 155
    LDL cholesterol, 153–56, 158–60, 162–63, 165, 168
    statins for, 156–58
    tests for, 153–54
chondroitin, 196
chromium, 342–43
chronotherapy, 45
The Circadian Code (Panda), 48
circadian rhythm, 22, 44–45, 206–8. *see also* light; sleep
cleaning products, for home, 218
cleansers, for personal use, 99, 126–27
clothing, 49, 82, 107, 319–20
cobalt poisoning, 342–43
coconut oil, 105
coenzyme Q10, 159, 182, 350
cognitive behavioral therapy (CBT)
  for anxiety, 61–63
  for insomnia (CBT-I), 49–50
  for pain, 173, 181
  for PTSD, 269–71
cognitive processing therapy (CPT), 270, 271
colchicine, 160
cold air, 218
colds and viral infections, 13–26
  flu, Tamiflu for, 21
  flu vaccine and, 21–22
  herbal medicines for, 16–18
  herpes, 22–25, 26
  historic background, 14–15
  nasal decongestion and, 20
  1918 Spanish Flu, 15
  nutrition for, 14–15
  rapid recovery for, 25–26
  saunas for cold prevention, 20–21
  supplements for, 19
  symptoms of, 13–14
  Your Rapid Recovery Toolkit, 388–90
cold therapy, 329–30, 341, 391
Commonwealth Fund, 1–2
ComPaRe long Covid e-cohort, 286–87
Composite Scale of Morningness (CSM), 45
compression socks, 82
constipation. *see* gut
contact dermatitis, 104
Conti, Paul, 268
continuous glucose monitoring (CGM), 212–13
conventional medicine, integrative medicine and, 5–6
cool-down exercises, 92
core strength, 84

coronary angiography, 154–55
coronary artery calcium score, 154
coronary artery disease (CAD), 347. *see also* heart surgery
corticosteroids, 64, 189, 216, 226–27
cortisol, 237
cosmetics, 108, 373
Courageous Women Fearless Living retreat, 371–72
Covid-19, 287. *see also* long Covid
cramps, menstrual, 121–22
cramps, muscle, 93–94
cranberries and cranberry juice, 124
C-reactive protein, 249
Crestor (rosuvastatin), 157–58
cromolyn, 226–27
Cummings, Matt, 72
curcumin. *see* turmeric
cytokines, 237

dairy, 98, 238–39, 365–66, 395
dancing, 260, 371–72
Daube, Hannes, 77, 78, 85
Da Vinci Surgical System, 376
daylight saving's time, 42
decongestion, 20
deep-breathing exercises, 276
Defense Department, 271
deglycyrrhizinated licorice (DGL), 32, 388
dendritic cells, 14
denosumab, 235
depression, 246–65
  causes of, 248–50
  diet and, 253–57
  exercise for, 259–60
  internal felt state of, 246–48
  light and, 260–62
  medications, 249, 251–53
  sleep and, 260
  suicide and, 97, 247, 252, 254, 267
  supplements for, 257–60
  testing for, 249, 250, 263–64
  treatment-resistant depression (TRD), 263–64
  whole-body hyperthermia and, 262–63
dermatitis, 103–9
DeVault, William, 339, 341
diabetes mellitus, 200. *see also* type 2 diabetes
Diabetes Prevention Program (DPP), 201
diarrhea. *see* gut
diet. *see also* vegetables and fruit; *individual names of foods*
  abdominal surgery and, 380–81
  anti-inflammatory foods, 365
  asthma and, 221–22

biochemical individuality and, 7
bone health and, 236–40
breast cancer and, 364–68, 370
Change Your Diet, Change Your Mind (Ede), 256
for cold and flu, 15–16
depression and, 253–57
Dietary Approaches to Stop Hypertension (DASH), 162
elimination diet, 29–31, 36–37, 396–99
fasting, 193
fasting-mimicking diet (FMD), 193–94
fruits and vegetables in, and benefits from, 8–9
hair and, 110
heart health and, 151–52, 156, 161–64
heart surgery and, 347, 356–57
for herpes, 23
ITIS diet, 194
keto diet, 163, 180, 197, 203, 256–57
low-FODMAP diet, 36–37
meal size and frequency, 32, 48
Mediterranean diet, 162, 203, 394–96
menopause and, 144–45
nutrition therapy (NT), intravenous, 356
for PMS and urogenital health, 120–21, 124, 127–28
post-op surgery, 332–35
protein in, 237, 256, 308–9, 333–34
RA pain and, 192
skin and, 98–99
surgery prehab and nutritional assessment, 308–10, 311
time-restricted eating, 151–52, 164, 206–8, 366–67
type 2 diabetes and, 199–200, 202–4, 206–9
vegan diet, 162, 199–200, 202, 239–40
dilation and curettage (D&C), 306
disease-modifying anti-rheumatic drugs (DMARDS), 192
D-limonene, 34
doctor-patient relationship, 383–84
dogs, 284
douching, 126–27
dreaming, 44
dust mites, 217
dynamic stretching, 92
dyspareunia, 370

echinacea, 17, 389
eczema (atopic dermatitis), 103–9, 114
Ede, Georgia, 256
eggs, 395
elderberry, 17–18

electrical stimulation devices, 88, 185, 303, 330
electrolytes, 93
elimination diet, 29–31, 36–37, 396–99
emotion, assessment of, 351. *see also* mind-body connection
endometrium and endometrial cancer, 140
English National Opera (ENO) Breathe, 293
Enhanced Recovery After Surgery (ERAS) protocols, 304–5, 310, 331
enteric nervous system (ENS), 28
environment
  breast cancer and, 372–73
  cleaning products, 218
  heart health and, 167–68
  menopause and, 145–47
  pain and, 179
  skin health and, 106–8
  for sleep, 46
Environmental Working Group (EWG), 108, 372–73
EPIC-Oxford study, 239
epithelium, 4
essential oils, 111–12, 320, 324, 388
estrogen. *see also* menopause; premenstrual syndrome (PMS) and urogenital health
  breast cancer and, 361, 364, 365, 367, 371–72
  creams, 124–25, 371
ethnicity, bone health and, 231
European Environmental Agency, 167
exercise
  for anxiety, 66–67
  benefits from, 8–9
  for bone health, 242–44
  breast cancer surgery and, 369–70, 371–72
  for depression, 259–60
  exercise-induced bronchoconstriction, 218, 219, 222
  for heart health, 156, 165–66
  heart surgery and, 348, 355–56
  long Covid and, 292
  for menopause, 143–44
  moderate exercise, measuring, 165–66
  for musculoskeletal pain, 92
  OA pain and, 190
  post-op surgery, 333, 335
  type 2 diabetes and exercising after meals, 208–9
extracorporeal shock wave therapy (ESWT), 82
eye movement desensitization and reprocessing (EMDR), 271–72
ezetimibe (Zetia), 158, 160

failed back surgery syndrome, 344
fasting, 193. *see also* time-restricted eating

fasting blood sugar, 153
fasting-mimicking diet (FMD), 193–94
fat (body). *see* weight
fat (dietary), menopause and, 144
Ferly app, 372
Fezolinetant, 147
fiber, 121, 256, 334–35
fibroids, 376–79
fight or flight, 58
fish, fatty cold-water, 255
fish oil, 160, 369, 392–93. *see also* omega-3 fatty acids
Fitbit, 48
five-finger (starfish) breathing, 400
flaxseed, 367
flu. *see* colds and viral infections
foam rollers, 86, 92, 94, 391
Food and Drug Administration, U.S. (FDA)
   function of, 401
   treatments tested/approved by, 71, 112, 113, 122, 141, 147, 168, 179, 180, 211, 235, 273, 280, 283, 325, 330, 343
food intolerance, 30
forehead cooling devices, 147
4-7-8 breathing, 7, 399–400
fracture risk, 232–33
fragrance, asthma and, 218
frailty, 307
Frankl, Victor, 59
freeze response, 272
fruit. *see* vegetables and fruit
furans, 146

gait, re-alignment of, 187
gallbladder surgery, 381
GammaCore, 71, 95, 179, 283–84
Gardner, Christopher, 162
garlic, 14, 15–16, 159, 389
gastroesophageal reflux disease (GERD), 27–28, 31–35, 388
gender and health. *see* men's health; women's health
general anesthesia, 322–25
genetics and genetic testing, 153–54, 231, 263, 322, 362
genital herpes, 22–25, 26
German Commission E, 129
German Surgical Society, 375
ginger, 324, 391
Global Mind Project, 255
Global Sauna Survey, 194–95
glucagon-like peptide-1 (GLP-1) receptor agonists, 211–12
glucosamine sulfate and chondroitin, 196

glucose, 253
glutamine, 184
glycemic index (GI), 98, 204–5
glyphosate, 145
Gokhale, Esther, 176, 379
Gokhale method, 85, 95, 172, 176, 379
Goop, 127
gratitude journal, 52
green light, 180–81
green tea, 100–101, 367
guided imagery, 301–2, 313–15, 316–17, 328–29
Guma, Monica, 194
gum disease, 192
gum health, 160–61
gut, 27–40
   bowel movement, post-op, 333, 346–47, 378
   elimination diet for, 29–31, 36–37, 396–99
   fasting and, 193
   gastroesophageal reflux disease (GERD), 27–28, 31–35, 388
   general upset stomach, 28–29
   gut-brain axis, 28, 255
   inflammatory bowel disease (IBD), 380
   irritable bowel syndrome (IBS), 35–39
   leaky gut, 3
   long Covid and, 292
   microbiome, 215–16
   post-op surgery, 326
   recovery and healing by, 4
   Your Rapid Recovery Toolkit, 390–91

Hackenmiller, Suzanne Bartlett, 379
hair loss, 109–13. *see also* skin and hair
Hall, Kevin, 204
handwashing, 14
Harper, Lyndsey, 372
Harris, Dan, 74
Harvard University, 255, 365
hatha yoga, 67, 275
headaches, 177–82
Heal Faster (Maizes), 8–9
Healing Back Pain (Sarno), 170–71
Healing (Bierman), 331–32
healing ceremony prior to surgery, 362–63
health, expectations for, 1–2
Healthy Living app, 108, 372–73
heartburn (GERD), 27–28, 31–35, 388
heart health, 151–68
   calcium and, 241
   cholesterol-lower medications for, 156–58
   environmental toxins and, 167–68
   exercise for, 156, 165–66
   heart disease reversal diet, 161–64
   hormone therapy and, 134–38, 140

medical research about, 116
Ornish program for, 7
plaque and, 152, 154–55, 156–58, 160–61, 164
POTS, 291
risk of heart disease, 155–56
stress and, 166
supplements and medications for, 158–60
tachycardia, 67–68
testing for heart disease, 152–55
time-restricted eating for, 151–52, 164
heart surgery, 346–58
   acupuncture following, 346–47
   blood transfusion, 347–48
   bypass surgery, 347–48, 350, 353–56
   cognitive issues and, 354–55
   depression and, 353–54
   diet and, 347, 356–57
   exercise and, 348, 355–56
   positive outlook for, 351
   post-operative expectations, 351–53
   supplements and medications prior to, 348–49, 350
   valve surgery, 341, 346, 348, 353, 355, 356
heat therapy, 87, 329–30, 391
heavy metals, 167–68
hemoglobin A1C, 153, 201, 206, 209, 212–13, 340
Heracles, 72
herbal medicines. *see also* vitamins and vitamin supplements
   for cold and flu, 16–18
   for herpes, 24–25
   for PMS and urogenital health, 117, 119–20, 130
herpes (HSV0a, HSV-2), 22–25, 26
hexing, 331
high-sensitivity C-reactive protein (hs-CRP), 153
Hippocrates, 27, 39
hip replacement, 338–42
Hoag Memorial Hospital, 332, 380
holy basil, 70
homeostasis activation, 2–5, 384
home preparation for surgery, 317–19
homocysteine, 154
honey, 16, 388
hops, 143
hormones. *see also* estrogen; premenstrual syndrome (PMS) and urogenital health
   androgens, 97
   cortisol, 237
   hormone therapy for menopause, 124–25, 134–41
   melatonin, 315
   oxytocin, 284
   parathyroid hormone, 235
   skin and, 98
   sleep and, 44, 54–55
   testosterone, 232
   thyroid, 250
Horowitz, Mark, 252
Horwitz, Randy, 217, 222, 227
hospital, packing for, 319–20
hot flashes and night sweats, 133–34, 147. *see also* menopause
Huddleston, Peggy, 302, 314–15, 316–17
Hutterites, asthma and, 215
hyaluronic acid, 189
hydration, 93, 123–24, 310, 323
hyperbaric oxygen therapy (HBOT), 185–86
hypertension, 155
hypnosis, 25, 37–38, 329
hypothyroidism, 250
hysterectomy, 135, 137, 140, 376–79

Iberogast, 34
ibogaine, 279, 282
ibuprofen, 121–22
Imperial College Healthcare NHS Trust, 293
Improve-It trial, 158
Indiana University, 222
Indigenous populations, psychedelics and, 282–83
infection, asthma and, 218
infection prevention, post-op, 325–26
inflammation
   anti-inflammatory foods, 365
   bone health and, 232, 237
   depression and testing for, 249
   heart health and, 156, 164
   inflammatory bowel disease (IBD), 380
   "itis," defined, 103–4
   OA and, 188–90
   rheumatoid arthritis (RA) and other inflammatory arthritis conditions, 190–97
inositol, 69
Insight Timer app, 51, 66, 71
insomnia. *see* sleep
insulin. *see* type 2 diabetes
integrative medicine, defined, 5–8. *see also* recovery from longstanding conditions; recovery from short-lived conditions; recovery from surgery
intensive care units (ICUs), 351–52
Interheart study, 155–56, 166
intermittent fasting. *see* time-restricted eating

International Agency for Research on Cancer, 145
International Olympics Committee, 94
International Osteoporosis Foundation, 240
intestines. *see* gut
intrinsic tremor response, 274
Irish Longitudinal Study on Ageing, 67
irrigation systems (nasal), 20
irritable bowel syndrome (IBS), 35–39
isoflavones, 365
"itis," defined, 103–4
ITIS diet, 194

Johns Hopkins University, 221, 264
joint toxicity, 342–43
Jolie, Angelina, 362
journaling (expressive writing), 52, 224–25, 276–77
Joyner-Kersee, Jackie, 217

Kabat-Zinn, Jon, 62, 173
Kaplan, Bonnie, 255, 257, 281
kava kava, 68–69, 368, 387–88
Kegel exercises, 378
Kennard, Anne, 377
ketamine, 185, 264, 279–81
ketogenic (keto) diet, 163, 180, 197, 203, 256–57
Keys, Ancel, 253
King's College Hospital, 348
knee replacement, 338–42
Kominos, Vivian, 158, 163
Kundalini yoga, 275

Lactobacillus, 19, 101, 124, 128–29, 258
lactose, 30
laparoscopic surgery, 375–76
La Roche, Loretta, 270
laughter therapy, 354
laundry products, 107
lavender, 69
LDL cholesterol, 153–56, 158–60, 162–63, 165, 168
leafy greens, 237
leaky gut, 3
"lean diabetes," 202
Lebensohn, Patricia, 90–91
lemon balm, 24–25
Levine, Peter, 272
licorice
    deglycyrrhizinated (DGL), 32, 388
    gargling, 315, 324
    gel, 105–6
    tea, Egyptian, 32, 390
lidocaine patches, 183
life expectancy, 2

lifestyle habits
    five specific habits and benefits from, 8–9
    heart health and, 152
    making change to, 384–85
    surgery and changes to, 341–42
Lifestyle Heart Trial, 161
ligament injuries, 78–81
light
    depression and, 260–62
    green light, 180–81
    laser therapy for hair growth, 112
    photo-biomodulation therapy (PBMT), 94, 112, 180
    sleep and, 42, 44, 46, 51, 261
liniments, 88
lion's mane mushroom, 184
lipids, abnormal, 155
Lipitor (atorvastatin), 157–58
lipoprotein(a) genetic test, 153–54
little t events, 268
liver, healing of, 4
Lloyd-Jones, Donald, 156
long Covid, 286–98
    alcohol and, 296
    causes, 287–88
    Covid-19, defined, 287
    diagnosing, 290
    exercise and, 292
    gut and, 292
    medications for, 289, 291, 295–96
    mind-body tools for, 293
    pacing recovery for, 297–98
    prevention, 288–89
    supplements for, 293–95
    symptoms of, 286–87, 290–91
    vaccine for, 288, 289
longstanding conditions, recovery from. *see* recovery from longstanding conditions
Lotsa Helping Hands, 313
Lover app, 372
loving kindness meditation (Metta), 65–66
low-dose naltrexone (LDN), 175
lower-back pain, 83–84, 87
low-FODMAP diet, 36–37
L-theanine, 69
lubricants, 370–71
lumpectomy (breast), 359–64, 374
lungs, healing of, 4. *see also* asthma
lymphedema, 363, 369
Lyon Heart Study, 162
lysine, 22–24

macrophages, 14

magnesium, 55, 70, 119, 159–60, 181, 210, 237, 350
Maimonides, 16
Maizes, Victoria, 8–9, 122, 385
Mandela, Nelson, 278
massage, 330, 364
mast-cell stabilizers, 294, 296
mastectomy, 361–64, 372
Maté, Gabor, 268–69
mattress pads, 147
McDougall, John, 199–200, 202
McGill, Stuart, 85, 95
McKenzie method, 85, 95
McMaster University, 348
MDMA, 279–80, 282
meal size and frequency, 32, 48
meat, in diet, 240, 366, 395
medical research about women, 116–17
medications (pharmaceutical)
   acyclovir, 22, 24–26
   antidepressants, 249, 251–53
   anxiety and, 64, 73–74
   for asthma, 64, 216, 226–27
   bone health and, 230, 232, 233–36
   for hair, 112–13
   for heart health, 156–60
   heart surgery preparation and, 348–49, 350
   hormone therapy for menopause, 124–25, 134–41
   for long Covid, 289, 291, 295–96
   medical research about, 116–17
   for musculoskeletal pain, 87–89
   opioid risk, reducing, 331–32
   for pain, 175, 188–89
   PMS and urogenital health, 121–23, 125
   pre-surgery review of, 311
   for PTSD, 273
   skin and, 97, 108–9
   surgery and, 341
   tapering off of, 252–53
   for type 2 diabetes, 211–12
Medicines and Healthcare Products Regulatory Agency, 343
meditation
   for back pain, 173–74
   for heart health, 166
   for long Covid, 293
   tummo, 262
Mediterranean diet, 9, 102, 110, 113, 114, 144, 148, 162, 168, 194, 196, 198, 203, 207, 213, 222, 228, 239, 248, 254, 255, 265, 355, 356, 258, 387, 394–96
melatonin, 34, 44, 54–55, 315
menopause, 133–48

diet and, 144–45
environmental triggers and, 145–47
estrogen creams, 124–25, 371
exercise for, 143–44
hormone therapy for, 124–25, 134–41
hot flashes and night sweats, 133–34, 147
supplements for, 141–43
Traditional Chinese Medicine for, 143
men's health
   bone health and, 231, 232, 241
   suicide risk and, 254
   UTIs and, 123
mental health, improving. *see* anxiety; depression; mind-body connection; post-traumatic stress disorder (PTSD); *individual types of therapy*
mental health, research about, 116–17
metabolic syndrome, 166
metformin, 211, 257, 289
methylfolate, 259
METS (metabolic equivalent of tasks), 355–56
Metta (loving kindness meditation), 65–66
microbiome, 215–16
micronutrients, 309–10. *see also* vitamins and vitamin supplements
migraines, 177–82
milk thistle, 324–25
Miller, Emmett, 328
Miller, Lisa, 249–50
mind-body connection. *see also* breathing exercises; exercise; writing and journaling; yoga
   for anxiety, 62–63
   aromatherapy, 320, 324, 327
   for asthma, 224–25
   guided imagery, 303, 328–29
   heart surgery and, 351
   for long Covid, 293
   mindfulness-based stress reduction for pain, 173
   mindset and psychedelics, 282–83
   for orthopedic surgery, 340
   positive outlook for surgery, 301–2, 313–15, 316–17
   skin health and, 99–100
mineral supplements. *see* vitamins and vitamin supplements
minimally invasive surgery, 375–82
   abdominal surgery, 380
   gallbladder surgery, 381
   gynecologic surgery, 376–79
   laparoscopic surgery, inception of, 375–76
Minnesota Starvation Experiment, 253
minoxidil, 112–13

Mirkin, Gabe, 79
mitochondria, 294–95
moisturizers, skin, 104–5
mold, 218
Monash University, 36
monoamine oxidase inhibitors (MAOIs), 249, 263
moral injury vs. PTSD, 269
Morgenstern, Julie, 50
Morningness-Eveningness Questionnaire (MEQ), 45
Morningness-Eveningness Stability Scale improved (MESSi), 45
Mühe, Erich, 375, 376
Multidisciplinary Association for Psychedelic Studies (MAPS), 279
multi-mineral multivitamins (MMMVs), 257, 350, 368
muscle loss, surgery and, 311
muscle sprains, 83–90
musculoskeletal pain, 77–95
   alignment and, 77–78
   broken bones, 90–91
   ligament injuries, 78–81
   muscle and tendon sprains, 83–90
   plantar fasciitis, 81–83
   weekend warrior success and, 91–94
   Your Rapid Recovery Toolkit, 391–92
mushrooms
   lion's mane, 184
   medicinal, 14, 16, 389–90
   psilocybin in, 264, 279, 282
music, 327–28
myomectomy, 379
My Stroke of Insight (Taylor), 10
The Myth of Normal (Maté), 268–69

N-acetyl Cysteine (NAC), 325
Naparstek, Belleruth, 305, 306, 315, 328
napping, 52–53
nasal breathing, 219–220
nasal decongestion, 20
National Aeronautics and Space Administration (NASA), 53
National Cancer Institute, 370
National Institutes of Health (NIH), 51, 135, 162, 204, 288, 402
National Osteoporosis Foundation Guide, 232–33
nausea, post-op surgery, 324
negativity, challenging, 10
NeilMed Sinus Rinse, 389
nerve pain, 182–86
nervous system, 58–59, 67. *see also* brain

nervous system reset class, 275–76
Nestor, James, 220
neti pots, 20
neural circuit pain, 170–71
neuraminidase, 21
neuroplasticity, 171
neurotransmitters, 28, 117–20, 170, 180, 279, 280, 327. *see also* anxiety; depression
NicAzel, 102
nicotinamide, 101
1918 Spanish Flu, 15
NNH (number needed to harm), 233
NNT (number needed to treat), 71, 233
nonpharmaceutical interventions. *see* herbal medicines; mind-body connection; vitamins and vitamin supplements
nonsteroidal anti-inflammatory drugs (NSAIDs), 188–89, 190
The Noonday Demon (Solomon), 246–47
North American Menopause Society, 137
NREM sleep, 43
Nurses' Health Study, 242, 369
NutriNet-Santé, 204
nutrition therapy (NT), intravenous, 356
nuts, 238

obesity. *see* weight
obstructive sleep apnea (OSA), 53, 219
oligosaccharides, 221
olive oil, 395
omega-3 fatty acids
   for anxiety, 68
   for arthritis (OA and RA), 195–96
   for asthma, 221–22
   for bone health, 238
   for breast cancer, 368
   for depression, 255, 258
   for heart health, 160
   for skin, 102
   sources of, 395
   surgery and, 310, 350
   Your Rapid Recovery Toolkit, 392–93
omega-6 foods, 221–22
omega-3 index, 154
Oncotype DX test, 361
opioid risk, reducing, 331–32
oral health, gums, 160–61, 192
oral hormone therapy, 138
organic food, 204, 255, 365–66
Ornish, Dean, 7, 161
orthopedic surgery, 337–45
   for back pain, 175
   back surgery, 343–45
   hip or knee replacement, 338–42

INDEX

joint toxicity and, 342–43
    for OA pain, 190
    prehab for, 337 (*see also* prehab for surgery)
    stem cells and, 343
osteoarthritis (OA), 90, 186–90, 195–96
osteopenia, 231–34, 239, 241
osteoporosis, 226, 231–41, 244. *see also* bone health
ovaries and oophorectomy, 137, 377
Oxford University, 16, 163
oxytocin, 284

pain signals, deactivating, 169–98
    back pain and, 172–77
    central sensitization (CS), 169–70, 174, 178
    migraines and tension headaches, 177–82
    nerve pain, 182–86
    neural circuit pain, 170–71
    opioids for pain, 331–32
    osteoarthritis (OA), 186–90, 195–96
    rheumatoid arthritis (RA) and other inflammatory arthritis conditions, 190–97
Paltrow, Gwyneth, 127
Panda, Satchin, 48
parasympathetic nervous system (SNS), 58
parathyroid hormone, 235
Paxlovid, 289, 295–96
PCBs, 146
PEACE and LOVE method, 79–80
pellet implant hormone therapy, 139–40
pelvic-floor physical therapy, 378–79
Pennebaker, James, 276
Penn State, 238
peppermint, 38–39, 180, 324
periodontal (gum) disease, 160–61, 192
pesticides, 146
pets. *see* animals
pharmacodynamics, 263
pharmacokinetics, 263
phosphorous, 237
photo-biomodulation therapy (PBMT), 94, 112, 180–81
phthalates, 146, 372
physical activity. *see* exercise
physical therapy, 339–40, 341, 344
physical therapy, pelvic-floor, 378–79
Physicians Committee for Responsible Medicine, 145
Pilates, Joseph and Pilates method, 86, 95, 172, 230, 244, 260, 302
piperine, 3
plantar fasciitis, 81–83
plant milks, fortified, 239

plaque, 152, 154–55, 156–58, 160–61, 164, 347
plastics, 106–7, 146, 147, 167
platelet-rich plasma (PRP) therapy, 89–90, 189
Plesio Health, 72
pollen, 217
polyphenols, 254, 367
polysaccharides, 18
post-op surgery experience, 322–36
    anesthesia recovery, 322–25
    anxiety, 327–28
    diet and, 332–35
    exercise and, 333, 335
    guided imagery for, 328–29
    heart surgery and expectations, 351–53
    infection prevention, 325–26
    opioid risk, 331–32
    pain reduction, 329–31
    sleep and rest, 323, 326–27, 331
postprandial glucose level, 205, 208–9, 211
post-traumatic stress disorder (PTSD), 266–85
    common treatments for, 269–73
    dogs for, 284
    medications for, 273
    moral injury vs., 269
    post-traumatic growth (PTG) and, 277–78
    psychedelics for, 278–81, 282–83
    symptoms and causes of, 266–67
    trauma, defined, 268–69
    trauma-releasing exercises, 273–77
    vagus nerve stimulation for, 283–84
    vitamins and minerals for trauma, 281
posture, 84, 176–77
POTS (postural orthostatic tachycardia syndrome), 291
pranayama, 65, 220, 293, 399. *see also* breathing exercises
prebiotics, asthma and, 221
Predimed study, 161–62
prednisone, 227
prehab for surgery, 306–21
    example of, 306–7
    fasting before surgery, 310
    frailty and, 307
    home preparation and, 317–19
    hospital comfort items, 319–20
    medications and supplements, reviewing, 311
    melatonin and licorice, 315
    nutritional status assessment for, 308–10, 311
    positive outlook for surgery, 301–2, 313–15, 316–17

prehab for surgery (cont.)
   prehab (prehabilitation), defined, 302
   social support for, 312–13, 318–19
   successful surgery, setting up for, 301–5
premenstrual syndrome (PMS) and urogenital health, 116–32
   medical research about women and, 116–17
   PMS, defined, 117–18
   PMS management and, 118–23
   urinary-tract infections (UTIs), 123–25
   vaginitis (vulvovaginitis), 125–31
Prepare for Surgery, Heal Faster (Huddleston), 302, 314–15, 316–17
probiotics
   for cold and flu, 19
   for depression, 258
   for gut health, 38
   for post-op surgery, 326
   for skin, 101–2, 108
   for urogenital health, 124, 128–31
   usprobioticguide.com, 130–31
   vaccines and, 22
progesterone. *see* menopause; premenstrual syndrome (PMS) and urogenital health
Prolon Five-Day Program, 193–94
prolonged-exposure therapy, 270–71
propolis, 22, 25
protein, 237, 256, 308–9, 333–34
proton pump inhibitors (PPIs), 33, 34
prunes, 238
psychedelic medicines, 264, 278–81, 282–83
pumpkin seed oil, 111

quercetin, 223, 294

radiation therapy, 364
Raison, Charles, 262
Rao, Naresh, 77, 79, 89, 91, 92
Raskin, Elizabeth, 332, 380
RECOVER (Researching COVID to Enhance Recovery) Initiative, 288
recovery, 1–10
   affirmation for, 386
   challenging negativity for, 10
   expectations for health and, 1–2
   Heal Faster (Maizes) for, 8–9
   integrative medicine approach to, 5–8
   recovery reflex and homeostasis activation, 2–5
   "Your Rapid Recovery Toolkit" for, 9
recovery from longstanding conditions, 9, 149–298. *see also individual names of conditions*
   asthma, 215–29
   bone health, 230–45
   depression, 246–65
   heart health, 151–68
   long Covid, 286–98
   pain signals, deactivating, 169–98
   post-traumatic stress disorder, 266–85
   type 2 diabetes, 199–214
recovery from short-lived conditions, 9, 11–148. *see also individual names of conditions*
   anxiety, 57–76
   colds and viral infections, 13–26
   gut, 27–40
   menopause, 133–48
   musculoskeletal pain, 77–95
   PMS and urogenital health, 116–32
   skin and hair, 96–115
   sleep, 41–56
recovery from surgery, 9, 299–383. *see also post-op surgery experience; prehab for surgery; individual names of surgeries*
   breast surgery and breast cancer, 359–74
   heart surgery, 346–58
   minimally invasive surgery, 375–82
   orthopedic surgery, 337–45
   post-op experience, 322–36
   recovery reflex and healing from, 4
   success, setting up for, 301–5
   surgical prehab, 306–21
recovery napping, 52–53
red yeast rice, 158–59
reflexology, 83
rehab, cardiac, 352–53, 355–56
Remo, Benjamin, 353–54
REM sleep, 43–44
resorption, 230–31
restorative yoga, 275–76
retinoids, 103
Reveri app, 51
rheumatoid arthritis (RA), 190–97
riboflavin, 181–82
Robinson, William, 188
robotic surgery, 376
Rossman, Martin L., 328
rosuvastatin (Crestor), 157–58
Rosy app, 372
Rucklidge, Julia, 281

S-adenosyl-L-methionine (SAMe), 196, 259
safety, in home, 317–18
saffron, 120
salicylic acid, 102–3
Salk Institute, 207
salves, 88

Salzberg, Sharon, 66
Sarno, John, 170–71, 172
sauna, 20–21, 194–95, 262–63
saw palmetto oil, 111
schedule. *see* light; sleep; time-restricted eating (TRE)
Schubiner, Howard, 170–71
Sea-Band, 390–91
seasonal affective disorder (SAD), 260–61
seborrheic dermatitis, 104
sedatives, 349
seeds, 238
selective serotonin reuptake inhibitors (SSRIs), 73, 122, 249, 251, 263, 273
semaglutides, 211–12
Semm, Kurt, 375, 376
Sensate, 71
serotonin-norepinephrine reuptake inhibitors (SNRIs), 73, 249
service dogs, 284
set and setting, for psychedelics, 282–83
Sethi, Gulshan, 312–14, 351, 354
sexual desire, breast cancer and, 370–72
shakes, protein, 309
Sheinberg, Rosie, 353
shift work, 207, 369
shingles, 182–83
short-lived conditions, recovery from. *see* recovery from short-lived conditions
side benefits, of integrative medicine, 7, 86, 118, 119, 120, 123, 166, 168, 184, 195, 196, 203, 212, 238, 259, 367, 384, 394
skin and hair, 96–115
　acne, 97–103
　dermatitis, 103–9
　hair loss, 109–13
　recovery reflex and healing of, 4
　skin layers, 96–97
sleep, 41–56
　anxiety and, 64
　apps for, 50, 51
　avoiding caffeine and alcohol before bed, 46–48
　body temperature and, 48–49
　breast cancer and, 368–69
　camping and, 55
　circadian rhythm, 22, 44–45, 206–8
　cognitive behavioral therapy for insomnia (CBT-I), 49–50
　depression and, 260
　eating before bed, 48
　for gut health, 32, 34
　healthy sleep components, 45–46
　importance of, 41–43
　long Covid and, 290–91
　meds and supplements for, 53–55
　pain and, 179
　post-op surgery, 323, 326–27, 331
　recovery napping, 52–53
　spiritual practices and, 51–52
　stages of, 43–45
　trackers for, 47–48
slippery elm, 34–35
SMILES trial, 254
smoking
　abstention, benefits from, 8–9
　asthma and, 217
　bone health and, 232
　heart disease and, 155
　RA pain and, 191
social support
　anxiety and, 59–60
　for surgery, 312–13, 318–19, 351–52
Sockwell, 82
sodium, bone health and, 240
Solomon, Andrew, 246–47
somatic experiencing, 272
sore throat, post-op, 315, 324
soy foods, 144–45, 238, 365
Spiegel, David, 51
spiritual practices. *see also* yoga
　anxiety and, 65–66
　Ayahuasca, 279, 282, 283
　breast cancer and, 373
　depression and, 249–50
　sleep and, 51–52
spironolactone, 103
sprains
　ligament, 78–81
　muscle and tendon, 83–90
St. John's wort, 142, 257–58
Stanford Medicine, 203
State University of New York at Stony Brook, 224
statins, 156–58
stem cells, 343
Stoner, Tamara, 280
Streisand, Barbra, 59
strength training, 243
stress
　asthma and, 218–19
　eczema and, 104
　heart health and, 156, 166
　menopause and, 146–47
　pain and, 171, 181 (*see also* pain signals, deactivating)
　RA pain and, 194
　viral infections and, 18, 22, 23, 26

stress test, 154
successful surgery, setting up for, 301–5
sugar. *see also* type 2 diabetes
   heart health and, 164
   menopause and, 144
   PMS and urogenital health, 120–21, 127, 217–128
suicide. *see also* depression
   among men, 254
   risk factors, 97, 247, 252, 267
sunburn, 390
supplements. *see also* vitamins and vitamin supplements; *individual names of supplements*
   for anxiety, 67–70
   for asthma, 222–23
   breast cancer surgery and, 368
   choosing, 401–2
   for depression, 257–60
   for heart health, 158–60
   heart surgery preparation and, 348–49, 350
   for herpes, 24–25
   for long Covid, 293–95
   for menopause, 141–43
   for musculoskeletal pain, 87–89
   for OA and RA, 195–96
   for PMS, 118–19
   pre-surgery review of, 311
   for sleep, 53–55
   tapering off of, 35
   for trauma, 281
   for type 2 diabetes, 209–10
Supreme Court, U.S., 282
surgery, recovery from. *see* recovery from surgery
sympathetic nervous system (SNS), 58–59, 67, 272
sympathomimetics, 349

tachycardia, 67–68
tai chi, 67
Tamiflu, 21
Taylor, David, 252
Taylor, Jill Bolte, 10
Taylor, Shelley, 59
tea tree oil, 100
Tedeschi, Richard, 277
telogen effluvium, 110–12
temperature
   cooking and heart health, 163–64
   menopause and, 146
   sleep and body temperature, 48–49
   whole-body hyperthermia, 262–63
tend and befriend pattern, 59–60
tendon sprains, 83–90

tennis balls, 72
10% Happier (Harris), 74
tension headaches, 177–82
Tension & Trauma-Releasing Exercises, 274
testing
   A1C, 153, 201, 206, 209, 212–13, 340
   Atherosclerotic Cardiovascular Disease (ASCVD) Risk Estimator, 157, 168
   breast cancer, 361, 362
   cholesterol, 153–54
   cobalt and chromium poisoning, 343
   depression, 249, 250, 263–64
   Fracture Risk Assessment Tool (FRAX), 232
   genetic, 153–54, 263
   heart disease, 152–55
   long Covid, 290
   Morningness-Eveningness Stability Scale improved (MESSi), 45
   of nutritional status prior to surgery, 308
testosterone, 232
texter's thumb, 84
Throat Coat Tea, 389
Time Management from the Inside Out (Morgenstern), 50
time-restricted eating (TRE), 151–52, 164, 206–8, 366–67
topical calcineurin inhibitors (TCIs), 108–9
trackers, sleep, 47–48
traditional Chinese medicine, 18, 143. *see also* acupuncture
transcutaneous electrical nerve stimulation (TENS), 88, 303, 330
transdermal hormone therapy, 139
transversus abdominus (TA) holds, 378–79
trauma, defined, 268–69. *see also* post-traumatic stress disorder
trauma-sensitive yoga, 275
treatment-resistant depression (TRD), 263–64
tremor response, 274
trigger points, 82
T-score, 232
Tsinghua University, 110
tummo meditation practice, 262
turmeric (curcumin), 120, 195, 294, 393–94
type 2 diabetes, 199–214
   aspirin and blood sugar, 210
   continuous glucose monitoring (CGM) for, 212–13
   as diabetes mellitus, 200
   exercising after meals for, 208–9
   glycemic index (GI) and, 204–5
   heart disease and, 155
   medication for, 211–12
   orthopedic surgery and, 340

reversal through diet, 199–204
supplements for, 209–10
time-restricted eating for, 206–8
type 1 diabetes vs., 200
vinegar and blood sugar, 205

UC San Diego Health, 207
UK Biobank, 42, 87, 208, 261
ultra-processed foods, 145, 204, 255–56, 395
University of Arizona, Andrew Weil Center for Integrative Medicine. *see* Andrew Weil Center for Integrative Medicine
University of Arizona, College of Medicine, 244
University of Washington, 173
Unwin, David, 202–3
Unwin, Jen, 203
Unwinding Anxiety app, 71
upset stomach, general, 28–29
urinary-tract infections (UTIs), 123–25
urogenital health of women. *see* premenstrual syndrome (PMS) and urogenital health
usprobioticguide.com, 130–31
uterine cancer, 377

vaccines
  Covid, 288, 289
  flu, 21–22
vaginal dryness, 370
vaginal hormone therapy, 124–25, 139
vagus nerve stimulation
  for PTSD, 283–84
  VNS devices, 71, 179, 283–84, 285
valerian, 54, 142
valve surgery, 341, 346, 348, 353, 355, 356
Van der Kolk, Bessel, 272, 274
vegan diet, 162, 199–200, 202, 239–40
vegetables and fruit
  asthma and, 221
  bone resorption inhibitory food items (BRIFI), 237
  breast cancer and, 365–66
  for cold and flu, 15–16
  depression and, 253–55
  fruit and diabetes, 205
  prioritizing, 395
Veterans Administration (VA), 185, 271
Viking Bath, 263
vinegar, 205
virtual reality, 330
vitamin D
  for asthma, 222–23
  for bone health, 236
  for depression, 258–59

for heart health, 159, 350
for joint pain, 196
for long Covid, 293
surgery and, 310, 350
for type 2 diabetes, 209
Your Rapid Recovery Toolkit, 393
vitamins and vitamin supplements. *see also* vitamin D
  A, 309
  B2, 181–82
  B3, 101
  B6, 119
  B8, 69
  B complex, 68, 281, 325
  B9 (methylfolate), 259
  C, 14, 19, 237, 325, 389
  for cold and flu, 14, 19
  for herpes, 24–25
  K, 237
  multi-mineral multivitamins (MMMVs), 257, 350, 368
  for PTSD, 281
  for trauma, 281
  zinc, 19, 101, 119, 129, 259, 293–94, 309, 389
vomiting, post-op surgery, 324

Walker, Matthew, 45–46
walking
  backwards, 176, 379
  daily, 7
  post-op, 323
  speed of, 208–9
weekend warrior success, 91–94. *see also* musculoskeletal pain
weight
  abdominal obesity, 155
  bone health and, 231
  "lean diabetes," 202
  maintenance of, 8–9
  menopause and, 144
  metabolic syndrome and, 166
  osteoarthritis and, 188
  rheumatoid arthritis and, 191–92
weight-bearing aerobic exercise, 243
weighted blankets, 71
Weil, Andrew, 186–87, 394. *see also* Andrew Weil Center for Integrative Medicine
Weill Cornell Medicine-Qatar, 201–2
Weintraub, Jill, 192
Western medicine, 5–6
wheat, gluten intolerance, 30
white blood cells, increased, 18
whole-body hyperthermia, 262–63

Why We Sleep (Walker), 45–46
Wiggins, Doreen, 364
Willett, Walter, 241
Winfrey, Oprah, 278
women's health. *see also* bone health; breast surgery and breast cancer; menopause; premenstrual syndrome (PMS) and urogenital health
   depression and perimenopause, 250
   medical research about women, 116–17
   tend and befriend pattern, 59–60
Women's Health Initiative (WHI), 135–36, 138, 239, 365, 371
Women's Study for the Alleviation of Vasomotor Symptoms (WAVS), 145
World Health Organization, 241, 271
Wright, Kenneth, 55
writing and journaling, 52, 224–25, 276–77

xenoestrogens, 372

Yale Cancer Center, 370
Yale Paxlovid for Long COVID (PAX LC) trial, 296
yeast infections, 126–29
YMCA, 201
yoga. *see also* meditation
   hatha yoga, 67
   heart health and, 166
   for long Covid, 293
   for musculoskeletal pain, 83
   pranayama, 65, 220, 293, 399 (*see also* breathing exercises)
   for PTSD, 274–76
   yoga nidra for sleep, 52
yoni practice, 127
Your Rapid Recovery Toolkit, 9, 387–400
Yuka app, 108

Zetia (ezetimibe), 158, 160
zinc, 19, 101, 119, 129, 259, 293–94, 309, 389
ZOE trial, 145
Z-score, 232
Zyrtec (cetirizine), 390

About the Author

Dr. Victoria Maizes is an internationally recognized leader, change agent, and innovator in the field of integrative medicine. As the founding executive director of the Andrew Weil Center for Integrative Medicine at the University of Arizona—where she also serves as a professor of medicine and public health—she has dedicated her professional life to transforming health care by educating physicians and empowering individuals to live healthier lives.

Dr. Maizes stewarded the growth of the program in integrative medicine from a small organization that trained four doctors each year into a world-renowned center of excellence. Under her leadership, the center developed premier national and international educational programs that now train more than 1,000 doctors, nurses, medical students, residents, and other health professionals annually. Collectively these integratively trained clinicians provide care to millions of people worldwide.

Named one of the world's "25 Intelligent Optimists" by *Ode* magazine, Dr. Maizes is a highly sought-after speaker and the cohost of the acclaimed podcast *Body of Wonder* with Dr. Andrew Weil. Dr. Maizes has received many honors and awards including the Inaugural Andrew Weil Endowed Chair in Integrative Medicine, the Bravewell Distinguished Service Award, and the Integrative Healthcare Symposium Leadership Award.

Dr. Maizes wrote *Heal Faster: Unlock Your Body's Rapid Recovery Reflex* to provide the tools for people to reclaim their health. She is also the editor of the Oxford University Press textbook *Integrative Women's Health* and the author of *Be Fruitful: The Essential Guide to Maximizing Fertility and Giving Birth to a Healthy Child.*

A summa cum laude graduate of Barnard College, Dr. Maizes received her medical degree from the University of California San Francisco Medical School, completed her family medicine residency at the University of Missouri, and her integrative medicine fellowship at the University of Arizona. You can learn more about her on her website: DrVictoriaMaizes.com.